Recent Advances in

Withdrawn

Paediatrics
23

Recent Advances in Paediatrics 22
Edited by T.J. David

ISBN 1-85315-597-7

ISSN 0-309-0140

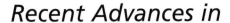

Recent Advances in

Paediatrics
23

Edited by

Timothy J. David MB ChB MD PhD FRCP FRCPCH DCH
Professor of Child Health and Paediatrics,
University of Manchester;
Honorary Consultant Paediatrician,
Booth Hall Children's Hospital, Manchester, UK

© 2006 Royal Society of Medicine Press Ltd

Published by the Royal Society of Medicine Press Ltd
1 Wimpole Street, London W1G 0AE, UK
Tel: +44 (0)20 7290 2921
Fax: +44 (0)20 7290 2929
Email: publishing@rsm.ac.uk
Website: www.rsmpress.co.uk

British Library Cataloguing in Publication Data
A catalogue record for this book is available from the British Library

ISBN 1-85315-652-3

Distribution in Europe and Rest of World:

Marston Book Services Ltd
PO Box 269
Abingdon
Oxon OX14 4YN, UK
Tel: +44 (0)1235 465500
Fax: +44 (0)1235 465555
Email: direct.order@marston.co.uk

Distribution in the USA and Canada:

Royal Society of Medicine Press Ltd
c/o BookMasters Inc
30 Amberwood Parkway
Ashland, OH 44805, USA
Tel: +1 800 247 6553/+1 800 266 5564
Fax: +1 419 281 6883
Email: order@bookmasters.com

Distribution in Australia and New Zealand:

Elsevier Australia
30-52 Smidmore Street
Marrikville NSW 2204, Australia
Tel: +61 2 9517 8999
Fax: +61 2 9517 2249
Email: service@elsevier.com.au

Editorial services and typesetting by GM & BA Haddock, Ford, Midlothian, UK

Printed in Great Britain by Bell & Bain, Glasgow, UK

Contents

Contents

Preface

The aim of *Recent Advances in Paediatrics* is to provide a review of important topics and help doctors keep abreast of developments in the subject. The book is intended for the practising clinician, those in specialty training, and doctors preparing for specialty examinations. The book is sold very widely in Britain, Europe, North America and Asia, and the contents and authorship are selected with this very broad readership in mind. There are 14 chapters which cover a variety of general paediatric, neonatal and community paediatric areas. As usual, the selection of topics has veered towards those of general, rather than special, interest.

The final chapter, an annotated literature review, is a personal selection of key articles and useful reviews published in 2004. Comment about a paper is sometimes as important as the original article, so when a paper has been followed by interesting or important correspondence, or accompanied by a useful editorial, this is also referred to. As with the choice of subjects for the main chapters, the selection of articles has inclined towards those of general, rather than special, interest. There is, however, special emphasis on community paediatrics and medicine in the tropics, as these two important areas tend to be less well covered in general paediatric journals. Trying to reduce to an acceptable size the short-list of particularly interesting articles is an especially difficult task. Each topic in the literature review section is asterisked in the index, so selected publications on (for example) child abuse can be identified easily, as can any parts of the book that touch on the topic.

I am indebted to the authors for their hard work, prompt delivery of manuscripts and patience in dealing with my queries and requests. I would also like to thank my secretaries Angela Smithies and Valerie Smith, and Gill Haddock of the RSM Press, for all their help. Working on a book such as this makes huge inroads into one's spare time, and my special thanks go to my wife and sons for all their support.

2005

Professor Timothy J. David
University Department of Child Health
Booth Hall Children's Hospital,
Manchester M9 7AA, UK
E-mail: t.david@netcomuk.co.uk

Julie A. Edge

1

Cerebral oedema in diabetic ketoacidosis

Cerebral oedema is a rare complication of diabetic ketoacidosis in children, but it has a significant morbidity and mortality. It occurs in only around one in a hundred episodes of diabetic ketoacidosis, but is the commonest cause of death and neurological disability in children with diabetes.

The pathophysiology of cerebral oedema still remains unclear, and it is possible that several different processes may be involved, resulting in a final common pathway of brain swelling. More recent case-control studies have started to unravel some of the contributions made by various patient and treatment factors to the overall risk of cerebral oedema, and use of newer imaging techniques has started to shed some light on the pathophysiology.

Cerebral oedema still frequently presents with respiratory arrest, which has an almost universally poor outcome, even if treatment with mannitol is instituted. There is increasing evidence that some of these episodes could be recognised at an earlier stage and treated before the severe neurological deficits occur. Thus, all medical staff looking after children with diabetic ketoacidosis need to be alert to the possible presenting features of cerebral oedema throughout the management of diabetic ketoacidosis.

EPIDEMIOLOGY

Cerebral oedema is the commonest cause of death in children with diabetes, being responsible for 80% of diabetic ketoacidosis-related deaths in children aged under 12 years between 1990 and 1996 in the UK.[1] Most episodes of cerebral oedema are not fatal so the incidence cannot be established merely by examining deaths; therefore, large population studies are required. The UK prospective study of the incidence of both fatal and non-fatal cerebral oedema

Julie A. Edge MD MRCP FRCPCH
Consultant in Paediatric Diabetes and Endocrinology, John Radcliffe Hospital, Headington, Oxford
OX3 9DU, UK. E-mail: julie.edge@paediatrics.ox.ac.uk

showed that cerebral oedema occurs with an overall likelihood of 7 per 1000 episodes of diabetic ketoacidosis.[2] Two different studies from the US have also reported very similar incidence figures – 1%[3] and 0.7%.[4] Cerebral oedema is more common in younger children, but rarely occurs in adults with diabetic ketoacidosis.

The largest case-series (a description of 69 cases reported by Rosenbloom[5] in the US) suggested that cerebral oedema was more likely to occur in children whose diabetic ketoacidosis occurred at the presentation of diabetes, rather than in children with already known diabetes who develop diabetic ketoacidosis. This suspicion has been confirmed in the UK population-based survey, where the incidence of cerebral oedema was found to be 11.9 per 1000 episodes diabetic ketoacidosis in newly diagnosed diabetes and 3.8 per 1000 in known diabetes.[2]

MAKING THE DIAGNOSIS

The clinical signs of cerebral oedema are variable. The child may actually present with signs of cerebral oedema before the diabetic ketoacidosis is treated,[6] there may be a deterioration and worsening of coma from admission, or, more commonly, a gradual improvement in the child's general condition, followed by a deterioration.[5] This deterioration may be gradual with reduced level of consciousness with headache, or sudden, with loss of consciousness, appearance of fixed dilated pupils or respiratory arrest once brain stem herniation is occurring. Symptoms can include confusion, irritability, behaviour change, headache and fits. Reduced conscious level alone, particularly on admission, may purely be a result of reduced pH, but this would tend to improve gradually. The timing of development of cerebral oedema is also variable, with most cases occurring between 4 and 12 h from

Table 1 Proposed criteria for the diagnosis of cerebral oedema – the combination of one diagnostic criterion, two major criteria, or one major and two minor criteria may be used to suggest the diagnosis, so that treatment can be given before respiratory arrest[8]

Diagnostic criteria
    Abnormal motor or verbal response to pain
    Decorticate or decerebrate posture
    Cranial nerve palsy (especially III, IV, and VI)
    Abnormal neurogenic respiratory pattern (*e.g.* grunting, tachypnea, Cheyne-Stokes respiration, apneusis)

Major criteria
    Altered mentation/fluctuating level of consciousness
    Sustained heart rate deceleration (decrease more than 20 beats/min) not attributable to improved intravascular volume or sleep state
    Age-inappropriate incontinence

Minor criteria
    Vomiting
    Headache
    Lethargy or not easily arousable
    Diastolic blood pressure > 90 mmHg
    Age < 5 years

the start of treatment, but it may present before the start of treatment, or up to 24 h afterwards.[5–7]

A detailed study of the medical notes of 24 cases of cerebral oedema has determined that it was possible to detect retrospectively, using a combination of clinical features, the majority of occurrences of cerebral oedema before the collapse. From this study a method of clinical diagnosis based on bedside evaluation of neurological state has been proposed (Table 1).[8] One diagnostic criterion, two major criteria, or one major and two minor criteria had a sensitivity of 92% and a false positive rate of only 4%, and theoretically allow for intervention before major collapse, although this has not yet been shown to be useful prospectively. It is important to recognise that cerebral oedema is a clinical, and not a radiological, diagnosis; a normal computed tomography (CT) scan up to several hours after the event does not exclude the diagnosis.[5,8]

In a large prospective UK study, we found that headache was a feature during treatment in one quarter of over 40 cases and none of 30 controls. The other particularly important feature was the heart rate, which fell by over 30% in 11 of 26 cases but only 2 of 60 controls at some time during the 6 h before the event.[9] However, these features were only found when retrospectively examining the notes for the study, and at no time did these features actually alert the treating paediatrician to the fact that cerebral oedema might be imminent. Therefore, the use of these 'early-warning systems' crucially depends on nursing staff being made aware of the importance and significance of some of these minor symptoms and alerting the medical staff immediately.

DIFFERENTIAL DIAGNOSIS

Other pathologies can present in a very similar way to cerebral oedema. These include sub-arachnoid haemorrhage, encephalitis, viral encephalitis, arterial thrombosis, spontaneous intracerebral haematomas, acute obstructive hydrocephalus and venous sinus thrombosis, all of which may present in a similar fashion. It has been suggested that up to 10% of instances thought to be cerebral oedema may be caused by alternative intracranial pathology,[5] and unless an accurate diagnosis is made, aetiological factors may be ascribed to cerebral oedema which are in fact related to other pathologies. Furthermore, specific treatment can be offered for some of these other conditions, *e.g.* venous sinus thrombosis.[10] Therefore, brain imaging (CT or MRI scan) should be carried out to look specifically for any alternative pathology and not to make the diagnosis of cerebral oedema, once the child is stabilised.

TREATMENT

The use of intravenous mannitol to increase plasma osmolality in the treatment of cerebral oedema was reported as early as 1970, but it was not universally successful. More recently, it has been suggested that, for maximum effect, mannitol should be given within 5 or 10 min of the initial deterioration in neurological function. However, in the study of Bello and Sotos,[4] 7 of 8 children given mannitol within 2 h survived, and 5 were normal neurologically. In addition, 3% (hypertonic) saline has been proposed and has been used in occasional case reports to good effect.[11]

Table 2 Measures which should be taken when cerebral oedema is suspected in a child with diabetic ketoacidosis

- Exclude hypoglycaemia as a possible cause of any behaviour change
- Give mannitol 1 g/kg stat (= 5 ml/kg mannitol 20% over 20 min) or hypertonic (3%) saline (5–10 ml/kg over 30 min). This needs to be given as soon as possible
- Restrict i.v. fluids to two-thirds maintenance and replace deficit over 72 h rather than 48 h
- The child will need to be moved to an intensive care unit (if not there already)
- Discuss with paediatric intensive care consultant (if assisted ventilation is required maintain $PaCO_2$ above 3.5 kPa)
- Once the child is stable, exclude other diagnoses by CT scan
- A repeated dose of mannitol should be given after 2 h if no response
- Document all events (with dates and times) very carefully in the medical records

From *British Society for Paediatric Endocrinology and Diabetes diabetic ketoacidosis guidelines* at <bsped.org.uk>.

Intracranial pressure monitoring and hyperventilation have also been proposed as soon as cerebral oedema is suspected, in addition to mannitol. However, the use of ventilation in diabetic ketoacidosis, where the $PaCO_2$ is already extremely low, may actually be dangerous. One of the factors associated with an adverse outcome in a large study was intubation with hyperventilation to a $PaCO_2$ less than 2.9 kPa.[7] It has, however, been suggested that, if intubation is necessary in a child with diabetic ketoacidosis, the $PaCO_2$ needs to be kept at a level (*i.e.* sufficiently low) which will not allow cerebral blood flow to increase suddenly, which may result in worsening of the situation.[12] Therefore, ventilation should only be used with extreme care in these children, and with the advice of a paediatric intensivist.

Practical measures in the management of a child with suspected cerebral oedema are shown in Table 2.

OUTCOME

Early studies reported high mortality rates of 60–90%, although it is possible that this was because only the more severe cases were being reported. In more recent population-based studies, mortality in all countries appears to be remarkably similar at around 20–25%.[2,6,13] Many survivors of cerebral oedema have, however, been left with severe neurological deficits which include hemiplegias, seizure disorder, short-term memory loss, learning problems and behavioural abnormalities in around 15–20% cases.[2,5–7] Diabetes insipidus and other pituitary hormone deficiencies have also been reported.

A particularly poor outcome is seen in those children who present with a respiratory arrest before any other signs or symptoms were present or recognised. In the UK study,[2] all of those who presented with a respiratory arrest either died or had severe neurological deficits. It is not entirely clear whether treatment influences outcome. In Rosenbloom's series,[5] 80% of the survivors in a good state had received 'early' treatment (before the onset of respiratory arrest) with mannitol and/or hyperventilation and dexamethasone, whereas this was the case in only 20% of those who died or were severely disabled. This may, however, be because they presented earlier with signs and symptoms of raised intracranial pressure before respiratory arrest, allowing intervention, rather than the good outcome being attributable to treatment.

CLINICAL RISK FACTORS

Until the cause(s) of cerebral oedema in diabetic ketoacidosis is understood, it will not be possible to design diabetic ketoacidosis guidelines which can reliably avoid the complication. Most information about this condition in the past has come from series of cases, where possible aetiological factors have been examined in groups of children who have presented with cerebral oedema. The traditional clinical risk factors will be discussed first, and then these will be examined in the light of three recently-reported case-control studies.

TRADITIONAL CONTRIBUTING FACTORS AND MECHANISMS

Fluids and sodium levels

The rate at which fluid is initially infused may be expected to relate to the speed of change of osmolality and electrolyte concentrations in the brain extracellular fluid relative to that within the brain cells, and thus to influence the development of cerebral oedema. Indeed, there have been case reports of cerebral oedema with huge infusions of fluid (initial rate 13 $l/m^2/day$), and one series of cases did suggest that 36 of 40 cases had received fluid rates of more than 4 $l/m^2/day$, but since there were no controls the significance of this finding is uncertain.[14] The largest case-series did not find any relationship between fluid rate and cerebral oedema.[5]

Change in osmolality of plasma and cerebrospinal fluid might also be expected to produce changes in brain cell size. In one early case-control study, the best predictors of cerebral oedema were duration of symptoms before admission and fall in serum osmolality; in particular, a fall in plasma sodium was more specific for the development of cerebral oedema than fall in blood glucose.[4] Two large studies of the fluid treatment of diabetic ketoacidosis have provided the most convincing evidence for an effect of plasma sodium concentration in the pathogenesis of cerebral oedema. In the first retrospective study of 219 episodes of diabetic ketoacidosis, 7 of whom developed cerebral oedema, all those with cerebral oedema had a plasma sodium level which fell during treatment, compared with only 50% of those with uncomplicated diabetic ketoacidosis.[3] The authors postulated that it was the failure of the plasma sodium level to rise as expected while the blood glucose fell that was a marker for excessive administration of free water, and thus for the development of cerebral oedema.

In a more recent publication, the same authors reported their prospective 5-year experience of 231 cases of diabetic ketoacidosis managed with a regimen in which plasma sodium was not allowed to fall (using fluid containing 75–125 mmol/l sodium).[15] They claimed that gradual rehydration can protect against cerebral oedema, since there were no cases of cerebral oedema in these patients (but see below). Further support for a relationship between falling plasma sodium concentration and cerebral oedema comes from a small study in very young children where 4 cases of cerebral oedema had progressively lower sodium levels during treatment than 10 controls.[16]

The type of fluid used may be expected to alter osmolality and therefore affect risk. In a British retrospective survey, cerebral oedema was more common an occurrence in units where 0.18% saline was routinely used in diabetic ketoacidosis treatment, than where greater concentrations of saline were used.[17] However, despite significant differences in the fluid management of diabetic ketoacidosis between the UK and the US (normal saline tended to be used for a much longer period in the UK), the incidence of cerebral oedema is remarkably similar,[2,4] suggesting that the fluid type used may have a limited impact on cerebral oedema risk. This is supported by an Australian study showing a similar incidence of cerebral oedema during two time periods where different fluid regimens were used.[18]

Rate of fall of blood glucose concentration

Although a rapid fall in blood glucose levels should be a risk factor if cerebral oedema was an osmotically-driven phenomenon, blood glucose levels and their rate of fall have been variously reported as higher or lower than in controls without cerebral oedema. A small case-control study found that control children had higher initial plasma glucose concentrations and a more rapid fall than did children who subsequently developed cerebral oedema.[16] None of the large case-series has implicated fall in blood glucose level as a risk factor.

Insulin dose

Early studies in hyperglycaemic rabbits and rats demonstrated that insulin may be required for the progression of the cerebral oedema, since those in whom glucose was lowered by peritoneal dialysis or saline alone did not develop the condition, whereas those treated with insulin and fluid rapidly developed brain swelling.[19,20]

Insulin may also affect cerebral cell volume by promoting influx of sodium, potassium and chloride into brain cells. One of the important plasma membrane transporters involved in cell volume regulation is the Na^+/H^+ exchanger, which is exquisitely sensitive to changes in cytosolic pH. It has been hypothesised that once treatment of diabetic ketoacidosis starts, the cytosol remains more acidotic, so that intracellular H^+ ions are exchanged for Na^+, thus favouring unopposed cellular accumulation of sodium and water, leading to oedema.[21] Furthermore, the exchanger is also activated by insulin and arginine vasopressin, so the high initial arginine vasopressin levels seen in diabetic ketoacidosis may potentiate this mechanism and contribute to the subclinical brain oedema present on admission. Thus oedema would be expected to become more pronounced after insulin treatment has begun, which is consistent with clinical experience.[22] However, none of the early case-series mentioned insulin dose as a risk factor for cerebral oedema.

Bicarbonate treatment

Bicarbonate infusion has also been implicated as a cause of cerebral oedema; full correction of metabolic acidosis in dogs using bicarbonate was associated with reduced cerebral spinal fluid oxygen tension, leading to the suggestion that brain hypoxia and cytotoxic brain swelling may result.[23] However, none of the large case-series could implicate bicarbonate infusion in the development of cerebral oedema.[5,14]

Role of ketones

β-Hydroxybutyrate and acetoacetate have been shown to alter the permeability of the vascular endothelium (effectively the blood–brain barrier) and to have direct effects on the production of the vasoconstrictor endothelin 1 in mouse brain endothelial cells.[24] More recent studies have shown that ketoacids can stimulate the Na–K–Cl transporter in brain cells, and thus the ketone bodies may be directly involved in the production of cerebral oedema.[25] This will no doubt be studied further.

RESULTS OF RECENT CASE-CONTROL STUDIES

It is difficult to tease apart all these possible predisposing factors, since those children who have the highest blood glucose levels are likely to be those who are the most severely dehydrated, receive the most fluids and have the greatest change in plasma osmolality and sodium during the first few hours, as well as being the most likely recipients of bicarbonate treatment. Furthermore, most of the studies reported up until the last 5 years were collections of cases which did not allow for comparison of those factors in children with diabetic ketoacidosis who did not develop cerebral oedema, and may, therefore, have ascribed risk factors erroneously. Three case-control studies have recently been reported which have used similar methodology and compared risk factors in groups of children with cerebral oedema compared to similar groups with diabetic ketoacidosis but with no cerebral oedema (Table 3).[6,13,26]

The main findings of the study from Glaser and colleagues[13] were that a higher plasma urea level and lower partial pressure of CO_2 were associated with significantly increased risk of cerebral oedema, both in the matched and

Table 3 Methodology of the three recent case-control studies

Study	Dates	Sample base	Cases (n)	Controls per case	Matching
Glaser et al. (2001)[13]	1982–1989	10 paediatric centres (9 US, 1 Australian)	61	6	3 random, 3 matched for severity
Edge et al. (2005)[26]	1995–1998	Entire UK, British Paediatric Surveillance Unit	43	4	Matched for age, sex, old/ new diabetes
Lawrence et al. (2005)[6]	1999–2001	Canadian Surveillance Unit	13	2	Unmatched

unmatched groups. Of all the therapeutic variables examined, only treatment with bicarbonate was associated with cerebral oedema. Neither fluid composition nor rate were implicated. However, despite this, plasma sodium levels fell to a greater extent in cases of cerebral oedema than in controls, suggesting that the fall in sodium may actually be a consequence of the cerebral oedema rather than a cause, owing perhaps to dysregulation of anti-diuretic hormone, or cerebral salt-wasting.[13]

The UK study of Edge and colleagues[26] also found that baseline patient variables present on admission were the greatest risk factors; these included more severe acidosis (with an odds ratio of 0.08–0.57; $P < 0.001$), and a high plasma urea level and high plasma potassium level, both possibly indicators of impaired renal function. Greater volumes of fluid over the first 4 h of treatment also conferred greater risk. Bicarbonate treatment was associated with a greater risk, but not when corrected for the degree of acidosis.[26]

Furthermore, another treatment variable was also implicated. If insulin was given to the child during the first hour of fluid treatment, this increased the risk of cerebral oedema with an odds ratio of 4.7 (95% CI 1.5–13.9; $P < 0.007$) when adjusted for baseline acidosis and matching criteria. Moreover, the dose of insulin during the first 2 h (but not after) was also related to increased risk. This suggests that a bolus of insulin, which is known not to be necessary in treatment of diabetic ketoacidosis, may actually be dangerous, and that it may be beneficial to delay the start of insulin therapy.[26] The mechanism by which insulin administration in the first hour could increase risk for cerebral oedema is unclear, but it could relate to rapid changes in electrolytes as described above. It may be that a short period of equilibration is needed once fluids are started, before insulin is added in, in order to prevent sudden changes in electrolyte concentrations within the brain cells.

The association of cerebral oedema with severity of illness was confirmed in the Canadian Surveillance Unit Study,[6] where lower initial bicarbonate level, higher plasma urea and higher blood glucose level were associated with cerebral oedema. However, there was no relationship with treatment factors, although there was a trend towards increased risk with greater volumes of fluid and bicarbonate treatment.[6] It may only have been the small size of the study which prevented these factors being significant.

Thus it seems that factors already present in the child at presentation of the diabetic ketoacidosis present the greatest risk for the development of cerebral oedema, with treatment variables have a lesser but still significant effect.

PATHOPHYSIOLOGY

The above discussion concentrates on the clinical risk factors, but do we know what is actually happening in the brain? Although the condition is described as 'cerebral oedema', there is no accepted definition of the condition, or any convincing description of a single process occurring in the brain.

IS THE MECHANISM OSMOTIC?

Classical thinking about the development of cerebral oedema is that it is related to the hypertonic conditions prevailing at the onset of diabetic ketoacidosis. The mechanisms of cell volume regulation in the brain are now well-documented.[27] The early stages of brain cell volume regulation (within 12 h of external osmolal changes) are characterised by changes in cytosolic electrolyte concentration, particularly K^+ and Cl^-, whose cellular concentrations are regulated by a variety of transport processes. More prolonged osmolal stress (more than 24 h) results in changes in cellular content of non-perturbing osmolytes, predominantly taurine and glutamine, myoinositol, and methylamines.[27] It is thought that these osmolytes dissipate slowly, and so it has been hypothesised that in the clinical situation of diabetic ketoacidosis, once rehydration is commenced, a rapid decline in plasma and cerebral spinal fluid osmolality favours net water movement into brain cells (Fig. 1). Certainly, in animals, the experimental evidence favours an osmotic phenomenon.[28]

SUB-CLINICAL CEREBRAL OEDEMA

It has been shown in several studies using CT scans, that the majority of children with diabetic ketoacidosis appear to have a degree of brain swelling without any symptoms of raised intracranial pressure,[29,30] although the universal presence of this entity has been challenged.[31] The reason why this sub-clinical brain swelling occurs is not clear, although the severity of subclinical brain swelling present before treatment has been shown to correlate with initial blood glucose concentration, implicating an osmolal mechanism.[22] In addition, although plasma osmolality was not related to the degree of subclinical cerebral oedema present on admission in 7 patients, the rate of change of the calculated effective osmolality correlated significantly with its progression.[22]

Therefore, there does appear to be some evidence that at least this subclinical brain swelling is osmotically-driven. However, the severe sudden clinical cerebral oedema may not be a simple extension of this process, and there is increasing evidence that other mechanisms besides changes in osmolality may be involved in the mechanism of its production.

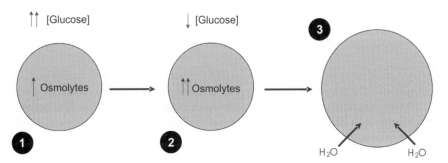

Fig. 1 Proposed theoretical osmotic mechanism for brain cell swelling in diabetic ketoacidosis. (1) Under conditions of increased extracellular osmolality due to increased glucose (and possibly sodium) concentrations, brain cells actively accumulate 'idiogenic osmoles' (now known to be inert osmolytes such as taurine and myoinositol). (2) When the diabetic ketoacidosis is treated and plasma glucose concentrations fall, brain cells remain relatively hyperosmolar owing to relatively higher concentrations of osmoles. (3) This results in movement of water into the cells and to cell swelling. 2006 © John Wiley & Sons Limited; reproduced with permission.[42]

IS THE MECHANISM ISCHAEMIC? LESSONS FROM NEWER IMAGING TECHNIQUES

The first descriptions of cerebral oedema in diabetic ketoacidosis were by Dillon and colleagues[32] and Young and Bradley[33] who believed that the post-mortem changes may have been caused by cerebral anoxia resulting from the reduced blood volume and haemoconcentration, leading in turn to increased capillary permeability. The areas of the brain affected (basal areas first, with a predeliction for the basal ganglia) would certainly be consistent with a hypoxaemic process.[34] Furthermore, risk factors found in the various case-control studies would lend support to the ischaemic hypothesis, since both hypocapnia, which causes cerebral vasoconstriction, and extreme dehydration, would be likely to lead to underperfusion of the brain.[13]

It has only been possible relatively recently to look closely at the brain substance with techniques that can examine osmolal mechanisms and blood flow in detail. A recent study in a small number of children with diabetic ketoacidosis used diffusion and perfusion MRI scans to assess the extracellular and intracellular spaces together with cerebral blood flow and cerebral blood volume.[35] The conclusions were that the patients had sub-clinical cerebral oedema, which was consistent with a vasogenic (rather than cytotoxic) mechanism, as it was associated with an expanded extracellular space, and that there was increased cerebral perfusion. The authors postulated that this may represent reperfusion of previously hypoperfused tissues with the administration of fluid during the treatment.[35]

A further study reported details of brain MRI and magnetic resonance spectroscopy data from 8 diabetic children with hyperglycaemia with or without ketoacidosis. All children, regardless of the severity of their clinical condition, showed the same qualitative findings over the first week after presentation; an increased brain tissue volume, and abnormal signal changes in the frontal region, consistent with oedema, and increased levels of myoinositol and taurine.[36]

The results from these two studies seem at odds, in that one suggests an osmolal mechanism for the brain swelling, but the other postulates vasogenic oedema. However, the taurine and myoinositol in the latter study persisted for up to 4 days, whereas accumulated organic osmolytes are thought to dissipate within 24 h. Increased taurine levels have been found following ischaemic stroke and traumatic brain injury and can remain elevated for more prolonged periods.[37] This may, therefore, suggest that in these children, the reason for the raised taurine levels may have been ischaemia. Thus both studies may suggest an ischaemic mechanism for the subclinical cerebral oedema of hyperglycaemia and diabetic ketoacidosis.

A very recent study in rats has provided further evidence for the hypoxic hypothesis. The Na–K–Cl co-transporter of brain microvascular endothelial cells (the cells which make up the blood–brain barrier) and astrocytes is a major participant in ischaemia-induced cerebral oedema in stroke. Bumetanide, an inhibitor of this transporter, was shown to abolish the development of cerebral oedema in rats made ketoacidotic.[25]

WHY DOES IT OCCUR IN CHILDREN AND NOT ADULTS?

This is one of the most intriguing questions of all. There may be several reasons why children might be at greater risk (Table 4), but little research has examined

Table 4 Speculation as to cause of increased susceptibility to cerebral oedema of children compared with adults

- Relatively greater brain volume
- Relatively greater oxygen requirement
- More rapid changes in plasma osmolality
- Lack of sex steroids
- Less (or more) developed mechanisms for brain cell volume regulation
- Differences in taurine (or other non-perturbing osmolyte) metabolism
- Differences in blood–brain barrier efficiency (*e.g.* aquaporin channels)

such differences. It has been shown that young rats adapt to brain cell volume perturbations by accumulating greater quantities of taurine than adult rats,[38] but there is no information in humans. Whether or not brain cell transport mechanisms differ in their actions in children and adults is not well understood, but there is some evidence that young women are more susceptible to cerebral oedema as a result of hypernatraemia than are males, because of efficiency differences in their cerebral sodium pump function. Thus it is possible that sex hormone production at puberty may affect such cellular pump mechanisms. If ischaemia is one of the mechanisms, then the high oxygen requirement of children's brains compared to adults may suggest that they would be more vulnerable.[34] The brains of starving children also take up ketones at a rate 4–5 times those of adults, and the regional uptake of ketones within the brain corresponds with the areas affected earliest in symptomatic cerebral oedema in diabetic ketoacidosis.

CAN CEREBRAL OEDEMA BE PREVENTED?

Despite the fact that some studies have suggested that the development of cerebral oedema may be related to the treatment of diabetic ketoacidosis, there are no intervention studies with a large enough power to detect a real reduction in the incidence of cerebral oedema because of the rarity of the condition. The report of Harris and Fiordalisi[15] suggested that cerebral oedema could be prevented by that the use of a fluid regimen which ensured a rise in the calculated plasma sodium level during treatment of diabetic ketoacidosis. However, in their report there were still 6 children in whom behaviour change or increasing obtundation were treated with mannitol.[15] Thus, it may be that diligent monitoring with early recognition of the neurological features of cerebral oedema, rather than prevention, was the cause of the improved outcome in this study.

Changes in diabetic ketoacidosis management protocols over the past 20 years have all aimed to reduce the incidence of cerebral oedema, and a recent international Consensus Working Group has produced evidence-based advice on the treatment of diabetic ketoacidosis.[39,40] It is now recommended that fluid replacement is carried out at a slow rate (without large volumes of resuscitation fluid) over 48 h. In addition, it may be sensible to recommend that the start of insulin therapy is delayed for at least an hour after intravenous fluid is commenced. Bicarbonate treatment has been shown to be unnecessary in all but the most severe acidosis, and is not recommended unless the pH is below 6.9 with evidence of myocardial compromise (British Society for Paediatric Endocrinology and Diabetes guidelines <www.bsped.org.uk>).

However, despite 'improvements' in diabetic ketoacidosis management, there is no evidence that the incidence of cerebral oedema has fallen either in the UK or in the US. The only way to prevent cerebral oedema categorically is to prevent diabetic ketoacidosis itself, especially at the onset of diabetes. In one area of Italy, it has been shown that this is possible; an education programme aimed at health professionals, school teachers and the general public to alert to the recognition of the signs and symptoms of diabetes in children, resulted in complete prevention of diabetic ketoacidosis.[41]

CONCLUSIONS

Cerebral oedema is a rare, unpredictable complication of diabetic ketoacidosis which has a high morbidity and mortality. Since the cause or causes are still obscure, it is difficult to design guidelines for the management of diabetic ketoacidosis that can avoid the complication. A high-risk population can be defined, and early recognition of the signs and symptoms of cerebral oedema may be possible with increased vigilance, allowing for intervention and possible improved outcome.

Key points for clinical practice

- Cerebral oedema occurs in around 1% of diabetic ketoacidosis episodes; it is more likely to occur in younger children and if the diabetes is newly-diagnosed.

- Children with diabetic ketoacidosis are at greater risk of developing cerebral oedema if they are severely acidotic, *i.e.* with a low pH or bicarbonate level (particularly if the $Paco_2$ is low), and have a high urea and high potassium concentration, suggesting severe dehydration and a degree of renal impairment.

- Management of diabetic ketoacidosis should be carried out according to one of the national or international guidelines (<bsped.org.uk> and <ispad.org>). One of the risk factors in treatment may be large volumes of fluid; therefore, large bolus volumes for resuscitation should be avoided.

- It may be prudent to delay insulin treatment for at least an hour after starting fluids when treating diabetic ketoacidosis, and bolus insulin doses should not be given. Bicarbonate treatment is not necessary in the majority of children and may be dangerous.

- It is particularly important to monitor children with diabetic keto-acidosis very closely during treatment. Subtle neurological changes may not be picked up with Glasgow Coma Scores, but should be noted and reported. Nurses should be aware of the importance of headache as a symptom of cerebral oedema, and that a bradycardia, even transient, may warn of impending brain stem herniation.

- Symptoms and signs include irritability, confusion, headache, behaviour change, reduced conscious level, fits, pupil abnormalities, slowing of the heart rate with or without raised blood pressure, and respiratory arrest. Clinical criteria for the diagnosis have been devised in retrospect and may be helpful in making the diagnosis, although this has yet to be proven.

Key points for clinical practice *(continued)*

- Mannitol or hypertonic saline should be given as soon as cerebral oedema is suspected, as there is some evidence that it may improve the outcome. Fluid rate should also be reduced, and the child moved to a paediatric intensive care unit.

- Cerebral oedema is a clinical rather than a radiological diagnosis, and a normal CT scan even several hours after the event does not exclude the diagnosis. CT scanning should only be done once the child is stable, and is done primarily to rule out other pathology which may present in the same way.

- The pathophysiology of cerebral oedema is still poorly understood although there is increasing evidence that ischaemic mechanisms may contribute to the clinical picture.

- Mortality is around 20%, and 30% of survivors are left with significant neurological sequelae.

- Prevention of diabetic ketoacidosis is currently the only way to prevent the occurrence of cerebral oedema.

References

1. Edge JA, Ford-Adams ME, Dunger DB. Causes of death in children with insulin dependent diabetes 1990–96. *Arch Dis Child* 1999; **81**: 318–323.
2. Edge JA, Hawkins MM, Winter DL, Dunger DB. The risk and outcome of cerebral oedema developing during diabetic ketoacidosis. *Arch Dis Child* 2001; **85**: 16–22.
3. Harris GD, Fiordalisi I, Harris WL, Mosovich LL, Finberg L. Minimizing the risk of brain herniation during treatment of diabetic ketoacidemia: a retrospective and prospective study. *J Pediatr* 1990; **117**: 22–31.
4. Bello FA, Sotos JF. Cerebral oedema in diabetic ketoacidosis in children. *Lancet* 1990; **336**: 64.
5. Rosenbloom A. Intracerebral crises during treatment of diabetic ketoacidosis. *Diabetes Care* 1990; **13**: 22–33.
6. Lawrence SE, Cummings EA, Gaboury I, Daneman D. Population-based study of incidence and risk factors for cerebral edema in pediatric diabetic ketoacidosis. *J Pediatr* 2005; **146**: 688–692.
7. Marcin JP, Glaser N, Barnett P, McCaslin I, Nelson D, Trainor J *et al*. Factors associated with adverse outcomes in children with diabetic ketoacidosis-related cerebral edema. *J Pediatr* 2002; **141**: 793–797.
8. Muir AB, Quisling RG, Yang MC, Rosenbloom AL. Cerebral edema in childhood diabetic ketoacidosis: natural history, radiographic findings, and early identification. *Diabetes Care* 2004; **27**: 1541–1546.
9. Edge JA, Flint J, Roy Y, Dunger DB. Can cerebral oedema be identified before the reduction in conscious level? *Pediatr Diabetes* 2004; **5**: 48.
10. Keane S, Gallagher A, Ackroyd S, McShane MA, Edge JA. Cerebral venous thrombosis during diabetic ketoacidosis. *Arch Dis Child* 2002; **86**: 204–205.
11. Curtis JR, Bohn D, Daneman D. Use of hypertonic saline in the treatment of cerebral edema in diabetic ketoacidosis (DKA). *Pediatr Diabetes* 2001; **2**: 191–194.
12. Tasker RC, Lutman D, Peters MJ. Hyperventilation in severe diabetic ketoacidosis. *Pediatr Crit Care Med* 2005; **6**: 405–411.
13. Glaser N, Barnett P, McCaslin I *et al*. Risk factors for cerebral edema in children with diabetic ketoacidosis. *N Engl J Med* 2001; **344**: 264–269.
14. Duck SC, Wyatt DT. Factors associated with brain herniation in the treatment of diabetic ketoacidosis. *J Pediatr* 1988; **113**: 10–14.
15. Harris GD, Fiordalisi I. Physiologic management of diabetic ketoacidemia. A 5-year prospective pediatric experience in 231 episodes. *Arch Pediatr Adolesc Med* 1994; **148**: 1046–1052.

16. Hale PM, Rezvani I, Braunstein AW, Lipman TH, Martinez N, Garibaldi L. Factors predicting cerebral edema in young children with diabetic ketoacidosis and new onset type I diabetes. *Acta Paediatr* 1997; **86**: 626–631.

17. Edge JA, Dunger DB. Variations in the management of diabetic ketoacidosis in children. *Diabet Med* 1994; **11**): 984–986.

18. Mel JM, Werther GA. Incidence and outcome of diabetic cerebral oedema in childhood: are there predictors? *J Paediatr Child Health* 1995; **31**: 17–20.

19. Tornheim P. Regional localization of cerebral edema following fluid and insulin therapy in streptozotocin-diabetic rats. *Diabetes* 1981; **30**: 762–766.

20. Arieff AI, Kleeman CR. Studies on mechanisms of cerebral edema in diabetic comas. Effects of hyperglycemia and rapid lowering of plasma glucose in normal rabbits. *J Clin Invest* 1973; **52**: 571–583.

21. Van der Meulen JA, Klip A, Grinstein S. Possible mechanisms for cerebral oedema in diabetic ketoacidosis. *Lancet* 1987; **2**: 306–308.

22. Durr JA, Hoffman WH, Sklar AH, El Gammal T, Steinhart CM. Correlates of brain edema in uncontrolled IDDM. *Diabetes* 1992; **41**: 627–632.

23. Bureau MA, Begin R, Berthiaume Y, Shapcott D, Khoury K, Gagnon N. Cerebral hypoxia from bicarbonate infusion in diabetic acidosis. *J Pediatr* 1980; **96**: 968–973.

24. Isales CM, Min L, Hoffman WH. Acetoacetate and beta-hydroxybutyrate differentially regulate endothelin-1 and vascular endothelial growth factor in mouse brain microvascular endothelial cells. *J Diabetes Complications* 1999; **13**: 91–97.

25. Lam TI, Anderson SE, Glaser N, O'Donnell ME. Bumetanide reduces cerebral edema formation in rats with diabetic ketoacidosis. *Diabetes* 2005; **54**: 510–516.

26. Edge JA, Roy Y, Widmer B *et al*. The UK prospective study of cerebral oedema complicating diabetic ketoacidosis. *Arch Dis Child* 2005; **90 (Suppl 2)**: A2–A3.

27. Trachtman H. Cell volume regulation: a review of cerebral adaptive mechanisms and implications for clinical treatment of osmolal disturbances. I. *Pediatr Nephrol* 1991; **5**: 743–750.

28. Levitsky LL. Symptomatic cerebral edema in diabetic ketoacidosis: the mechanism is clarified but still far from clear. *J Pediatr* 2004; **145**: 149–150.

29. Krane EJ, Rockoff MA, Wallman JK, Wolfsdorf JI. Subclinical brain swelling in children during treatment of diabetic ketoacidosis. *N Engl J Med* 1985; **312**: 1147–1151.

30. Hoffman WH, Steinhart CM, el Gammal T, Steele S, Cuadrado AR, Morse PK. Cranial CT in children and adolescents with diabetic ketoacidosis. *AJNR Am J Neuroradiol* 1988; **9**: 733–739.

31. Smedman L, Escobar R, Hesser U, Persson B. Sub-clinical cerebral oedema does not occur regularly during treatment for diabetic ketoacidosis. *Acta Paediatr* 1997; **86**: 1172–1176.

32. Dillon ES, Riggs HE, Dyer WW. Cerebral lesions in uncomplicated fatal diabetic acidosis. *Am J Med Sci* 1936; **192**: 360–365.

33. Young E, Bradley RF. Cerebral edema with irreversible coma in severe diabetic ketoacidosis. *N Engl J Med* 1967; **276**: 665–669.

34. Muir A. Therapeutic controversy. Cerebral edema in diabetic ketoacidosis; a look beyond rehydration. *J Clin Endocrinol Metab* 2000; **85**: 509–513.

35. Glaser NS, Wootton-Gorges SL, Marcin JP *et al*. Mechanism of cerebral edema in children with diabetic ketoacidosis. *J Pediatr* 2004; **145**: 164–171.

36. Cameron FJ, Kean MJ, Wellard RM, Werther GA, Neil JJ, Inder TE. Insights into the acute cerebral metabolic changes associated with childhood diabetes. *Diabet Med* 2005; **22**: 648–653.

37. Glaser NS, Buonocore MH. Cerebral metabolic alterations in children with diabetic ketoacidosis. *Diabet Med* 2005; **22**: 515–516.

38. Trachtman H, Yancey PH, Gullans SR. Cerebral cell volume regulation during hypernatremia in developing rats. *Brain Res* 1995; **693**: 155–162.

39. Dunger DB, Sperling MA, Acerini CL *et al*. European Society for Paediatric Endocrinology/Lawson Wilkins Pediatric Endocrine Society consensus statement on diabetic ketoacidosis in children and adolescents. *Pediatrics* 2004; **113**: e133–e140.

40. Dunger DB, Sperling MA, Acerini CL *et al*. ESPE/LWPES consensus statement on diabetic ketoacidosis in children and adolescents. *Arch Dis Child* 2004; **89**: 188–194.

41. Vanelli M, Chiari G, Ghizzoni L, Costi G, Giacalone T, Chiarelli F. Effectiveness of a prevention program for diabetic ketoacidosis in children. An 8-year study in schools and private practices. *Diabetes Care* 1999; **22**: 7–9.

42. Edge JA. Cerebral oedema during treatment of diabetic ketoacidosis: are we any nearer finding a cause? *Diabetes Metab Res Rev* 2000; **16**: 316–324.

Davide Martino Russell C. Dale

2

Post-streptococcal autoimmune brain disorders

Post-infectious illnesses linked to Group A β-haemolytic streptococcal (GABHS) infections, particularly rheumatic fever, may present with a complex array of neurological and psychiatric manifestations. These neuropsychiatric syndromes seem typically related to a dysfunction in the cortico-striato-thalamo-cortical circuitry, which controls motor, emotional and cognitive functional domains. The nosographic classification of post-streptococcal neuropsychiatric diseases is, however, still incompletely resolved, and comprises two recognised nosological entities and a spectrum of other conditions, the nosological definitions of which are currently debated.

WELL-DEFINED POST-STREPTOCOCCAL NEUROPSYCHIATRIC DISEASES

Sydenham's (rheumatic) chorea

Sydenham's chorea has been the first neurological disease to be causally linked to GABHS infection. It was described by Thomas Sydenham in 1686, who labelled it St Vitus's Dance, involuntarily heralding some later confusion between the currently acknowledged post-streptococcal illness and epidemic 'dancing mania', a phenomenon of mass hysteria observed in the past during large religious gatherings.[1] Descriptions of large 19th century European paediatric cohorts suggested its inclusion among the major clinical manifestations of acute rheumatic fever.[2]

Davide Martino MRCP
Department of Neuroinflammation, Institute of Neurology, Queen Square, London WC1N 3BG, UK
and Department of Neurological and Psychiatric Sciences, University of Bari, Bari, Italy

Russell C. Dale PhD (for correspondence)
Department of Neuroinflammation, Institute of Neurology, Queen Square, London WC1N 3BG,
London and Neurosciences Unit, Great Ormond Street Hospital NHS Trust, London, UK
E-mail: rdale@ion.ucl.ac.uk

The annual incidence of Sydenham's chorea is 0.2–0.8 per 100,000 in industrialised countries although outbreaks are still encountered world-wide.[3] Its prevalence is much higher in non-industrialised countries and in particular developing communities, *e.g.* the Aborigines of northern Australia. Sydenham's chorea occurs in 10–40% of the patients with rheumatic fever, displaying strong geographical variability. Children aged 5–15 years are most commonly affected, with a female-to-male ratio ranging from 3:1 to 7:1. A family history of rheumatic fever and Sydenham's chorea is considered a predisposing factor.[3]

Sydenham's chorea is diagnosed primarily on clinical grounds when at least two among involuntary movements, hypotonia and behavioural disorders occur with an acute/subacute onset.[1] In addition, there should be a temporal association with streptococcal pharyngitis, diagnosed either by positive culture from pharyngeal swab or raised titres of antistreptococcal antibodies. Moreover, given the long latency between infection and onset of chorea (1–6 months), other causes of chorea need to be excluded.[1] Acute Sydenham's chorea is associated with cardiac involvement (overt carditis or pathological silent valvular regurgitation) in 50–80% of cases, whereas rheumatic arthritis occurs in 20–40%. Sydenham's chorea is an isolated phenomenon in about 30% of cases. Sydenham's chorea may have an episodic or persistent (> 2 years) course.[3] In 10–40% of cases, its course is relapsing-remitting, with the first recurrence following the initial episode after 3 months or up to 10 years or more.[4] Recurrences may not be associated with other signs of active rheumatic fever, and may be triggered by non-specific infections, pregnancy or oral contraceptives.[4]

Choreic movements are the typical involuntary movements in Sydenham's chorea, and may involve the whole body, particularly distal extremities, although they may remain unilateral in up to 30% of cases. In the acute phase, patients progressively display a continuous flow of involuntary contractions, characterised by swift, purposeless, asynchronous and unsuppressible movements, which may affect dexterity and normal gait, and may initially be misjudged as 'clumsiness' or 'restlessness'. Typically, incapacity to keep still is observed in these children (motor impersistence), whereas movements cease during sleep. Speech is abnormal in a third of cases, sounding intermittent, explosive and reduced in fluency.[3] Decreased muscle tone, often associated with hyporeflexia, is present in the majority of cases, seemingly of central origin;[5] when hypotonia is severe, the course is prolonged and patients appear prostrated and dehydrated (chorea paralytica).[3] Less common neurological features observed in Sydenham's chorea are hypometric saccades, oculogyric crises, bradykinesia, tics, hemiballism and migraine.[3,6]

Behavioural abnormalities are known to occur in Sydenham's chorea since Thomas Sydenham's seminal description, although their spectrum has been analysed in detail only in the last 15 years.[7] Obsessive-compulsive symptoms and obsessive-compulsive disorder during the acute phase of Sydenham's chorea have been consistently reported in 20–40% of cases without a previous history of obsessionality. Their symptoms overlap typical childhood-onset obsessive-compulsive disorder, including contamination fears, aggressive and somatic obsessions, checking, repeating, hoarding, counting and washing rituals. Obsessive-compulsive behaviour may precede chorea by weeks and display an acute course, disappearing before the cessation of involuntary movements. Symptoms of separation anxiety, generalised anxiety, social phobia, major depression and enuresis occur in 10–40% of patients. Additionally, children who develop Sydenham's chorea, especially the persistent type, are more likely to have a history of attention deficit/hyperactivity disorder than those with rheumatic fever without chorea.[8]

The identification of a pathological phenotype of Sydenham's chorea is hindered by the paucity of post-mortem reports of the condition, secondary to its generally benign course and favourable outcome. Available pathological descriptions are, therefore, likely to be biased towards the most severe forms, presenting with neuronal loss, gliosis, hyperemia, perivascular lymphocytic infiltration, and petechial haemorrhages, all predominantly involving striatal and thalamic nuclei.[3]

Structural abnormalities on CT or MRI may be present during the active phase of the illness, and seem reversible in parallel to the clinical picture. However, conventional MRI is usually normal. When abnormalities exist, MRI structural changes include oedematous swelling on T_1-weighted images (especially during the initial episode) and high-signal T_2-weighted lesions of caudate, putamen and globus pallidus. In about 20% of cases, permanent striatal changes may be observed, especially in clinically persistent forms. Occasionally, newly appearing lesions may be found at follow-up, without any clinical correlates. Gadolinium-enhanced basal ganglia lesions are an exceptional finding. In one case, a reduced N-acetylaspartate peak on MR proton spectroscopy could be detected suggesting neuronal loss. SPECT and PET studies showed hyperperfusion and glucose hypermetabolism of the striatum and thalamus particularly in the acute phase, which may be explained either by active inflammation in these structures, or by enhanced striatal activity secondary to increased corticostriatal inputs.[3]

Post-streptococcal acute disseminated encephalomyelitis and an encephalitis lethargica-like variant

The second well-defined post-streptococcal neuropsychiatric illness is post-streptococcal acute demyelinating encephalomyelitis (ADEM), accounting for about 10% of cases of ADEM. This is by definition a paediatric post-infectious (post-viral, post-bacterial or post-vaccinal) acute monophasic inflammatory CNS disorder mainly involving the white matter, although cortical and/or subcortical grey matter lesions occur in almost 30% of cases. The diagnosis is based on clinical, laboratory and neuroradiological grounds. Dale and associates[9] showed that the post-streptococcal form of ADEM is clinically different from other forms, due to a higher frequency of movement disorders, particularly dystonia. Of these children, 70% show also a behavioural syndrome, comprising emotional lability, inappropriate laughter, separation anxiety, confusion and hypersomnolence.[9] Although most of these patients have a monophasic illness, post-streptococcal multiphasic disseminated encephalomyelitis has been reported, with a recurrence occurring within 4 weeks from initial manifestation.[10] In 80% of cases, hyperintense basal ganglia lesions are present on T_2-weighted MRI images, whereas only 18% of non-streptococcal ADEM cases present with basal ganglia lesions.[9]

Another acute-subacute encephalitic illness, linked to streptococcal infection, has been described, which resembles encephalitis lethargica.[11] This is a syndrome which appeared in an epidemic form throughout Europe and North America between 1916 and 1927, striking people of all ages, and was observed only sporadically afterwards. Encephalitis lethargica presents with abnormalities of consciousness and sleep, associated with Parkinsonism, hyperkinesias, eye-movement abnormalities (ophthalmoplegia, nystagmus, oculogyric crises), and psychiatric features (obsessive-compulsive disorder, mutism, apathy, conduct disorders). One-third of encephalitis lethargica patients developed long-standing Parkinsonism. Brain pathology revealed lymphocytic and plasma cell infiltrates in perivascular spaces and neuronal loss, mainly in the basal ganglia and brainstem (including substantia nigra and locus coeruleus). The contemporaneous occurrence of this epidemic and the influenza pandemic of 1918 suggested a common infectious cause; however, this was recently excluded by molecular biological examination of archival tissue samples from victims of both epidemics. Interestingly, diplococci were detected in the throats of encephalitis lethargica patients during the epidemic, and dogs vaccinated with diplococci developed a similar illness. Also, during the epidemic, encephalitis lethargica was more incident in late winter, similar to the seasonal variability of streptococcal pharyngitis. Recently, a new series of 20 patients (18 children) with a very similar presentation was reported: 55% of them had had pharyngitis in the preceding weeks. Of these, 40% showed T_2 hyperintensities in the basal ganglia and brainstem. Anti-streptolysin-O titres were significantly elevated; CSF showed lymphocytic pleocytosis, elevated protein content and oligoclonal bands in the majority of these patients.[11] An encephalitis lethargica-like illness might be a variant of post-streptococcal ADEM, confirming the specific tropism for the basal ganglia exhibited by post-streptococcal CNS disease.

POST-STREPTOCOCCAL NEUROPSYCHIATRIC DISEASES IN PROGRESS OF DEFINITION

Post-streptococcal obsessive-compulsive disorder and tic disorder (the PANDAS phenotype)

Obsessive-compulsive symptoms and tics temporally linked to streptococcal infections have been postulated to occur in children who do not fulfil diagnostic criteria for Sydenham's chorea or manifest an acute inflammatory cerebral illness. This is consistent with a relatively selective damage to the basal ganglia, the possible pathophysiological substrate of post-streptococcal CNS diseases. Obsessive-compulsive disorder and tics are thought to be secondary by structural and functional abnormalities of the basal ganglia (mainly, caudate and putamen). It is not, therefore, surprising that also obsessive-compulsive and tics which are temporally linked to streptococcal infections often occur together.

Post-streptococcal obsessive-compulsive symptoms/tics may present, however, in a peculiar manner, which is distinguishable from classical paediatric obsessive-compulsive disorder or Tourette's syndrome, and have been temporarily labelled PANDAS (paediatric autoimmune neuropsychiatric

Table 1 Operative criteria for the diagnosis of paediatric autoimmune neuropsychiatric disorders associated with streptococcal infections (PANDAS)[12]

> - Presence of obsessive-compulsive disorder and/or tic disorder (meeting DSM-IV criteria)
>
> - Prepubertal symptom onset
>
> - Episodic course characterised by acute, severe onset and dramatic symptom exacerbations
>
> - Temporal relationship between GABHS infections and symptom exacerbations (ascending and descending titres of anti-streptococcal antibodies should be observed in parallel with clinical exacerbations and remissions)
>
> - Neurological abnormalities (*e.g.* choreiform movements) present during symptom exacerbations

disorders associated with streptococcal infections). The five operational criteria for diagnosis of PANDAS are listed in Table 1.[12] PANDAS obsessive-compulsive symptoms do not differ from those in childhood-onset obsessive-compulsive disorder, as much as tics in PANDAS overlap those observed in chronic tic disorders in respect to their phenomenology. However, the age at symptom onset in PANDAS is about 3 years younger than in childhood-onset obsessive-compulsive disorder and about 2 years younger than in Tourette's syndrome. The most characteristic feature of PANDAS is their relapsing-remitting course, temporally associated with an immune response triggered by streptococcal infections. Typically, symptoms occur 'out of the blue', often overnight, abruptly peaking in severity within the first 1 or 2 days, and lasting for several weeks. The core symptoms may be accompanied by attentional difficulties, emotional lability, hyperactivity, separation anxiety and urinary frequency or enuresis. Although a frank chorea needs to be absent in order to support diagnosis, mild choreiform movements elicited during neurological examination for soft signs are often present, and may affect handwriting.[12]

One of the main hurdles in the recognition of the PANDAS phenotype as a distinct nosological entity is the difficulty demonstrating clear exacerbations of obsessive-compulsive disorder and Tourette's syndrome with streptococcal throat infections, all highly prevalent conditions in paediatric years. Recent controlled studies, in which prospective follow-up of children with streptococcal infections or tic and/or obsessive-compulsive disorder was performed, provided inconsistent results. A robust, population-based, retrospective, case-control study showed that patients with obsessive-compulsive disorder or tic disorder recruited from out-patient facilities were about 2-fold more likely to have had prior streptococcal infection in the 3 months before onset date, with a higher risk for children with multiple streptococcal infections within 12 months.[13] Other prospective reports, however, failed to detect a clear and significant association between the exacerbation of tics/obsessive-compulsive symptoms and streptococcal infections. Overall, taking into account these discrepancies, PANDAS may exist as a distinct nosological entity, although their incidence and prevalence might be lower than expected, hindering their discrimination from the overall population of the highly prevalent tic and obsessive-compulsive disorders.

To some extent, the PANDAS phenotype clinically overlaps Sydenham's chorea. A recent long-term observation of South African Sydenham's chorea patients showed that 12% of cases developed a chronic tic disorder, and 14% manifested the PANDAS phenotype over the years following the first episode of chorea, and a significantly higher frequency of behavioural problems was recorded in these patients with long-term complications.[14] However, it is still debated whether the PANDAS phenotype falls within the spectrum of rheumatic fever. Although preliminary reports suggested a higher proportion of echocardiographic valvular abnormalities in children with post-streptococcal tic disorder, a recent cross-sectional study on patients strictly fulfilling PANDAS criteria showed that 59 of 60 patients did not manifest any valvular abnormality on 2-dimensional echocardiography, suggesting PANDAS is purely a brain disorder without multi-organ involvement.[15]

The strong clinical similarity between the PANDAS phenotype and TS or childhood-onset obsessive-compulsive disorder suggested the possibility that a subgroup of children with the latter two conditions might have a pathogenic link to streptococcal infections, despite the absence of the typical relapsing-remitting course which characterises PANDAS. These studies are reviewed below.

Other forms of post-streptococcal movement disorders

Other types of movement disorders shortly following GABHS infection have been reported in the last few years. In a cohort of 40 UK children presenting with movement disorders following streptococcal pharyngitis (defined by pharyngeal culture and/or serology), a notable variety of hyperkinetic movement disorders was observed. Although chorea and tics (respectively fulfilling diagnostic criteria for Sydenham's chorea and PANDAS) were the most frequent neurological signs in these children, dystonia, tremor, stereotypies, or myoclonus were reported in up to 12% of cases.[16] Other notable case reports include generalised dystonia associated with infantile bilateral striatal necrosis,[17] a case of paroxysmal dystonic choreoathetosis and two cases with transient restless legs syndrome-like symptoms following GABHS infection.[18] Finally, a few anecdotal reports described cases of generalised and isolated abdominal myoclonus apparently triggered by streptococcal infection.[19]

Other forms of post-streptococcal behavioural abnormalities

Psychiatric symptoms have been observed also in patients affected by rheumatic fever without chorea; obsessive-compulsive symptoms or disorder were reported in 35% of these patients, 15% had an anxiety disorder, and 15% reported enuresis.[8] In a clinical series of British children presenting with movement disorders following streptococcal pharyngitis, acute emotional and/or behavioural alteration occurred in 82.5% of patients, supporting the hypothesis that an autoimmune process directed to the basal ganglia very often presents with a wide array of behavioural features. The most frequent changes were emotional lability (32.5%), anxiety (27.5%), obsessions and/or compulsions (22.5%), depression (17.5%), aggressive, oppositional, or disruptive behaviours (14%), and attention deficit (17.5%). Within this cohort

Table 2 Summary of the predominant clinical features of post-streptococcal neuropsychiatric disturbances and their occurrence in the three main characterised post-streptococcal CNS illnesses

Hyperkinetic movement disorders
  Chorea[a,b]
  Dystonia[b]
  Tics[a,b,c]
  Oculogyric crises[a,b]
  Facial grimacing[a,b]
  Hemiballism[a]
  Paroxysmal choreoathetosis
  Myoclonus

Hypokinetic movement disorders
  Bradykinesia[a,b]
  Rest tremor[b]
  Rigidity[b]
  Postural instability[b]

Psychiatric features
  Mutism[b]
  Anxiety/depression[a,b,c]
  Apathy[a,b]
  Obsessive-compulsive behaviour[a,b,c]
  Catatonia[b]
  Agitation[a,b]
  Confusion[b]
  Aggressiveness[b,c]
  Disinhibition[b,c]

[a]Present in Sydenham's chorea.
[b]Present in post-streptococcal acute disseminated encephalomyelitis (or in its encephalitis lethargica-like variant).
[c]Present in the PANDAS phenotype.

of 40 subjects, ICD-10 psychiatric diagnoses of emotional disorders occurred in 47.5%, including obsessive-compulsive disorder (27.5%), generalised anxiety (25%), and depressive episode (17.5%).[16]

Summary of clinical findings

Despite the apparent diversity of clinical findings in post-streptococcal brain disorders, the spectrum of disease generally conforms to extrapyramidal movement disorders (chorea, tics, dystonia, Parkinsonism and myoclonus) and a broad range of psychiatric disorders (particularly emotional disorders). Associated sleep disorders (insomnia in hyperkinetic disorders and hypersomnolence in hypokinetic disorders) are sometimes described, and occasionally other dysfunction of the CNS (encephalopathy and disseminated CNS dysfunction). The basal ganglia appears to be the most vulnerable brain region clinically and radiologically (Table 2).

Treatment

The therapeutic options for neuropsychiatric post-streptococcal disturbances fall within three main categories – symptomatic, immunomodulatory and antibiotic.[20] The involuntary movements exhibited by these patients, predominantly chorea and tics, traditionally respond to the same medications used in other well-known choreatic and tic disorders. In Sydenham's chorea, the first-choice drugs are valproic acid and carbamazepine, whereas antidopaminergic agents, such as pimozide and haloperidol, are used in patients who do not respond to valproate or those with chorea paralytica.[21] In addition, the use of neuroleptics in Sydenham's chorea patients is hindered by their sensitivity to develop tardive Parkinsonism and dystonia.[21] Symptomatic treatment of tics and obsessive-compulsive symptoms in patients with the PANDAS phenotype does not differ from the treatment approach in classical Tourette's syndrome or paediatric obsessive-compulsive disorder.

Immunomodulatory treatments comprise corticosteroids, intravenous immunoglobulins (IVIG) and plasma exchange. Trials of immunomodulatory agents are justified by the assumption of an immune-mediated brain damage, characteristic of all post-infectious syndromes. Corticosteroids are generally used in children with severe Sydenham's chorea refractory to symptomatic therapies or antibiotics, or in those who develop tardive movement disorders following the use of neuroleptics. In this scenario, aggressive treatment (25 mg/kg/day of methylprednisolone for 5 days) followed by 1 mg/kg/day of prednisone proved to be well-tolerated and more effective than simple long-term treatment with low doses of oral prednisone.[21] A recent randomised-entry controlled trial on 18 patients showed that IVIG and plasma exchange were slightly more effective than prednisone in reducing chorea severity; this finding needs to be confirmed by larger randomised trials.[22] Further evidence for the autoimmune nature of post-streptococcal neuropsychiatric disorders came from a double-blind randomised trial which compared plasma exchange with IVIG and sham IVIG for the treatment of tics and obsessive-compulsive symptoms in 29 children fulfilling the PANDAS criteria. Both treatments significantly improved emotional symptoms and global functioning. Plasma exchange produced a beneficial effect within 1 week of treatment, whereas IVIG-induced symptom amelioration not before the third week. Moreover, the benefit induced by IVIG was of smaller entity than the one obtained with plasma exchange, in keeping with the hypothesis of a predominantly antibody-mediated disorder.[23] Nevertheless, this small, albeit encouraging trial raised a few methodological points of debate, and its results are yet to be confirmed by other studies on larger clinical cohorts and with longer follow-up periods.

GABHS remains uniquely sensitive to long-term, low-dose penicillin, which may be administered orally or parenterally. The minimum treatment period for patients with one or more episodes of Sydenham's chorea without carditis is generally 5 years, or up to 18 years of age. Alternative agents are sulphadiazine or macrolides (erythromycin, azithromycin).[24] A recent double-blind, randomised, controlled trial on 23 patients with the PANDAS criteria showed that penicillin and azithromycin were both effective in decreasing streptococcal infections and neuropsychiatric symptom exacerbations.[25] Nevertheless, at present, guidelines regarding the use of antibiotic prophylaxis in the PANDAS phenotype are lacking. This decision should, therefore, be based on clinical indications in each individual after clinical follow-up.

IMMUNOPATHOGENESIS OF POST-STREPTOCOCCAL CNS DISORDERS

Hypothesis

The immunopathogenesis of post-streptococcal brain disorders is incompletely defined. However, what is clear is that in post-streptococcal CNS disorders, GABHS does not typically cause bacteraemia, nor does the intact organism gain access to the CNS. It is, therefore, apparent that CNS dysfunction must be secondary to toxin-mediated or immune-mediated disease. A number of different immunopathogenic abnormalities are possible. For example, GABHS is capable of producing vasculitis (particularly with skin involvement). However, there is little imaging evidence of small or large vessel vasculitis or stroke-like episodes in Sydenham's chorea or PANDAS. Along the same lines, cell-mediated immunity, cytokine activation or superantigen-mediated disease is possible and will be considered below. However, most attention has been focused on a B-cell or antibody-mediated hypothesis (discussed below). This is partly due to the landmark paper by Husby, finding anti-neuronal antibodies in Sydenham's chorea compared to controls. A popular, yet unproven, hypothesis is termed molecular mimicry, and states that the host forms an immune response against the bacteria which cross-reacts with the host tissues, in this case brain. Although popular, the molecular mimicry hypothesis remains unproven. Molecular mimicry could become a real pathogenic mechanism if there was a breakdown of immune tolerance, due to specific or non-specific immune activation. The antibody hypothesis is also popular due to the apparent clinical reversibility of many of the clinical syndromes. The complete recovery of some Sydenham's chorea and PANDAS patients and the normal imaging makes vasculitic or cytotoxic cell-mediated pathogenesis less likely (although not impossible). Finally, it is possible that the diseases we call Sydenham's chorea and PANDAS may have a number of different immune aetiologies. It is also possible that a number of different variables are aetiologically important in the development of post-streptococcal CNS syndromes including the age of onset, neurochemical variables and streptococcal serotypes.

Cellular immunopathogenesis

Very little focus has been given to cellular autoimmunity, partly because investigation is more complex and time-consuming. Indirect methods to assess the role of cellular autoimmunity have been done by measuring cytokine deviation in serum or CSF.

Cytokines

There are many cytokines and chemokines that have a variety of pro-inflammatory or anti-inflammatory actions, and even have direct effects on neuronal function and survival. Investigations of cytokines in serum and CSF can define whether there is a trend towards a Th1 (cell-mediated) or Th2 (humoural) autoimmunity. Church and co-workers[26] found elevated interleukin (IL)-4 and IL-10 levels, and normal interferon-γ in the CSF and serum of acute Sydenham's chorea, and proposed a Th2 response is more likely. However, Teixera found increased interferons (CXCL9 and CXCL10) in the serum of Sydenham's chorea suggesting Th1 (cell-mediated) mechanism may be involved in the pathogenesis of Sydenham's chorea.[27]

Superantigens

GABHS, like *Staphylococcus aureus*, is capable of inducing superantigen-mediated disease, and GABHS superantigens are capable of non-specifically stimulating vast numbers of lymphocytes with consequent excessive cytokine and antibody release plus cell-mediated tissue destruction. This immunopathogenic mechanism is currently hypothesised, due to GABHS recognised superantigen potential, rather than any specific data supporting this hypothesis. Indeed, the very modest cytokine alterations seen in acute Sydenham's chorea do not support this hypothesis.[26] However, further investigation is certainly warranted in the superantigen hypothesis.

Adhesion molecules

Adhesion molecules such as soluble intercellular adhesion molecule-1 (sICAM-1), vascular cell adhesion molecule-1 (VCAM-1) and E-selectin are molecules whose role includes the cellular transport of activated lymphocytes across the vascular endothelium and, therefore, blood–brain barrier. These molecules are overexpressed in a number of neuro-inflammatory disorders. We have recently reported increased levels of sICAM-1 (but not VCAM-1 or E-selectin) in Sydenham's chorea and PANDAS.[28] These findings do not provide specific understanding regarding the immune pathogenesis, although they do provide support to the neuro-inflammatory process. Interestingly, VCAM-1 and E-selectin were significantly elevated in patients with Tourette's syndrome compared to neurology and healthy controls supporting an immune pathogenic hypothesis in Tourette's syndrome.[28]

Antibodies and the B-lymphocyte hypothesis

Activated B-lymphocytes become plasma cells and produce antibodies. For antibodies to gain access to the brain in significant number, it would be necessary for there to be a breach of the blood–brain barrier, which may occur during systemic inflammation (such as in rheumatic fever). However, recent evidence indicates that activated lymphocytes (T- and B-) are capable of gaining access to the brain across an intact blood–brain barrier. Lymphocytes survey the brain (at low levels) all of the time, and are rarely problematic.[29] However, if they recognise self-proteins, a pro-inflammatory cascade is possible with further cell recruitment. Therefore, lymphocytes (if activated) can gain access to the brain even through a intact blood–brain barrier. The blood–brain barrier in post-streptococcal CNS disorders has not been investigated and its integrity is, therefore, unknown. It is theoretically possible that activated B-lymphocytes could produce serum autoimmunity, and gain access to the CNS through an intact blood–brain barrier and produce intrathecal autoantibodies in the CNS. Antineuronal antibodies have been a focus of investigation in Sydenham's chorea and PANDAS. In 1976, Husby demonstrated, using an indirect immunofluorescent technique, antibodies that bound to caudate and subthalamic neurones (basal ganglia) in 46% of Sydenham's chorea patients ($n = 30$) compared to 14% of rheumatic fever (without chorea; $n = 50$) and only 4% of controls ($n = 203$).[30] The staining pattern was to the cytoplasm of axons, and antibody reactivity was reduced after pre-incubation with GABHS cell-wall preparations.[30] Furthermore, Bronze leant support to a molecular mimicry hypothesis by showing antibody cross-reactivity between streptococcal and neuronal epitopes.[29] Further examination of Sydenham's chorea cohorts and PANDAS cohorts using immunofluorescence found increased antibodies in patients compared to controls, although the specificity was significantly less impressive (patients 80–91%, controls 33–50%).[31] In two separate studies, Kotby and Church found significantly improved specificity in cohorts of Sydenham's chorea using immunofluorescence (acute Sydenham's chorea patients 95–100%, controls 0–13%).[32,33]

Church expanded upon these findings by using the semi-quantitative ELISA technique and Western blotting. Western blotting causes some disruption of the protein structure but allows separation of protein to allow demonstration of common antibody–antigen interaction. Using Western blotting, Church found that autoantibodies against brain autoantigens of molecular weight 40 kDa, 45 kDa (doublet) and 60 kDa are found in 90–100% of Sydenham's chorea, PANDAS, post-streptococcal ADEM and post-streptococcal Parkinsonism (encephalitis lethargic-like) patients but only 0–13% of controls,[29,33,34] and proposed that they may represent a useful disease marker. In addition, the same antibody findings have been found in the CSF of a limited number of patients tested.[29] However, a number of reports from Singer's group have cast doubt on the specificity of these antibodies.[35] It should be noted that there are significant differences in the methodologies between the two groups, most importantly in the detection methods. Singer uses low antigen concentrations, and enhanced chemiluminesence detection of antibody binding. Enhanced chemiluminesence is very sensitive and can demonstrate low titre of probably insignificant autoantibodies (an array of autoantibodies are present in all individuals and are of no significance). Singer's group employ enhanced chemiluminesence and then complex analysis methods to interpret their findings.[35] Church used a detection method of reduced sensitivity (colormetric), thereby avoiding detection of low-titre autoantibodies of dubious significance.[33] Using enhanced chemiluminesence, Singer found Western blotting revealed increased antineuronal antibodies in acute Sydenham's chorea versus controls, but not in PANDAS.[29,35] The discrepancies between the investigating groups highlight the difficulties involved in autoimmune models and the importance of standardised methodologies.

Two significant papers have expanded upon the antineuronal antibody hypothesis and defined putative neuronal autoantigens. Kirvan et al.[36] demonstrated a cross-reactive antibody response between Streptococcus N-acetyl-β-D-glucosamine and neuronal lysoganglioside GM-1. They also showed potential antibody pathogenicity (increased intracellular signalling.[36] These findings were only from one patient and further examination of the specificity of these antibodies in patient cohorts is required.

Expanding on the work by Church, we have been able to define the 40 kDa, 45 kDa and 60 kDa neuronal antigens as neuronal isoforms of the glycolytic enzymes aldolase C, neuron-specific enolase and pyruvate kinase M1.[37] These enzymes are involved in energy production in the cytoplasm of neurones, but also exist on the neuronal cell membrane as receptors and additionally provide energy support to ion channels. The antigens are, therefore, theoretically available to antibody binding without disruption of the cell integrity. Interestingly, these proteins also exist on the cell surface of GABHS and there is high level of homology between the streptococcal and neuronal enzymes. These findings are interesting, yet it is still unknown whether the antibodies are pathogenic or just markers. Another question that arises is 'why are the basal ganglia specifically involved?' as these neuronal glycolytic enzymes are not basal ganglia specific. One possible explanation is that the basal ganglia are vulnerable due to their huge metabolic demand (basal ganglia vulnerability is seen in mitochondrial cytopathy, neonatal hypoxic ischaemia and hypoglycaemia). Basal ganglia GABAergic spiny neurones have the highest resting potential of any neurons and have been shown to be the most vulnerable neuronal population to energy failure.[38]

In conclusion, anti-neuronal antibodies are found in some post-streptococcal CNS cohorts, although the findings are controversial. More work is required to determine the use of antineuronal antibodies as markers of these disorders. Demonstrating the presence of antibodies does not mean that they are pathogenic. Removing the antibodies (with plasmapheresis) has been performed in one study and produced improvement in PANDAS patients compared to controls.[23] This small study needs to be reproduced and the methodology has been criticised.[29] Further pathogenic potential has been investigated by infusing patient antibody into rat brains. Two studies demonstrated increase in abnormal movements or behaviours, whereas one study failed to demonstrate a difference.[29] Employing a different method, Hoffman et al.[29] induced disease in rats after immunisation with an M6 streptococcal homogenate, and showed IgG deposition in the brain.

Although there is evidence of antineuronal antibodies (and possible pathogenicity), the findings are controversial and, in some cases, conflicting. Further investigation is required before these disorders can be considered autoantibody mediated.

D8/17 B-lymphocyte marker

A surface marker D8/17 on B-lymphocytes was found to be overexpressed in patients with rheumatic fever and Sydenham's chorea.[39] Studies in the 1990s suggested this was a useful marker of disease in Sydenham's chorea and PANDAS.[29] However, subsequently there have been problems with test-retest agreement[29] and further methodological problems have cast doubt on D8/17 as a marker. Although CD19 B-lymphocytes are overexpressed in Sydenham's chorea and PANDAS, D8/17 is not proving reliable as a disease marker.[29,39]

ROLE OF POST-STREPTOCOCCAL AUTOIMMUNITY IN COMMON NEUROPSYCHIATRIC SYNDROMES

The fact that GABHS can induce immune-mediated brain syndromes resulting in tics and emotional disorders such as obsessive-compulsive disorder, has lead to speculation that idiopathic disorders such as Tourette's syndrome and obsessive-compulsive disorder are secondary to post-streptococcal autoimmunity. Unfortunately, as the exact immune mechanism in Sydenham's chorea and PANDAS has not been defined, it could be considered premature to attempt to examine cohorts of obsessive-compulsive disorder and Tourette's syndrome for markers of post-streptococcal autoimmunity. As a consequence, it is not surprising that the results are inconsistent.

Evidence of recent streptococcal infection or colonisation in Tourette's syndrome or obsessive-compulsive disorder

A number of groups have compared streptococcal serology in cohorts of Tourette's syndrome with healthy controls. Some of these groups have found a positive association (elevated streptococcal serology in Tourette's syndrome) whereas others have found no association.[39] The largest single study tested 300 children (150 with tics and 150 without tics) for streptococcal serology at one time point, and found a significantly higher ASO titre in tic patients compared to controls. They also found a relationship between the severity of tic disorder and the magnitude of streptococcal antibody response.[40]

Mell et al.[13] recently published the first epidemiological study examining this hypothesis. Between 1992 and 1999, children receiving their first diagnosis of obsessive-compulsive disorder, Tourette's syndrome or tic disorder were assessed for recent streptococcal infection.[13] The cases were matched with controls for age, gender, locality and propensity to seek healthcare. The obsessive-compulsive disorder, tic, and Tourette's syndrome patients were more likely to have had prior streptococcal infection in the 3 months before onset. In addition, having multiple infections with GABHS within a 12-month period was associated with an increased risk of Tourette's syndrome (odds ratio 12.6; 95% CI, 1.93–51.0). This study was the most robust examination of a possible association to date.[13]

Anti-neuronal antibodies in idiopathic obsessive-compulsive disorder or Tourette's syndrome

In the same vein, there are some conflicting findings regarding the presence of antineuronal antibodies. Interestingly, Singer's group were one of the first to find anti-neuronal antibodies in Tourette's syndrome compared to controls (including proposing a 60 kDa autoantigen, similar to Church).[29,39] Subsequent studies by Singer's group have found no evidence of autoantibodies in Tourette's syndrome patients against the neuronal proteins proposed by Church and Dale to be autoantigens in post-streptococcal CNS disease and Tourette's syndrome.[33,35,37] We have looked at 100 adults and children with Tourette's syndrome, and 50 children with obsessive-compulsive disorder and found increased antineuronal antibodies in patients compared to controls (23% in Tourette's syndrome, 42% in obsessive-compulsive disorder, versus 2–10% of control groups.[29,39] In addition, we identified the same brain autoantigens (40 kDa, 45 kDa and 60 kDa) as those seen in Sydenham's chorea and PANDAS were involved in autoantibody binding. We speculated that a subgroup of idiopathic Tourette's syndrome and obsessive-compulsive disorder may be secondary to post-streptococcal autoimmunity. However, because of the discrepancy in results between different groups, further examination is clearly required before this potentially revolutionary thinking can be accepted in these common disorders.

D8/17 as a marker in idiopathic Tourette's syndrome and obsessive-compulsive disorder

Despite the initial excitement that D8/17 was a significantly elevated in patients with obsessive-compulsive disorder and Tourette's syndrome,[31,39] the same concerns to those described earlier regarding D8/17 specificity have been recently raised.[29] The role of D8/17 as a marker in obsessive-compulsive disorder and Tourette's syndrome remains uncertain at present.

CONCLUSIONS

Post-streptococcal autoimmune brain disorders usually present with a range of extrapyramidal and psychiatric disorders. The pathophysiology appears to be immune-mediated although the exact disease mechanism remains to be elucidated. These disorders remain an intriguing model of common movement and psychiatric disorders in children.

Key points for clinical practice

- Post-streptococcal brain disorders are still present in industrialised countries and are endemic in non-industrialised countries.
- Development of disease is probably multifactorial with genetic, neurochemical and microbiological variables.
- Classic clinical phenotypes include an array of extrapyramidal movement disorders such as chorea, tics, dystonia and Parkinsonism.
- Psychiatric disorders are classic accompaniments, particularly emotional disorders such as obsessive-compulsive disorder. The psychiatric disorders can occur as a post-streptococcal disorder in isolation.
- MRI is normal in conventional imaging, although inflammatory changes are seen, particularly in the dystonic or Parkinsonian phenotypes.
- The clinical phenomenology, imaging and pathology all point to vulnerability of the basal ganglia.
- The immune mechanisms are incompletely defined. Most investigation has been into the role of antineuronal antibodies.
- The role of post-streptococcal autoimmunity in common neuropsychiatric syndromes such as Tourette's syndrome and obsessive-compulsive disorders has lead to conflicting results.
- Treatment of Sydenham's chorea and established PANDAS should be with prophylactic antibiotics. The use of other immunosuppression is, as yet, inadequately supported by scientific evidence.

References

1. Swedo SE. Sydenham's chorea. A model for childhood autoimmune neuropsychiatric disorders. *JAMA* 1994; **272**: 1788–1791.
2. Martino D, Tanner A, Defazio G *et al*. Tracing Sydenham's chorea: historical documents from a British paediatric hospital. *Arch Dis Child* 2005; **90**: 507–511.
3. Cardoso F. Infectious and transmissible movement disorders. In: Jankovic JJ, Tolosa E. (eds) *Parkinson's Disease and Movement Disorders*, 4th edn. Philadelphia, PA: Lippincott Williams and Wilkins, 2002; 584–595.
4. Korn-Lubetzki I, Brand A, Steiner I. Recurrence of Sydenham chorea. Implications for pathogenesis. *Arch Neurol* 2004; **61**: 1261–1264.
5. Cardoso F, Dornas L, Cunningham M, Oliveira JT. Nerve conduction study in Sydenham's chorea. *Mov Disord* 2005; **20**: 360–363.
6. Teixeira Jr AL, Meira FC, Maia DP, Cunningham MC, Cardoso F. Migraine headache in patients with Sydenham's chorea. *Cephalalgia* 2005; **25**: 542–544.
7. Swedo SE, Leonard HL, Schapiro MB *et al*. Sydenham's chorea: physical and psychological symptoms of St Vitus dance. *Pediatrics* 1993; **91**: 706–713.
8. Mercadante MT, Busatto GF, Lombroso PJ *et al*. The psychiatric symptoms of rheumatic fever. *Am J Psychiatry* 2000; **157**: 2036–2038.
9. Dale RC, Church AJ, Cardoso F *et al*. Poststreptococcal acute disseminated encephalomyelitis with basal ganglia involvement and auto-reactive antibasal ganglia antibodies. *Ann Neurol* 2001; **50**: 588–595.
10. Hartel C, Schilling S, Gottschalk S, Sperner J. Multiphasic disseminated encephalomyelitis associated with streptococcal infection. *Eur J Paediatr Neurol* 2002; **6**: 327–329.
11. Dale RC, Church AJ, Surtees RA *et al*. Encephalitis lethargica syndrome: 20 new cases and evidence of basal ganglia autoimmunity. *Brain* 2004; **127**: 21–33.
12. Swedo SE, Leonard HL, Garvey M *et al*. Pediatric autoimmune neuropsychiatric disorders associated with streptococcal infections: clinical description of the first 50 cases. *Am J Psychiatry* 1998; **155**: 264–271.
13. Mell LK, Davis RL, Owens D. Association between streptococcal infection and obsessive-compulsive disorder, Tourette's syndrome, and tic disorder. *Pediatrics* 2005; **116**: 56–60.
14. Walker KG, Lawrenson J, Wilmshurst JM. Neuropsychiatric movement disorders following streptococcal infection. *Dev Med Child Neurol* 2005; **47**: 771–775.
15. Snider LA, Sachdev V, MaCkaronis JE, St Peter M, Swedo SE. Echocardiographic findings in the PANDAS subgroup. *Pediatrics* 2004; **114**: e748–e751.
16. Dale RC, Heyman I, Surtees RA *et al*. Dyskinesias and associated psychiatric disorders following streptococcal infections. *Arch Dis Child* 2004; **89**: 604–610.
17. Dale RC, Church AJ, Benton S *et al*. Post-streptococcal autoimmune dystonia with isolated bilateral striatal necrosis. *Dev Med Child Neurol* 2002; **44**: 485–489.
18. Matsuo M, Tsuchiya K, Hamasaki Y, Singer HS. Restless legs syndrome: association with streptococcal or mycoplasma infection. *Pediatr Neurol* 2004; **31**: 119–121.
19. Smyth P, Sinclair DB. Multifocal myoclonus following group A streptococcal infection. *J Child Neurol* 2003; **18**: 434–436.
20. Jordan LC, Singer HS. Sydenham chorea in children. *Curr Treat Options Neurol* 2003; **5**: 283–290.
21. Cardoso F. Chorea: non-genetic causes. *Curr Opin Neurol* 2004; **17**: 433–436.
22. Garvey MA, Snider LA, Leitman SF, Werden R, Swedo SE. Treatment of Sydenham's chorea with intravenous immunoglobulin, plasma exchange, or prednisone. *J Child Neurol* 2005; **20**: 424–429.
23. Perlmutter SJ, Leitman SF, Garvey MA *et al*. Therapeutic plasma exchange and intravenous immunoglobulin for obsessive-compulsive disorder and tic disorders in childhood. *Lancet* 1999; **354**: 1153–1158.
24. Neutze JM. The cardiac aspects of rheumatic fever. In: Weatherall DJ, Ledingham JGG, Warrell DA. (eds) *Oxford Textbook of Medicine*, vol. 2, 3rd edn. Oxford: Oxford Medical, 2000; 2432–2436.
25. Snider LA, Lougee L, Slattery M, Grant P, Swedo SE. Antibiotic prophylaxis with azithromycin or penicillin for childhood-onset neuropsychiatric disorders. *Biol Psychiatry* 2005; **57**: 788–779.

26. Church AJ, Dale RC, Cardoso F *et al*. CSF and serum immune parameters in Sydenham's chorea: evidence of an autoimmune syndrome? *J Neuroimmunol* 2003; **136**: 149–153.

27. Cardoso F. Tourette syndrome: autoimmune mechanisms. In: Fernandez-Alvarez E, Arzimanoglou A, Tolosa E. (eds) *Paediatric Movement Disorders. Progress in Understanding*. Montrouge, France: John Libbey Eurotext, 2005: 231–246.

28. Martino D, Church AJ, Defazio G *et al*. Soluble adhesion molecules in Gilles de la Tourette's syndrome. *J Neurol Sci* 2005; **234**: 79–85.

29. Dale RC. Post-streptococcal autoimmune disorders of the central nervous system. *Dev Med Child Neurol* 2005; **47**: 785–791.

30. Husby G, van de Rijn I, Zabriskie JB, Abdin ZH, Williams Jr RC. Antibodies reacting with cytoplasm of subthalamic and caudate nuclei neurons in chorea and acute rheumatic fever. *J Exp Med* 1976; **144**: 1094–1110.

31. Williams KA, Grant JE, Schlievert P, Kim SW. Exploring the pathophysiology of PANDAS: streptococcus, Sydenham's, and superantigens. In: Fatemi SH. (ed) *Neuropsychiatric Disorders and Infection*. London: Taylor and Francis, 2005: 162–170.

32. Kotby AA, El Badawy N, El Sokkary S, Moawad H, El Shawarby M. Antineuronal antibodies in rheumatic chorea. *Clin Diagn Lab Immunol* 1998; **5**: 836–839.

33. Church AJ, Cardoso F, Dale RC, Lees AJ, Thompson EJ, Giovannoni G. Anti-basal ganglia antibodies in acute and persistent Sydenham's chorea. *Neurology* 2002; **59**: 227–231.

34. Church AJ, Dale RC, Giovannoni G. Anti-basal ganglia antibodies: a possible diagnostic utility in idiopathic movement disorders? *Arch Dis Child* 2004; **89**: 611–614.

35. Singer HS, Hong JJ, Yoon DY, Williams PN. Serum autoantibodies do not differentiate PANDAS and Tourette syndrome from controls. *Neurology* 2005; **65**: 1701–1717.

36. Kirvan CA, Swedo SE, Heuser JS, Cunningham MW. Mimicry and autoantibody-mediated neuronal cell signaling in Sydenham chorea. *Nat Med* 2003; **9**: 914–920.

37. Dale RC, Candler PM, Church AJ, Wait R, Pocock JM, Giovannoni G. Neuronal surface glycolytic enzymes are autoantigen targets in post-streptococcal autoimmune CNS disease. *J Neuroimmunol* 2006; In press.

38. Calabresi P, Centonze D, Bernardi G. Cellular factors controlling neuronal vulnerability in the brain: a lesson from the striatum. *Neurology* 2000; **55**: 1249–1255.

39. Murphy TK, Herbstman DM, Edge PJ. Infectious trigger in obsessive-compulsive and tic disorders. In: Fatemi SH. (ed) *Neuropsychiatric Disorders and Infection*. London: Taylor and Francis, 2005: 135–153.

40. Cardona F, Orefici G. Group A streptococcal infections and tic disorders in an Italian pediatric population. *J Pediatr* 2001; **138**: 71–75.

Titus K. Ninan

3

Brittle asthma

Brittle asthma was a term coined by Turner Warwick in 1976.[1] She described a group of adult patients with wide variability in peak expiratory flow rates with difficult-to-control asthma. This distinct phenotype with severe asthma had chaotic, unpredictable, peak expiratory flow rate variability that put them in a different category. It soon became apparent that this category of patients shared marked intragroup heterogeneity and that different clinicians labelled them differently.[2,3] However, most studies on severe asthma phenotypes have been done in adult populations over the age of 15 years.[2-5] This review will, therefore, look at evidence of similar phenotypes in childhood, and suggest best-management strategies.

TERMINOLOGY

Clinicians who manage adults and children with difficult-to-manage asthma refer to this cohort using a number of terms: difficult to treat asthma, difficult acute asthma, chronic persistent asthma, therapy-resistant asthma, corticosteroid-resistant asthma, life-threatening asthma, near fatal and fatal asthma, asthma beyond the guidelines, brittle asthma, refractory asthma.[2,4-8]

In 2002, the European Respiratory Society Task Force sought an all-encompassing inclusive, rather than exclusive, definition for this cohort of patients and coined the term difficult/therapy-resistant asthma.[6] The age group covered by the European Respiratory Society Task Force included all children over the age of 5 years. An American Thoracic Society Workshop in 2000 used the term refractory or severe asthma to identify this cohort of patients.[7] The American Thoracic Society Workshop agreed to a set of major

Titus K. Ninan FCP FRCPCH
Consultant Paediatrician, Heartlands Hospital, Heart of England NHS Foundation Trust, Bordesley Green East, Birmingham B9 5SS, UK
E-mail: titus.ninan@heartofengland.nhs.uk

33

Table 1 Refractory asthma: workshop consensus for typical clinical features

Major characteristics

In order to achieve control to a level of mild/moderate persistent asthma:

- Treatment with continuous or near continuous (= 50% of year) oral corticosteroids
- Requirement for treatment with high-dose inhaled corticosteroids

Minor characteristics

- Requirement for daily treatment with a controller medication in addition to inhaled corticosteroids (*e.g.* long-acting β-agonist, theophylline, or leukotriene antagonist)
- Asthma symptoms requiring short-acting β-agonist use on a daily or near daily basis
- Persistent airway obstruction (FEV_1 < 80% predicted; diurnal PEF variability > 20%)
- One or more urgent care visits for asthma per year
- Three or more oral steroid 'bursts' per year
- Prompt deterioration with ≤ 25% reduction in oral or inhaled corticosteroid dose
- Near-fatal asthma event in the past

and minor criteria (2 major and 7 minor) as summarised in Table 1. They define severe or refractory asthma as the presence of one or both major criteria and at least two minor criteria. This definition is applicable only when other conditions have been ruled out (Table 2), exacerbating factors optimally treated and poor adherence not a confounding issue.

Both groups excluded children under the age of 5 years because the phenotypic characterisation of pre-school wheeze is different.[9,10] Their response to therapy is variable and there is significant overlap between the various phenotypes.

PATTERN RECOGNITION IN DIFFICULT ASTHMA

Clinicians over the years have used a temporal sequence of events (*i.e.* symptom exacerbations, chronicity and rapidity of onset, response to treatment) to describe 'patterns of asthma'. These descriptions come from personal observations of

Table 2 Diagnoses that may masquerade as difficult/therapy-resistant asthma

- Obliterative bronchiolitis
- Vocal cord dysfunction
- Bronchomalacia
- Inhaled foreign bodies
- Cystic fibrosis
- Recent aspiration (particularly in handicapped children)
- Developmental abnormalities of the upper airway
- Immunoglobulin deficiencies
- Primary ciliary dyskinesia

astute clinicians in small group of patients. Clearly, there is considerable overlap between these cohorts. To obtain validity of these patterns, they have to be verified in larger cohorts. Uniformity in approach to pattern recognition, investigations, treatment and follow-up will help with disease understanding and, therefore, better management of these cohorts with a more favourable long-term outcome.

TYPES OF BRITTLE ASTHMA

Paediatricians now manage teenagers and young adults (up to 19 years of age) in many centres. It is likely that they will come across patients with brittle asthma. Two distinct types have been recognised in patients over the age of 15 years.[3]

Type 1 patients showing a peak expiratory flow rate variability of more than 40% diurnal variation for more than 50% of the time over at least 150 days despite being on maximal inhaled therapy as per the Scottish Inter-Collegiate Network/British Thoracic Society (SIGN-BTS) guidelines.[11]

Type 2 patients who developed acute severe attacks invariably occurring in less than 3 h but appear well controlled between attacks.

EPIDEMIOLOGY

Surprisingly, very little is known about the exact prevalence of brittle or severe asthma. The adult West Midlands database suggest a value of around 0.05% of the adult asthmatic population.[12]

Patients with type 1 brittle asthma show a female preponderance, whereas those of type 2 show no sex predilection. There is, however, an increased risk of death or being admitted to an intensive care unit in both of these groups. The risk factors commonly identified are shown in Table 3. It is also clear that patients with severe asthma have other co-morbid factors such as on-going eczema, dysfunctional breathing, or significant side effects of therapy especially from oral corticosteroids. The economic impact is significant. In the US, 40% of the cost of asthma is believed to be associated with emergency room use, hospitalisation and death. In Europe, the average cost per patient with severe asthma is 6 times that of someone with mild asthma.

Table 3 Factors that may contribute to loss of control in asthma

- Poor compliance/adherence to therapy
- Psychological and emotional factors
- Inadequate medical facilities
- Poor access to medical facilities
- Inadequate treatment
- Exposure to allergens
- Viral respiratory tract infections
- Indoor/outdoor pollution
- Gastro-oesophageal reflux
- Genetic factors

DIAGNOSIS

The diagnosis of brittle or difficult-to-treat asthma is established from a good clinical history and evidence of variable and reversible airways obstruction. Increasingly, one is looking for evidence of persistent airway inflammation by measuring exhaled nitric oxide,[13,14] examining for inflammatory cells in induced sputum and bronchial alveolar lavage and, finally, histopathology of the airways looking for the typical changes of asthma.[15,16] However, alternative diagnoses that mimic asthma have to be ruled out (Table 2). Some of these conditions co-exist with bronchial asthma and may contribute to the worsening of asthma. Vocal cord dysfunction can occur in isolation or in conjunction with severe asthma. Vocal cord dysfunction is often regarded as a psychological condition; this is not always the case and vocal cord dysfunction can occur as a consequence of hyper-responsiveness of the upper airways.[17,18] Diagnosis is usually established using flow volume loops and laryngoscopy.

AETIOLOGICAL ASSOCIATIONS

GENETICS

No single genotype has been consistently isolated. Adult patients with brittle asthma as well as patients with severe asthma report losing a relative from acute severe asthma more frequently than those with less severe asthma.[19] Loss of lung function and near fatal asthma has been reported in patients with mutations of the interleukin (IL)-4 gene and the IL-4 receptor gene.

ATOPY

More than 90% of type 1 brittle asthma adult patients show multiple positive skin test to inhaled and ingested allergens.[20] Many of these patients are continuously exposed to allergens at home which may be an exacerbating factor.[21]

AIR FLOW LIMITATION

Poor bronchodilator response to β-agonist is common in patients with severe or refractory asthma. This failure is attributed to a variety of reasons, such as down-regulation of β-receptors, structural alterations within the airways and unknown obstructive element or a different disease process altogether.[22,23]

AIRWAY HYPER-RESPONSIVENESS

The airway narrowing secondary to a provocative agent or stimuli appears to be exaggerated in patients with severe or brittle asthma.[24] Other authors have noted a failure to obtain a plateau-like response in the dose–response curve.[25] Both of these factors appear to play a distinct part in severe or brittle asthma.

PSYCHOSOCIAL FACTORS

Patients with severe or brittle asthma often have a poor quality of life and a greater number of asthma-related events.[26,27] They tend to be less capable of dealing with acutely worsening symptoms. This may be related to poor perception of lung dysfunction secondary to decrease in chemosensitivity to hypoxia. The response to hypercapnia is usually normal.[28]

FOOD ALLERGY/INTOLERANCE

Intolerance to a number of foods most notably dairy products, wheat, eggs, peanuts, citrus fruits and soya bean have been described.[29] Removal of the relevant food can produce dramatic improvements in some patients. Poor adherence leading to persistence of symptoms is common. An empirical exclusion of specific foods for at least 6–8 weeks must be regarded as the way forward if food intolerance is suspected.

PATHOLOGICAL CHANGES

Endobronchial and autopsy studies show an inflammatory pattern consistent with T-helper cell type 2 (Th2) paradigm.[30,31] Increases in eosinophil and lymphocytes along with Th2-type cytokines such as IL-4 and IL-5 have been described. In adult patients dying of status asthmaticus, the predominant cells are often the neutrophils.[32] Broncho-alveolar lavage (BAL) studies in intubated patients with severe asthma also support the neutrophil concept.[33] This may well be a reason why some of these patients are poorly responsive to steroids although this is speculative at the moment. The histopathology and BAL studies would, therefore, suggest at least two different subtypes of severe asthma – one with a predominantly eosinophilic inflammation and the other with a neutrophilic inflammation.[34]

CLINICAL EVALUATION AND MANAGEMENT

The preschool child presenting with acute severe asthma is a management challenge. The structural and physiological peculiarities that predispose to severe air flow obstruction in preschool children include disproportionately narrow peripheral airways, mucous gland hyperplasia, poor static elastic recoil of the lung and a highly compliant rib cage. The above-mentioned factors and the increased susceptibility to viral lower respiratory tract infections make these infants particularly vulnerable to severe lower airways obstruction and atelectasis.[35] The low birth-weight infant exposed to passive smoke who picks up a lower respiratory tract infection is a particularly vulnerable patient. In temperate climates with seasonal RSV epidemics, it is often difficult to distinguish between severe asthma and RSV infection, with the infection exacerbating the asthma. The mortality rate for asthma in this age group is about 5 per 100,000 population.[36]

Despite maximal therapy, the adolescent with severe asthma is frequently a management challenge. Often, there is a disconnection between expectation and outcome. Adherence to therapy is often poor and ranges from 30–70% resulting in poor symptom control.[37] The mortality rate for asthma in adolescents is generally higher than the rest of the paediatric age group. Possible reasons include psychological dysfunction, altered perception of disease severity, lack of adult supervision, poor compliance secondary to desire for increased autonomy and over reliance on inhaled β_2-agonists leading to delay in seeking appropriate treatment. Deaths from asthma are greatest amongst the least advantaged in society.

A protocol for evaluating severe/brittle asthma is useful. The European Respiratory Society Task Force on difficult asthma identified the need for 'integrated approach to define clinical phenotypes, evaluate risk factors, understand pathophysiology and find novel therapies'.[6] The diagnostic work-up of children should include symptom scores to assist severity, full pulmonary function tests including spirometry, flow volume loops, total lung capacity and residual volumes.[6,7] Daily peak expiratory flow rate charts to assess diurnal variability for a period of time (usually 6 weeks) is an additional valuable diagnostic tool.

Blood tests should include full blood count looking for eosinophilia, serum IgE, total immunoglobulins, and allergen-specific IgE.

Nitric oxide is a biomarker of airway inflammation and has been used to study both severity of asthma and the response to treatment. Using nitric oxide in children experiencing frequent symptoms despite being on high-dose inhaled corticosteroids, it has been possible to identify different subgroups of patients with difficult asthma.[13,14]

Radiological investigations should include chest X-ray looking for infiltration, interstitial and bullous lung disease. High-resolution computed tomography (CT) scans of the chest are useful to exclude primarily other pathologies of the lung especially obliterative bronchiolitis and bronchiectasis. The usefulness of this technique in assessing severe/brittle asthma remains unconfirmed.

A psychological assessment of the family dynamics is extremely useful to help progress with management.[26,27]

Heaney et al.[38] used a 'systemic evaluation protocol' in 73 adult subjects. In poorly controlled asthmatic subjects, they found a high prevalence of co-morbidity.[38] Dysfunctional breathlessness, vocal cord dysfunction and bronchiectasis are three of the conditions that are seen in childhood that they identified in their adult patients. Targeted treatment of identified co-morbidities unfortunately had a minimal impact on asthma-related quality of life in those patients with therapy-resistant disease.

THERAPY OPTIONS

Once the diagnosis is confirmed after an extensive history, physical examination and investigations, the treatment is holistic as is the case for anyone with severe complex asthma. The SIGN-BTS guidelines recommend that the cohort of patients be managed through a lead tertiary centre.[11] This centre will, in time, develop expertise in understanding the changing patterns of severe asthma. Appropriate pharmacological agents should be used and the side effects carefully looked for.

The corner stone of managing severe/brittle asthma is high-dose, high-potency inhaled corticosteroids. Generally, the treatment is combined with a long-acting bronchodilator, usually as separate inhalers to provide more flexibility of dosing schedules. Leukotriene receptor antagonists have been used in this population with some benefit.

Oral corticosteroids often have to be used and must be used in the smallest possible dose to achieve symptom control. If patients need 20 mg or more of prednisolone every alternate day, pharmacokinetic studies must be performed as they often provide useful information about absorption and elimination rates of corticosteroids. 'Steroid resistance' or 'steroid insensitivity' is defined as failure of bronchodilator response after 7 days of prednisolone (1 mg/kg/day) in children with a prebronchodilator FEV_1 of less than 70%. Adherence to treatment is an on-going issue in some of these children and depot preparation of corticosteroids administered i.m. may have to be resorted to.

Exhaled nitric oxide can be used to monitor response to treatment; if equipment is not easily available, the clinical parameters should be carefully monitored to assess response to therapy.

In some patients with severe/brittle asthma alternative T-cell immuno-modulator drugs have been used. Gold salts, cyclosporine, methotrexate and immunoglobulin infusions have all been used. The macrolides tacrolimus and sirolimus are similar to cyclosporine in their end effects. Brequinar sodium, mycophenolate mofetil, and leflunomde may be of benefit in patients with oral steroid-dependent asthma.[39] An anti-IgE monoclonal antibody is now available and early studies in carefully selected patients are encouraging. Some studies indicate the ability of some of these agents to decrease corticosteroid use by 50% but concurrent improvement in pulmonary function test is limited. The extensive and severe toxic effects of the alternative treatments preclude their long-term use.[6,7]

In adults, continuous subcutaneous infusion of terbutaline has shown to be effective in controlling peak expiratory flow variability and symptoms in 50% of patients. The development of subcutaneous abscesses and nodules limits its use.[40]

CONCLUSIONS

The phenotype of brittle asthma is a distinct entity amongst a heterogeneous condition that has been labelled by clinicians as refractory/therapy-resistant asthma/severe asthma. Although certain genetic polymorphisms have been loosely associated, further research is required to identify consistent genetic polymorphisms in this population for it to be of meaningful benefit to the patient. Information on the natural history and epidemiology of this condition at the moment is sparse.

Clinicians continue to label them differently although attempts to define them have been made at various workshops. The definitions have either been all-encompassing or very tight leading to poor agreement and uptake amongst clinicians. Although investigative approaches have been suggested, the lack of availability of these facilities across centres throughout the country make the identification of these cohorts into distinct subtypes difficult. Centralising care to fewer centres will help address a number of unanswered questions in this complex group of children who have significant morbidity, increased mortality and consume significant resources.

Key points for clinical practice

- Clinicians who manage children with difficult asthma recognise that it is a multifaceted disease.

- Brittle asthma is one such distinct phenotype in a larger heterogeneous group of difficult-to-manage asthma.

- In children over the age of 15 years, two distinct types of brittle asthma have been recognised based on their clinical profile.

- Co-morbid factors (such as eczema, vocal cord dysfunction and toxicity to some of the treatments) add to significant morbidity that these children experience.

- The economic impact of severe/brittle asthma is very significant. The average cost in Europe for a patient with severe asthma is 6 times that of someone with mild asthma.

- Diagnosis is established from a good history, evidence of reversibility, airway inflammation and looking for inflammatory markers in broncho-alveolar lavage or induced sputum.

- The preschool child with acute severe wheeze poses a different set of challenges to the adolescent.

- The mortality rate for adolescents with severe asthma is high; a number of risk factors have been identified.

- Systematic evaluation protocols are useful to define clinical phenotype, evaluate risk factors, understand pathophysiology and find effective treatments.

- High-dose, high-potency inhaled corticosteroids with add-on therapies are the mainstay of treatment. The treatment, however, has to be holistic for optimum benefit.

- A number of new treatments are being studied but their usefulness at the moment is limited by the extent of their toxicity.

References

1. Turner Warwick M. On observing patterns of airflow in asthma. *Br J Dis Chest* 1977; **71**: 73–86.
2. Ayres JG, Miles JF, Barnes PJ. Brittle asthma. *Thorax* 1998; **53**: 315–321.
3. Ayres JG. Severe asthma phenotypes – a case for more specificity. *J R Soc Med* 2001; **94**: 115–118.
4. Ten Brinke A, Zwinderman AH, Sterk PJ, Rabe KF, Bel EH. Factors associated with persistent airflow limitation in severe asthma. *Am J Respir Crit Care Med* 2001; **164**: 744–748.
5. Dragos D, Campbell D, Robinson DS, Chung KF. Significance of persistent airflow obstruction in patients with severe asthma. *Eur Respir J* 2002; **20**: 406s.
6. Chung KF, Godard P. (eds) European Respiratory Society Task Force Report on difficult therapy-resistant asthma. *Eur Respir Rev* 2000; **10**: 23–25.
7. Anon. Proceedings of the American Thoracic Society workshop on refractory asthma. *Am J Respir Crit Care Med* 2000; **162**: 2341–2351.

8. McGeehan M, Busse WW. Refractory asthma. *Med Clin North Am* 2002; **86**: 1073–1090.
9. Martinez FD, Wright AL, Taussig LM, Holberg, CJ, Halonen M, Morgan WJ. Asthma and wheezing in the first six years of life. The Group Health Medical Associates. *N Engl J Med* 1995; **332**: 133–138.
10. Martinez FD, Bonner A. Clinical diagnosis of wheezing in early childhood. *Allergy* 1995; **50**: 701–710.
11. Anon. British guidelines on the management of asthma. *Thorax* 2003; **58** (Suppl 1); 17–29.
12. Ayres JG, Jyothish D, Ninan T. Brittle asthma. *Paediatr Respir Rev* 2004; **5**: 40–44.
13. Thomas PS, Gibson PG, Wang H, Shah S, Henry RL. The relationship of exhaled nitric oxide to airway inflammation and responsiveness in children. *J Asthma* 2005; **42**: 291–295.
14. Pijnenburg MW, Bakker EM, Hop WC, De Jongste JC. Titrating steroids on exhaled nitric oxide in children with asthma: a randomized controlled trial. *Am J Respir Crit Care Med* 2005; **172**: 831–836.
15. Payne DN, Rogers AV, Adelroth E *et al*. Early thickening of the reticular basement membrane in children with difficult asthma. *Am J Respir Crit Care Med* 2003; **167**: 78–82.
16. Gibson PA, Norzila MZ, Fakes K, Simpson J, Henry RL. Pattern of airway inflammation and its determinants in children with acute severe asthma. *Pediatr Pulmonol* 1999; **28**: 261–270.
17. Newman KB, Mason UG, Schmaling KB. Clinical features of vocal cord dysfunction. *Am J Respir Crit Care Med* 1995; **152**: 1382–1386.
18. Ayres JG, Gabbot PL. Vocal cord dysfunction and laryngeal hyperresponsiveness: a function of altered autonomic balance? *Thorax* 2002; **57**: 284–285.
19. Ayres JG, Chung KF, Szczepura A *et al*. Patients with at risk asthma have a high frequency of reported asthma death in first degree relatives – evidence from the PARA UK database. *Thorax* 2001; **56**: S103.
20. Miles JF, Cayton RM, Tunnicliffe WS, Ayres JG. Increased atopic sensitization in brittle asthma. *Clin Exp Allergy* 1995; **25**: 1074–1082.
21. Tunnicliffe WS, Fletcher TJ, Hammond K *et al*. Sensitivity and exposure to indoor allergens in adults with differing asthma severity. *Eur Respir J* 1999; **13**: 654–659.
22. Larsen GL, Cherniack RM, Irvin CG. Pulmonary physiology of severe asthma in children and adults. In: Szefler SJ, Leung DYM. (eds) *Severe Asthma: Pathogenesis and Clinical Management*. New York: Marcel Dekker, 1996.
23. Cho SH, Seo JY, Choi DC *et al*. Pathological changes according to the severity of asthma. *Clin Exp Allergy* 1996; **26**: 1210–1219.
24. Ding DJ, Martin JG, Macklem PT. Effects of lung volume on maximal methacholine-induced bronchoconstriction in normal humans. *J Appl Physiol* 1987; **62**: 1324–1330.
25. Nielson CP, Crowley JJ, Vestal RE, Connolly MJ. Impaired beta-adrenoceptor function, increased leukocyte respiratory burst, and bronchial hyperresponsiveness. *J Allergy Clin Immunol* 1992; **90**: 825–832.
26. Garden GMF, Ayres JG. Psychiatric and social aspects of brittle asthma. *Thorax* 1993; **48**: 501–505.
27. Wamboldt MZ, Fritz G, Mansell A, McQuaid EL, Klein RB. Relationship of asthma severity and psychological problems in children. *J Am Acad Child Adolesc Psychiatry* 1998; **37**: 943–950.
28. Kikuchi Y, Okabe S, Tamura G *et al*. Chemosensitivity and perception of dyspnoea in patients with a history of near fatal asthma. *N Engl J Med* 1994; **330**: 1329–1334.
29. Baker C, Tunnicliffe WS, Duncanson R, Ayres JG. Double blind placebo controlled studies of food intolerance in brittle asthma. *J Am Dietet Assoc* 2000; **100**: 1361–1367.
30. Wenzel SE Szefler SJ, Leung DY, Sloan SI, Rex MD, Martin RJ. Bronchoscopy evaluation of severe asthma. Persistent inflammation associated with high dose glucocorticoids. *Am J Respir Crit Care Med* 1997; **156**: 737–743.
31. Leung DYM, Martin RJ, Szefler SI *et al*. Disregulation of interleukin 4, interleukin 5 and interferon gamma gene expression in steroid resistant asthma. *J Exp Med* 1995; **181**: 33–40.
32. James AL, Elliot JG, Abramson MJ, Walters EH. Time to death, airway inflammation and remodelling in fatal asthma. *Eur Respir J* 2005; **26**: 429–434.
33. Wenzel SE, Schwartz LB, Langnack EL *et al*. Evidence that severe asthma can be divided

pathologically into two inflammatory subtypes with distinct physiological and clinical characteristics. *Am J Respir Crit Care Med* 1999; **160**: 1000–1008.

34. Payne D, Bush A. Phenotype specific treatment of difficult asthma in children. *Paediatr Resp Rev* 2004; **5**: 116–123.
35. Nelson. In: Behrman, Kliegman, Jenson. (eds) *Text Book of Paediatrics*, 16th edn. New York: WB Saunders, 2000; 664–680.
36. Sly RM, O'Donnell R. Stabilization of asthma mortality. *Ann Allergy Asthma Immunol* 1997; **78**: 347–354.
37. Myers TR. Pediatric asthma epidemiology: incidence, morbidity, and mortality. *Respir Care Clin North Am* 2000; **1**: 1–14.
38. Heaney LG, Conway E, Kelly C *et al*. Predictors of therapy resistant asthma: outcome of a systematic evaluation protocol. *Thorax* 2003; **58**: 561–566.
39. Corrigan CJ. Asthma refractory to glucocorticoids: the role of newer immunosupressants. *Am J Respir Crit Care Med* 2002; **1**: 47–54.
40. Ayres JG, Fish DR, Wheeler DC, Wiggins J, Cochrane GM, Skinner C. Subcutaneous terbutaline and control of brittle asthma or appreciable morning dipping. *BMJ* 1984; **288**: 1715–1716.

Clare Pain   Eileen Baildam

4

Childhood-onset systemic lupus erythematosus

Systemic lupus erythematosus is a chronic relapsing and remitting multisystem disorder characterised by production of autoantibodies that leads to wide-spread inflammation of blood vessels and tissues. This can affect any organ system of the body leading to a multitude of different symptoms and signs and to a different presentation in nearly every patient.

Of patients with systemic lupus erythematosus, 15–20% develop the condition in childhood and adolescence.[1] The incidence of paediatric systemic lupus erythematosus is estimated to range from 0.36 to 0.9 per 100,000 children per year. Most children present during their teenage years and systemic lupus erythematosus is rare before 5 years of age. Girls tend to be affected approximately 5 times more often than boys.[2]

Lupus is a potentially life-threatening disorder and, whilst modern aggressive treatments have transformed the mortality rate, the 10-year survival of childhood onset disease is only 85.7%.[3] Children are more likely to die of active disease and they accrue more organ damage than adults.[3,4] In particular, children have more severe haematological and renal disease and an increased incidence of neurological disease.[1,5] For this reason, treatment should be undertaken in specialist paediatric rheumatology centres with expertise in treating this difficult disease and with access to the full range of paediatric subspecialties and intensive care.

Childhood-onset systemic lupus erythematosus occurs during a child's physical, emotional and intellectual development and so it is important to

Clare Pain BMBS BMedSci MRCPCH (for correspondence)
Paediatric Registrar, Makay-Gordon Centre, Royal Manchester Children's Hospital, Pendlebury, Manchester M27 4HA, UK. E-mail: clareypain@hotmail.com

Eileen Baildam MBChB FRCP FRCPCH MRCGP
Consultant Paediatric Rheumatologist, Royal Liverpool Children's Hospital, Alder Hey, Eaton Rd, Liverpool L12 2AF, UK. E-mail: eileen.baildam@rlc.nhs.uk

recognise the adverse effects the disease, treatment and prognosis can have on the individual and their family.

PATHOGENESIS

Systemic lupus erythematosus has a multifactorial aetiology. Differences in genetic make-up and immunological responses have been identified in patients with lupus and there are environmental triggers in some patients.

GENETICS

Siblings of patients with lupus have a 10–20-fold increased risk of developing the disease and twin studies have shown a 24% concordance rate in monozygotic twins compared with 2% in heterozygous pairs.[6] A family history of autoimmune disease is a risk factor for systemic lupus erythematosus and this increases with the number of first degree relatives affected by autoimmune disease.[6]

HLA haplotypes (especially HLA-DR2) have been associated with an increased susceptibility to develop systemic lupus erythematosus.[7]

HORMONAL INFLUENCES

It has been hypothesised that oestrogens play a role in the aetiology of lupus. This is supported by the peak presentation of systemic lupus erythematosus in women aged 15–40 years and by the alteration of the ratio of female to male patients; initially 4:1 in children under 10 years, increasing to 9:1 after puberty and dropping to 2:1 in post-menopausal women.[1]

IMMUNE DYSREGULATION

Disturbances in the immune system occur in systemic lupus erythematosus. These include a high ratio of CD4[+] to CD8[+] T cells, defects in immune cell tolerance, and abnormal signalling by immune cells. Immune tolerance is lost, leading to production of autoantibodies. These antibodies target antigens located in nuclei, cytoplasm and on cell surfaces. This leads to the formation of immune complexes and to complement activation and inflammation.

Dendritic cells
Abnormal activation of dendritic cells in systemic lupus erythematosus has been suggested to cause selection rather than deletion of T cells that have receptors to self-antigens.[6]

B cells and autoantibodies
Patients with lupus show hypergammaglobulinaemia and increased titres of autoantibodies in their serum. It has been shown that autoantibodies occur and increase in numbers prior to the clinical manifestations of systemic lupus erythematosus. Immune complexes containing anti-DNA and anti-RNP antibodies activate plasma dendritic cells to produce interferon (IFN)-α which induces differentiation of B cells into antibody-secreting plasma cells and activates monocytes and myeloid dendritic cells.[6] B cells themselves also secrete cytokines

and chemokines including interleukin (IL)-2, IL-6, IL-10, IFN-γ and tumour necrosis factor (TNF)-α and they are involved in antigen presentation to CD4$^+$ T cells.

T cells
T cells from patients with systemic lupus erythematosus appear to respond faster to antigenic triggers than healthy T cells. They also appear to be able to resist apoptosis by up-regulation of cyclo-oxygenase-2 expression.[6]

Cytokine alterations
The cytokines that have been reported as elevated in systemic lupus erythematosus include type-I interferon, IL-6, IL-10, IL-12 and IL-18. Levels also correlate with disease activity. Children with systemic lupus erythematosus have shown increased serum levels of TNF receptors.[6]

Apoptosis
The development of autoantibodies is thought to be due to impaired clearance of apoptotic cells. During apoptosis, plasma and nuclear antigens are displayed on the cell surface. This allows intracellular antigens to be targeted by lymphocytes that are immune-intolerant, creating autoantibodies.[8]

Lupus flares can be triggered by ultraviolet light and infection. Both these conditions are associated with increased apoptosis leading to release of large quantities of antigen, and subsequent production of antibodies and inflammation.[8]

Complement
Deficiency of any of the early components of the classical complement pathway (C1q, C2 and C4) predisposes to severe systemic lupus erythematosus early in life.[6,8]

ENVIRONMENTAL TRIGGERS

Systemic lupus erythematosus flares are associated with certain triggers including ultraviolet light, exercise, stress, pregnancy, infection and drugs such as antibiotics, anticonvulsants, hormones and non-steroidal anti-inflammatories.[9]

CLINICAL PRESENTATION

The most common clinical features of lupus in childhood at presentation are fever (68%), arthritis (74%), fatigue (74%), weight loss (58%) and malar rash (52%) (Table 1).[5] About 82% of children present with renal involvement.[10]

SKIN MANIFESTATIONS

Malar rash
The typical malar rash occurs on the cheeks and often on the eyelids, characteristically sparing the nasolabial folds. It is often photosensitive.

Oral and nasal ulcers
The ulcers that occur in systemic lupus erythematosus are typically painless and on the hard palate but may be painful and anywhere in the oral or nasal mucosa. Nasal ulcers may cause recurrent nosebleeds.

Table 1 Clinical features in childhood-onset systemic lupus erythematosus

Clinical features	Cumulative features in children with SLE (%)	References
Constitutional		
Fatigue	87	5
Fever	–	
Weight loss	71	5
Lymphadenopathy	36	5
Musculoskeletal		
Non-erosive arthritis	74–100	5,6
Tenosynovitis	–	
Myopathy	–	
Avascular necrosis	–	
Dermatological		
Malar rash	44-74	5,6
Alopecia	7–48	5,6
Oral ulcers	26–48	5,6
Photosensitivity	16–40	5,6
Discoid lesions	10–19	5,6
Renal		
Proteinuria	61	5
Glomerulonephritis	55–65	5,11
Hypertension	40	10
Renal failure	–	
Gastrointestinal tract		
Diffuse abdominal pain	–	
Oesophageal dysmotility	–	
Colitis	–	
Hepatosplenomegaly	58	5
Autoimmune hepatitis		
Pancreatitis		
Pulmonary		
Pleuritis	5-77	6
Pneumonitis	40–60	5,6
Pulmonary haemorrhage	1–10	5,6.12
Pulmonary embolism	2–3	6,12
Pleural effusions	30	6
Pulmonary hypertension	7	12
Interstitial lung disease	3–14	6,12
Shrinking lung syndrome	3–14	6,12
Cardiac		
Pericarditis	5–26	5,6,12
Libman-Sacks endocarditis	7	5
Myocarditis	3	12
Valvular lesions	–	
Conduction defects	3	12
Neuropsychiatric		
Headache	43–72	5,6,11
Seizures	26–51	5,6,11
Paresis	26	5
Organic psychosis	10–13	5,11
Cognitive impairment	55	6,11
Mood disorder	57	6,11
Cranial nerve and peripheral neuropathies	15–16	6,11
Chorea	7–9	6,11
Cerebrovascular disease*	12	6,11
Myelopathy	1	6,11

Table 1 *(continued)* Clinical features in childhood-onset systemic lupus erythematosus

Clinical features	Cumulative features in children with SLE (%)	References
Vascular		
Raynaud's phenomenon	26	5
Vasculitic lesions#	16–52	5,6
Thrombophlebitis	–	
Peripheral gangrene	–	
Thromboembolism	–	
Digital infarcts	–	
Haematological		
Anaemia	72–84	5,6
Coomb's positivity	58	5
Thrombocytopenia	8–74	5,6
Leucopenia	27–74	5,6
Lymphopenia	30–59	5,6
Antiphospholipid syndrome	–	
Ocular		
Retinopathy	20–35	6
Papilloedema	–	
Endocrine		
Hypo/hyperthyroidism	–	

*Cerebrovascular disease includes cerebral infarction, transient ischaemic attack, chronic multifocal disease, haemorrhage and sinus thrombosis.
#Vasculitic lesions include petechiae, purpura and vasculitic ulcers.

Alopecia

Children may suffer from alopecia although this may require direct questioning.

Discoid lupus

Discoid lesions appear as well-defined erythematous patches with adherent scales and follicular plugging. They tend to occur in sun-exposed areas and are exacerbated by ultraviolet light. Lesions can cause atrophic scarring[1] and hypo- or hyperpigmentation can occur as lesions resolve.[13]

Discoid lupus represents an almost separate disease entity to systemic lupus erythematosus. In adults with discoid lupus, 5–10% will develop systemic lupus erythematosus. Data from children have shown that 26% of paediatric patients with discoid lupus developed systemic lupus erythematosus in a 36-month follow-up period.[13] Discoid lupus without systemic disease is rare in children. Careful evaluation for systemic features should occur and laboratory investigations often precede clinical evidence of systemic lupus erythematosus.[1]

RENAL DISEASE

Up to 80% of children with systemic lupus erythematosus develop renal involvement during their disease course and of these 90% will do so within 2 years of disease onset.[1,10]

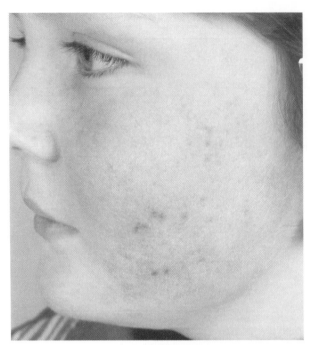

Fig.1 Typical malar rash with nasolabial sparing in child with systemic lupus erythematosus

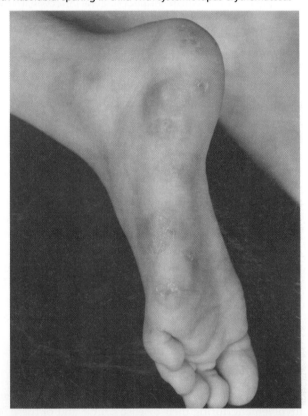

Fig.2 Cutaneous lupus lesions on soles of feet of child with systemic lupus erythematosus

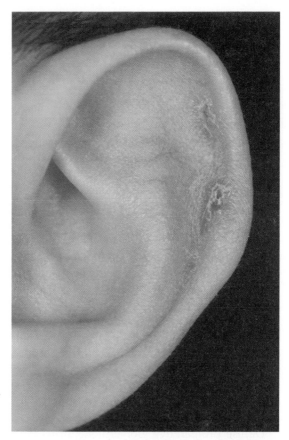

Fig. 3 Vasculitic lesions on ear of boy with systemic lupus erythematosus

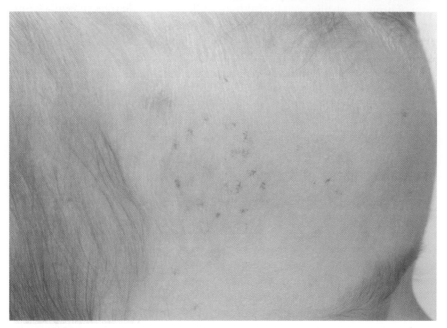

Fig. 4 Residual telangiectasia in infant with previous neonatal lupus

Table 2 The original World Health Organization classification of lupus nephritis with frequency of children affected[6,14]

Class	Type of nephritis	Frequency of children affected[6]
I	Normal glomeruli	7.5–8%
II	Mesangial nephritis	14–21%
III	Focal proliferative glomerulonephritis	2–36%
IV	Diffuse proliferative glomerulonephritis	40–65%
V	Membranous	5–20%

Despite improved diagnosis and treatment, lupus nephritis remains a major cause of morbidity and mortality in children.[2] Renal involvement most often presents with proteinuria and/or persistent microscopic haematuria. Hypertension occurs in around 40% of patients and some develop reduced renal function.[10]

The World Health Organization (WHO) classifies lupus nephritis according to renal biopsy appearance (Table 2), which helps aid treatment choice. This classification has been modified but the former system is still often used by pathologists.[14]

Long-term follow-up of affected patients has shown that those with focal or diffuse proliferative glomerulonephritis will go on to develop chronic renal failure if not treated with immunosuppressive therapies.[15]

Diffuse proliferative glomerulonephritis is the most common and severe form of lupus nephritis seen in children. Children with membranous nephritis tend to develop nephrotic syndrome. Mesangial nephritis has a good prognosis and is often controlled with minimal treatment, although progression of disease may occur.[1]

Hypertension is a significant risk factor for renal failure and children with hypertension should be treated.[10]

The treatment for end-stage renal failure includes dialysis and renal transplantation. The 5-year kidney survival rate in childhood-onset lupus nephritis ranges from 44–93%.[10]

NEUROPSYCHIATRIC SYSTEMIC LUPUS ERYTHEMATOSUS

The nervous system can become involved in lupus and clinical features can be psychiatric or neurological involving the central, peripheral and autonomic nervous system. The American College of Rheumatology revised classification criteria[16] only included seizures and psychosis as neuropsychiatric manifestations but further neuropsychiatric syndromes have since been defined to aid diagnosis and exclusion of potential non-lupus aetiologies.[17]

Retrospective studies of neuropsychiatric systemic lupus erythematosus in childhood-onset disease suggest it occurs in 20–30% of children with systemic lupus erythematosus. However, a prospective study found that it occurred in 95% of paediatric systemic lupus erythematosus patients using the American

Table 3 Neuropsychiatric syndromes in systemic lupus erythematosus as defined by the American College of Rheumatology

Central nervous system
        Aseptic meningitis
        Cerebrovascular disease
        Demyelinating syndrome
        Headache (including migraine and benign intracranial hypertension)
        Movement disorder (chorea)
        Myelopathy
        Seizure disorder
        Acute confusional state
        Anxiety disorder
        Cognitive dysfunction
        Mood disorder
        Psychosis

Peripheral nervous system
        Guillain-Barré syndrome
        Autonomic neuropathy
        Mononeuropathy
        Myasthenia gravis
        Cranial neuropathy
        Plexopathy
        Polyneuropathy

Adapted from the American College of Rheumatology nomenclature and case definitions for neuropsychiatric lupus syndromes.[17]

College of Rheumatology nomenclature.[11] Of those children that develop neuropsychiatric disease, 75–80% will do so within the first year.[1]

The presentation of neuropsychiatric lupus is variable and the life-time prevalence in one study was as follows: headache 72%, mood disorder 57%, cognitive disorder 55%, seizure disorder 51%, acute confusional state 35%, anxiety disorder 21%, peripheral nervous system 15%, cerebrovascular disease 12%, psychosis 12%, chorea 7%, demyelinating syndrome 4%, aseptic meningitis 1% and myelopathy 1%. Serious and life-threatening neuropsychiatric systemic lupus erythematosus occurred in 76% of their study group.[11]

Chorea is seen much more frequently in paediatric patients and is often associated with antiphospholipid antibodies.[1] Migranous or tension headaches are very common. Severe unremitting pain may indicate raised intracranial pressure and central vein thrombosis. Central vein thrombosis is most often seen in the presence of antiphospholipid antibodies.[1] Lupus can cause cognitive dysfunction but this is difficult to evaluate.

The diagnosis of neuropsychiatric lupus is difficult to make and must exclude other causes of central nervous system pathology including drug side effects, infection and metabolic disturbance.

Magnetic resonance imaging (MRI) is the investigation of choice to assess neuropsychiatric systemic lupus erythematosus both for cerebrovascular and spinal pathologies.

ARTHRITIS

Up to 90% of children with systemic lupus erythematosus will have arthritis, which tends to present as a symmetrical polyarthritis affecting both large and small joints. Unlike juvenile idiopathic arthritis, the arthritis tends to be painful and out of keeping with the clinical findings in the joints.[1]

CARDIAC

Pericarditis is the most common cardiac feature of systemic lupus erythematosus; however, lupus can affect every part of the heart producing myocarditis, coronary artery disease and also Libman-Sacks endocarditis where fibrous sterile vegetations are found on the valves.[6] Silent cardiac abnormalities are a common finding with 16–32% of children having asymptomatic abnormalities including valvular insufficiency, cardiomegaly and myocardial perfusion defects that may predispose to early-onset ischaemic heart disease, the major cause of premature deaths in adults with lupus.[18,19]

RESPIRATORY

The lungs are involved in 5–77% of children with systemic lupus erythematosus with the most common features being pleuritis, acute pneumonitis and chronic interstitial lung disease.[6,12] Children with systemic lupus erythematosus may have abnormal pulmonary function tests despite having no respiratory symptoms, with one study finding 40% had a restrictive lung impairment.[20] Pulmonary haemorrhage is a rare, but life-threatening complication of systemic lupus erythematosus with mortality approaching 90% despite intensive treatment.[6]

Patients that present with respiratory symptoms and signs should have a chest radiograph and spirometry performed. A high-resolution CT scan of the chest may also be helpful.

HAEMATOLOGY

Systemic lupus erythematosus can cause thrombocytopenia, leucopenia and lymphopenia. There may be anaemia due to chronic disease or secondary to Coomb's positive haemolytic anaemia.[5]

ANTIPHOSPHOLIPID SYNDROME AND CHILDHOOD SYSTEMIC LUPUS ERYTHEMATOSUS

Antiphospholipid or anticardiolipin syndrome was first described in systemic lupus erythematosus patients (secondary antiphospholipid syndrome) but can occur on its own (primary antiphospholipid syndrome). It is characterised by recurrent thrombosis, fetal loss and thrombocytopenia in association with anticardiolipin antibodies or lupus anticoagulant. Thrombotic events affect veins and arteries of all sizes and all locations.[21]

Treatment of antiphospholipid syndrome

Patients that have antiphospholipid antibodies but no clinical sequelae do not

Table 4 Preliminary criteria for the classification of antiphospholipid syndrome

CLINICAL CRITERIA
 Vascular thrombosis
 Adverse pregnancy outcome:
 • ≥ 1 unexplained pregnancy loss beyond 10 weeks' gestation
 • ≥ 3 unexplained, consecutive pregnancy losses before 10 weeks' gestation
 • ≥ 1 premature births of a normal neonate at or before 34 weeks' gestation because of pre-eclampsia, eclampsia or placental insufficiency

LABORATORY CRITERIA
 Moderate or high titres of IgG or IgM anticardiolipin antibodies
  (≥ 2 occasions at least 6 weeks apart)
 Circulating anticoagulant (≥ 2 occasions at least 6 weeks apart)

Adapted from Wilson et al.[22]

need any specific treatment although some clinicians treat with antiplatelet therapy such as aspirin as this can reduce thrombosis risk.

Those children who experience thrombosis need anticoagulation with heparin followed by warfarin. This needs to achieve an INR of 3.0–3.5 and should be life-long as the risk of recurrence is high.[21] Symptomatic patients, such as those with chorea and significantly raised antiphospholipid antibodies, should probably be treated if there is evidence on imaging of any changes even if not thought to be thrombotic. Long-term outcome studies on early prophylactic treatment are required but the condition is rare.

DRUG-INDUCED LUPUS

Drug-induced lupus has been associated with over 40 different medications. Unlike drug hypersensitivity reactions, drug-induced lupus takes months to years of treatment with an offending agent to develop and is dose-dependent.

The clinical and laboratory features of drug-induced lupus mimic systemic lupus erythematosus. It is often not until the drug is stopped that the clinician can diagnose drug-induced lupus. Symptoms resolve within days to weeks of ceasing the drug, although this can take up to a year.

Procainamide and hydralazine are the drugs associated with the highest incidence of drug-induced lupus. The most common implicated drugs used in childhood include carbamazepine, phenytoin, isoniazid, minocycline and sulphasalazine. A lupus-like syndrome has been associated with ingestion of high quantities of alfalfa.[9]

NEONATAL LUPUS

Neonatal lupus is associated with maternal autoantibodies anti-SSA/Ro and anti-SSB/La. The disease in the neonate is secondary to transplacental passage of IgG-mediated autoantibodies. Not all mothers who have infants with neonatal lupus have systemic lupus erythematosus.[23]

Congenital heart block

Only 2% of neonates born to mothers with anti-SSA/Ro or SSB/La antibodies develop congenital heart block although it carries a mortality of 15–30%. Of those children that survive the immediate neonatal period, 67% require permanent pacing. The recurrence rate in subsequent pregnancies is about 19%.[23]

Neonatal lupus rash

This rash is often photosensitive and appears as annular plaques with erythema and scaling. It occurs on the face and scalp with a preference for upper eyelids but can be seen all over the body. Lesions may be absent at birth, developing at several weeks of age, with resolution occurring at 6–8 months as mother's autoantibodies disappear from the baby's circulation.[23]

Other manifestations

Babies with neonatal lupus can present with liver impairment or thrombocytopenia.[23]

DIFFERENTIAL DIAGNOSIS

Because of the many ways in which systemic lupus erythematosus can present, the differential diagnosis is beyond the scope of this review. However, for those children who present with fever, weight loss, rashes and arthralgia the important differentials to rule out include viral infections (especially Epstein-Barr virus, cytomegalovirus, human parvovirus B19), streptococcal and post-streptococcal syndromes, Kawasaki's disease, malignancy (especially neuroblastoma, leukaemia and lymphoma), inflammatory bowel disease, sarcoidosis and other rheumatological diseases most notably juvenile dermatomyositis and systemic onset juvenile idiopathic arthritis. Unusual organ disease should raise the possibility of systemic lupus erythematosus especially if there is more than one system affected.

LABORATORY INVESTIGATIONS

AUTOANTIBODIES

In systemic lupus erythematosus, antinuclear antibodies are a good screening tool with high sensitivity of at least 95% but poor specificity of approximately 50%.[24,25] Anti-double stranded (ds) DNA antibodies are specific to systemic lupus erythematosus but are only positive in 60% of patients with systemic lupus erythematosus.[8,25] Testing for dsDNA by *Crithidia* is the gold standard being highly sensitive and specific. Other autoantibodies in lupus include antibodies to extractable nuclear antigens, the most important of which include antibodies to SSA/Ro, SSB/La, RNP and Smith (Sm). Anti-Sm is very specific for lupus but is only positive in 10–30% of lupus patients.[25]

Anticardiolipin antibodies are the most common form of antiphospholipid antibody and are present in up to 65% of paediatric patients with systemic lupus erythematosus.[1] The prevalence of anticardiolipin antibodies in healthy children is around 5–20% and they can be generated by bacterial and viral infections. The presence of anticardiolipin antibodies in children does not equate to antiphospholipid syndrome.[26]

Table 5 The American College of Rheumatology revised criteria for classification of systemic lupus erythematosus[16,24]

Criteria	Definition
Malar rash	Fixed erythema, flat or raised, over malar eminences, tending to spare nasolabial folds
Discoid lupus	Erythematous raised patches of adherent keratotic scaling and follicular plugging. Atrophic scarring may be seen in older lesions
Photosensitivity	Skin rash as a result of unusual reaction to sunlight
Oral or nasal ulceration	Oral or nasopharyngeal ulcers, usually painless, observed by a physician
Non-erosive arthritis	Non-erosive arthritis involving 2 or more peripheral joints, characterised by tenderness, swelling or effusion
Serositis	Pleuritis – pleuritic pain, rub heard or pleural effusion, or: Pericarditis – documented by ECG or rub or pericardial effusion
Nephritis	Persistent proteinuria > 0.5 g/day not > 3+. Cellular casts: red cell, haemoglobin, granular, tubular or mixed
Neurological	Seizures in the absence of offending drugs or metabolic derangement (e.g. uraemia, ketoacidosis, electrolyte imbalance), or: Psychosis in the absence of offending drugs or metabolic derangement (e.g. uraemia, ketoacidosis, electrolyte imbalance)
Haematological	Haemolytic anaemia with reticulocytes, or: Leucopenia < 4000 per mm^3 on 2 or more occasions, or: Lymphopenia < 1500 per mm^3 on 2 or more occasions, or: Thrombocytopenia < 100,000 per mm^3 in absence of offending drugs
Immunological	Anti-DNA antibody, or: Anti-Sm antibody, or: Anti-phospholipid antibodies: (i) abnormal anticardiolipin antibody IgG or IgM; (ii) positive lupus anticoagulant; (iii) false positive for syphilis for > 6 months
Anti-nuclear antibody	Abnormal titre of ANA at any point in absence of drugs known to be associated with drug-induced lupus

Abbreviations: ANA, anti-nuclear antibody; anti-DNA, antibody to native DNA; anti-Sm, antibody to Sm nuclear antigen; ECG, electrocardiogram; IgG, immunoglobulin G; IgM, immunoglobulin M.

INFLAMMATORY MARKERS

In children with systemic lupus erythematosus, erythrocyte sedimentation rate (ESR) seems to correlate well with disease activity. The C-reactive protein is usually normal or only slightly raised, although it can rise significantly in the presence of serositis. This discrepancy between ESR and C-reactive protein can be useful in the diagnosis of systemic lupus erythematosus. In a known patient with lupus, if the C-reactive protein is raised then the clinician should be considering infection especially in the acutely unwell child where it is sometimes difficult to make the distinction between an acute lupus flare and infection.[27]

COMPLEMENT

Deposition of immune complexes and activation of the inflammatory cascade leads to complement activation and consumption. Measuring C3 and C4 is helpful in the diagnosis of systemic lupus erythematosus as it is a condition of hypocomplementaemia; at disease presentation, 65% of children have low complement levels.[5,25]

COAGULATION

Lupus anticoagulant antibodies are antiphospholipid antibodies that interfere with phospholipid-dependent coagulation tests.[8] If lupus anticoagulant is asked for, clotting tests performed include kaolin clotting test, activated partial thromboplastin time and dilute Russell viper venom time.[21]

CLASSIFICATION CRITERIA

The American College of Rheumatology have 11 revised criteria for the classification of systemic lupus erythematosus (Table 5). If a patient has 4 out of 11 criteria, this gives 96% sensitivity and 96% specificity of the patient having systemic lupus erythematosus. The criteria do not all have to be present at a defined time and can be cumulative.[16,24]

MANAGEMENT

The management of children with systemic lupus erythematosus involves a multidisciplinary team encompassing paediatric rheumatologists, physiotherapists, occupational therapists, nurse specialists and social work support. Other specialists are often involved depending on the organ systems affected by the disease. Consultation with a paediatric nephrologist should occur early if renal involvement is present. Similarly, for paediatric neurology, psychiatry and dermatology shared care in combined clinics works well.

Chronic disease in childhood and adolescence affects the child's physical and emotional development. Time must be devoted to discuss with the family and the young person how the disease and its treatment affect these areas.

ASSESSMENT

When assessing the child with lupus, it is important to identify change in disease activity, any permanent organ damage and the effect of the disease on the patient's quality of life.[28] There are several assessment tools available to the clinician which are sensitive in evaluating children and can guide management and assess effectiveness of drugs in trials. These include the BILAG (British Isles Lupus Activity Group) and SLEDAI (systemic lupus erythematosus disease activity score) which both look at disease activity.[29] The SLICC/ACR (systemic lupus international co-operating clinics/American College of Rheumatology) damage index assesses permanent organ damage.[29] The Childhood Health Assessment Questionnaire (CHAQ) measures a child's functional ability in 8 activities of daily living and includes a parent's global assessment of the child's well-being on a 10-cm visual analogue scale (VAS; where 0 = very well and 10 = very poor).[28]

The routine methodical assessment of the child with lupus requires a careful history and examination of organ systems including cardiovascular, respiratory, neuropsychiatric, renal, gastrointestinal, skin, musculoskeletal and reticulo-endothelial systems, with investigations as appropriate. It is important to monitor growth, puberty and development.

Not all symptoms in the child with systemic lupus erythematosus are attributable to lupus activity. Some may be due to side effects of treatment or unrelated to lupus.

Together with clinical assessment, laboratory investigations can aid in assessing disease activity and damage. Monitoring serial anti-dsDNA titres and complement levels can be helpful as a surrogate for disease activity.[25]

Full blood count and white cell differential with Coomb's test and blood film, ESR and liver function tests should be checked regularly.[28] Renal disease in children with lupus is often silent and urinalysis, serum urea and electrolytes, albumin and blood pressure measurement must be performed at regular intervals. If proteinuria is present this should be quantified with an early morning urinary protein to creatinine ratio or equivalent.[10,28]

Thyroid function should be monitored and amylase checked in the presence of abdominal pain. Anticardiolipin antibodies and lupus anticoagulants need to be repeated at least at annual reviews. Regular bone density scans are needed in patients on corticosteroid treatment.

DRUG THERAPIES

Corticosteroids are needed initially in the majority of children with systemic lupus erythematosus to bring the disease under control. Steroid-sparing immunosuppressive therapy is used early to minimise steroid side effects and maintain remission. Different agents are used in different situations, as systemic lupus erythematosus is a heterogeneous disorder.

Favourable outcome in children and adolescents with systemic lupus erythematosus is related to rapid disease control and associated with aggressive initial treatment, proceeding to fast tapering of corticosteroids while keeping disease activity under control.[1]

Mild disease can be controlled with hydroxychloroquine, non-steroidal anti-inflammatory drugs and oral steroids, whilst severe lupus flares especially CNS or renal involvement require intravenous cyclophosphamide and methylprednisolone to induce remission. New regimens use monthly intravenous pulses of cyclophosphamide for 6 months and then change to azathioprine, mycophenolate mofetil or methotrexate depending on the organs involved.

The number of children requiring immunosuppressive medications in addition to corticosteroids reaches 58.8% in some series.[3] A balance is required between prevention of organ damage and treatment with potentially harmful drugs.

Corticosteroids

Most cases of systemic lupus erythematosus will require corticosteroids. In mild disease, oral prednisolone is often used, initially at 1–2 mg/kg; in more major organ disease, a short burst of high-dose steroids is often encouraged such as pulsed methylprednisolone at 20–30 mg/kg on 3 consecutive days, followed by a tapering dose of oral corticosteroid once disease activity is under control. Oral steroids may not be adequately absorbed if there is gut involvement.

Whilst corticosteroids are the main-stay of treatment of systemic lupus erythematosus, they are associated with numerous side effects including osteoporosis, Cushingoid facies, obesity, growth retardation, cataracts and possible risk of accelerated atherosclerosis. Corticosteroid use is one of the risk factors for damage in paediatric patients.[4]

Immunosuppressive therapy should be considered for a child with systemic lupus erythematosus in whom it is predicted that prednisolone would not otherwise be adequately reduced.[30]

Hydroxychloroquine

Hydroxychloroquine is used to treat mild disease, particularly affecting skin and joints. Recent studies have suggested that it may have a disease modifying role in more severe disease and may even have a lipid-lowering effect which could reduce atherosclerosis.[30] Patients on hydroxychloroquine who appeared to be in remission and subsequently stopped taking the drug had a higher rate of flares than those who continued to be on the drug.[31] There have been no studies of hydroxychloroquine efficacy in the paediatric population with systemic lupus erythematosus but it is generally used.[30]

Methotrexate

Methotrexate has been shown to be effective in controlling skin and joint disease in adults.[8] A study of 11 children with systemic lupus erythematosus showed initial good response but, after 7–23 months of treatment, 8 of the children had a flare of disease activity.[32]

A recent study has shown good results with combined i.v. cyclophosphamide and high-dose methotrexate in children with refractory lupus nephritis.[10]

Azathioprine

Azathioprine is used in paediatric systemic lupus erythematosus to control flares and maintain remission allowing tapering of steroid dose.[30] Paediatric patients with class IV nephritis treated at time of diagnosis with corticosteroids and azathioprine appear to have a similar or improved long-term survival when compared to usage of cyclophosphamide alone.[10]

Cyclophosphamide

Cyclophosphamide has made a huge impact on mortality from severe organ involvement in paediatric lupus. Cyclophosphamide is associated with increased susceptibility to infection, infertility, malignancy, haemorrhagic cystitis and alopecia. The effect on fertility is directly related to the total cyclophosphamide dose. Sustained amenorrhoea appears to be uncommon in those patients under 26 years of age treated with pulsed cyclophosphamide therapy but evidence of premature ovarian failure in adults exists. Pre-treatment use of gonadotrophin releasing hormone antagonists to stop periods may reduce this and should be discussed. Previous studies on prepubertal children have suggested that gonadal toxicity does not occur if the cumulative dosage does not exceed 200 mg/kg with males being more sensitive to damage than females.[10] Pretreatment storage of sperm should be considered but careful counselling for this needs to be done with the regional fertility service.

To date, no malignancies have been reported in those children treated with pulsed cyclophosphamide and the intravenous route is thought to be a lower risk for bladder tumours than the oral route. However, longer term follow-up is required to assess this risk fully.[10]

Mycophenolate mofetil

Mycophenolate mofetil inhibits purine synthesis, has antiproliferative effects on lymphocytes and attenuates production of autoantibodies by B cells.[15]

Studies in adults have shown that mycophenolate mofetil and steroids are as effective as intravenous cyclophosphamide and prednisolone in treating diffuse proliferative glomerulonephritis.[30] Furthermore, short-term therapy with i.v. cyclophosphamide followed by maintenance treatment with mycopheonlate mofetil or azathioprine appears to be more efficacious and safer than long-term therapy with i.v. cyclophosphamide.[15]

Studies on mycophenolate mofetil in children with systemic lupus erythematosus are limited to small series but suggest that if used in combination with corticosteroids or cyclophosphamide, it can reduce lupus activity and lead to tapering of steroid doses.[33] The results appeared more favourable in those patients with membranous glomerulonephritis.[33]

Cyclosporin A

This immunosuppressive agent has been used to treat lupus nephritis and may reduce proteinuria.[10]

Rituximab

Rituximab is a monoclonal antibody that binds specifically to B-cell surface antigen mediating B-cell lysis. It has been used in children with systemic lupus erythematosus refractory to conventional immunosuppression and has been shown to be effective and safe.[34]

Autologous bone marrow transplant

Children with severe systemic lupus erythematosus refractory to treatment have been successfully treated with autologous stem cell transplant. The reported transplant-related mortality rate for autoimmune disease is 5–10% and, therefore, must only be considered in those patients with life-threatening lupus who have failed conventional therapies.[35]

Treatments for cutaneous lupus

Management of cutaneous lesions begins with sun avoidance. Topical corticosteroids and hydroxychloroquine are standard treatments. Most lesions respond to the immunosuppressive therapies mentioned previously. Treatments specific for refractory cutaneous lesions include topical (retinoids and tacrolimus) and systemic treatments (thalidomide, dapsone, retinoids).[36]

SUN AVOIDANCE

Children should be prescribed sun-block with factor 50–60 as ultraviolet light can predispose to a lupus flare and cutaneous lesions are often photosensitive. As sunscreens do not block all ultraviolet light, patients should be advised to wear sun-protective clothing and minimise contact with direct sunlight.[36]

GROWTH

Growth assessment, monitoring of growth velocity and pubertal development are important in children with systemic lupus erythematosus who may experience growth failure, particularly with early-onset disease. This is due not only to disease activity but also to corticosteroid use. There is also an increased incidence of endocrine causes of growth failure in children with systemic lupus erythematosus including thyroiditis and growth hormone deficiency.[1]

OSTEOPENIA AND OSTEOPOROSIS

The risk factors for development of osteopenia in children with systemic lupus erythematosus include long-term steroid treatment, inflammation, arthritis, poor physical activity, suboptimal nutrition, lack of sun-exposure, renal disease and ovarian dysfunction.[1,37]

The frequency of osteopenia in patients with childhood onset systemic lupus erythematosus is significantly higher than in matched controls at around 40% and appears to correlate to cumulative steroid dose.[37]

Children on corticosteroids should have their dietary intake of calcium and vitamin D assessed regularly at clinic visits, with encouragement to avoid inactivity and excessive weight gain. Some studies have shown that the use of calcium and vitamin D supplements may help prevent bone loss.[38]

Those children who have had high cumulative steroid doses should have formal assessment of their bone mineral density. Dual-X-ray absorptiometry is the current gold standard.[38] Children with osteopenia and osteoporosis can be treated effectively with a bisphosphonate such as pamidronate.

INFECTION AND VACCINATION

Children with systemic lupus erythematosus are more prone to infections than healthy children because of disease-associated immune dysfunction and immunosuppressive treatments. Particular susceptibility to pneumococcal infection arises from functional asplenia, hypocomplementaemia and abnormal macrophage and neutrophil function.[1] Children with systemic lupus erythematosus should receive all routine childhood vaccinations and should receive pneumococcal and annual influenza immunisation, unless taking significant immunosuppressive treatments, where live vaccines are relatively contra-indicated.[1]

Before commencing a child on immunosuppressive therapy, it is useful to check varicella and measles immunity so that parents can be advised on a course of action if the child is exposed.

OUTCOME

Mortality rates for systemic lupus erythematosus are improving. In 1963, the 2-year survival rate was quoted at 58%, whereas in 1980–1990 the 5-year survival has been shown to be 85–93%.[5] Recently, survival has been shown to be 100% at 5 years and 85.7% at 10 years.[3]

This marked improvement in survival can be explained by earlier recognition of mild disease, availability of better treatments and earlier, and more aggressive management.[1]

Whilst adults tend to die secondary to complications of treatment and disease, children tend to die during acute lupus flares and from sepsis. As the treatment of systemic lupus erythematosus improves, we may expect to see more children surviving into adulthood and an increased mortality and morbidity from irreversible disease damage and treatment side-effects.[1]

Cumulative disease activity over time results in permanent organ damage; therefore, rapid control of disease activity should minimise damage. The early use of pulsed steroids with the introduction of steroid sparing drugs and quick tapering of oral steroid dose is advised.[4]

Brunner *et al.*[4] assessed paediatric patients with systemic lupus erythematosus using the SLICC/ACR (systemic lupus international co-operating clinics/American College of Rheumatology) damage index. They found that 61% had damage in at least one organ or system and this primarily affected the musculoskeletal (avascular bone necrosis), ocular, renal and neuropsychiatric systems.[4]

Some degree of long-term, and often permanent, organ dysfunction from either systemic lupus erythematosus or its treatments has been found in 88% of patients. Complications included hypertension (41%), growth retardation (38%), chronic pulmonary impairment (31%), ocular abnormalities (31%), permanent renal damage (25%), neuropsychiatric symptoms (22%), musculoskeletal damage (9%), and gonadal impairment (3%).[39]

ACCELERATED ATHEROSCLEROSIS

Accelerated atherosclerosis has been observed in systemic lupus erythematosus patients. Proposed pathogenesis includes disease-related factors (arterial vasculitis, immune-complex mediated endothelial damage, antiphospholipid antibodies) and treatment-related factors (steroid induced hyperlipidaemia and obesity), as well as hypertension.[40] A recent series in an adult population showed that patients aged 20–39 years had a 16-fold increased risk of death from coronary heart disease.[6] Children with systemic lupus erythematosus have ultrasonographic evidence of premature atherosclerosis. Risk of atherosclerosis appears to be related to severity of disease rather than disease duration.[40]

Studies in paediatric patients have shown abnormalities of lipid metabolism both secondary to disease itself and to corticosteroid therapy.[40] The Atherosclerosis Prevention in Pediatric Lupus Erythematosus (APPLE) study is currently underway to evaluate the role of statins in prevention of atherosclerosis in children with systemic lupus erythematosus.[6]

Key points for clinical practice

- Systemic lupus erythematosus is a potentially life-threatening disease; however, patients can do well if the disease is recognised early and treated aggressively.

- The production of autoantibodies (antibodies directed against self-antigens) is the hallmark of systemic lupus erythematosus. This leads to wide-spread inflammation of blood vessels and tissues, causing multisystem disease.

- Systemic lupus erythematosus is a heterogeneous disease and should be considered in any child with severe organ disease particularly if more than one system is affected.

- Children tend to have more severe manifestations of the disease at diagnosis and a more aggressive clinical course. In particular, children with renal or neuropsychiatric lupus have greater severity of disease and a poorer outcome than adults.

- Systemic lupus erythematosus, as any chronic disease, can affect a child's physical, emotional and intellectual development. It is important to recognise the effects the disease and its treatments can have on the child and young adult.

- The most useful investigations for diagnosing systemic lupus erythematosus are anti-nuclear antibody which is highly sensitive, anti-dsDNA which is highly specific and extractable nuclear antigens. Consider a *Crithidia* dsDNA if the dsDNA is unexpectedly negative when all other features fit the diagnosis. An ESR is often raised out of proportion with C-reactive protein. Full blood count may show features suggestive of lupus such as Coomb's positive haemolytic anaemia or thrombocytopenia. There is often hypocomplement-aemia and hypergammaglobulinaemia. Serial measurement of anti-dsDNA and complement levels are useful markers of disease activity.

- The child with lupus who is acutely unwell needs to be assessed to determine whether this deterioration is secondary to an acute disease flare or to infection. The symptoms of systemic lupus erythematosus and infections are very similar so a high index of suspicion for infection is required. Infections may be opportunistic in children on immunosuppressant therapy. A raised C-reactive protein in the absence of serositis may indicate infection.

- When assessing the child with lupus, it is important to identify current active disease, permanent organ damage and the effect of the disease on the patient's quality of life. There are several named assessment tools available to the clinician.

Key points for clinical practice (continued)

- Renal disease is a major cause of morbidity and mortality in children with systemic lupus erythematosus. It often presents silently; therefore, it is essential to monitor urinalysis and blood pressure regularly.

- Corticosteroids are needed initially in the majority of children with systemic lupus erythematosus to bring the disease under control. Steroid-sparing immunosuppressive therapy is used early to minimise steroid side-effects and maintain remission. Hydroxychloroquine is useful for milder symptoms whereas methotrexate, azathioprine and mycophenolate mofetil are used with more active disease. For life-threatening disease flares, a combination of intravenous corticosteroid and cyclophosphamide is commonly used.

- In refractory disease, the monoclonal antibody rituximab has been used successfully. Some children with severe refractory disease have been treated with autologous stem cell transplant, although this therapy confers a high mortality rate of 5–10%.

- The short- and long-term outcome for children with systemic lupus erythematosus has improved in recent years. As patients with systemic lupus erythematosus survive longer, there is significant morbidity from the disease and its treatments. It is difficult to balance minimising permanent organ damage with side effects from potentially harmful drugs.

- The complications of systemic lupus erythematosus include end-organ damage, osteoporosis, growth disturbance and accelerated atherosclerosis.

- Children with systemic lupus erythematosus tend to die from sepsis and from acute disease flares, particularly renal and central nervous system involvement. The increased susceptibility to infection is secondary to the disease and immunosuppressive therapies.

References

1. Klein-Gitelman M, Reiff A, Silverman ED. Systemic lupus erythematosus in childhood. *Rheum Dis Clin North Am* 2002; **28**: 561–577.
2. Petty RE, Cassidy JT. Systemic lupus erythematosus. In: Cassidy JT, Petty RE. (eds) *Textbook of Pediatric Rheumatology*. Philadelphia, PA: WB Saunders, 2001; 396–449.
3. Miettunen PM, Ortiz-Alvarez O, Petty RE *et al*. Gender and ethnic origin have no effect on longterm outcome of childhood-onset systemic lupus erythematosus. *J Rheumatol* 2004; **31**: 1650–1654.
4. Brunner HI, Silverman ED, To T, Bombardier C, Feldman BM. Risk factors for damage in childhood-onset systemic lupus erythematosus. *Arthritis Rheum* 2002; **46**: 436–444.
5. Rood JM, ten Cate R, van Suijlekom-Smit LW *et al*. Childhood-onset systemic lupus erythematosus. *Scand J Rheumatol* 1999; **28**: 222–226.
6. Stichweh D, Arce E, Pascual V. Update on pediatric systemic lupus erythematosus. *Curr Opin Rheumatol* 2004; **16**: 577–587.

7. Sestak AL, Nath SK, Harley JB. Genetics of systemic lupus erythematosus: how far have we come? *Rheum Dis Clin North Am* 2005; **31**: 223–244.
8. Gordon C, Salmon M. Update on systemic lupus erythematosus: autoantibodies and apoptosis. *Clin Med* 2001; **1**: 10–14.
9. Rubin RL. Drug-induced lupus. *Toxicology* 2005; **209**: 135–147.
10. Perfumo F, Martini A. Lupus nephritis in children. *Lupus* 2005; **14**: 83–88.
11. Sibbitt WL, Brandt JR, Johnson CR et al. The incidence and prevalence of neuropsychiatric syndromes in pediatric onset systemic lupus erythematosus. *J Rheumatol* 2002; **29**: 1536–1542.
12. Beresford MW, Cleary AG, Sills JA et al. Cardiopulmonary involvement in juvenile systemic lupus erythematosus. *Lupus* 2005; **14**: 152–158.
13. Moises-Alfaro C, Berron-Peréz R, Carrasco-Daza D et al. Discoid lupus erythematosus in children: clinical, histopathologic, and follow-up features in 27 cases. *Pediatr Dermatol* 2003; **20**: 103–107.
14. Weening JJ, D'Agati VD, Schwartz MM et al. The classification of glomerulonephritis in systemic lupus erythematosus revisited. *J Am Soc Nephrol* 2004; **15**: 241–250.
15. Contreras G, Pardo V, Leclercq B et al. Sequential therapies for proliferative lupus nephritis. *N Engl J Med* 2004; **350**: 971–980.
16. Hochberg MC. Updating the American College of Rheumatology revised criteria for the classification of systemic lupus erythematosus. *Arthritis Rheum* 1997; **40**: 1725.
17. American College of Rheumatology. The American College of Rheumatology nomenclature and case definitions for neuropsychiatric lupus syndromes. *Arthritis Rheum* 1999; **42**: 599–608.
18. Gazarian M, Feldman BM, Benson LN, Gilday DL, Laxer RM, Silverman ED. Assessment of myocardial perfusion and function in childhood systemic lupus erythematosus. *J Pediatr* 1998; **132**: 109–116.
19. Guevara JP, Clark BJ, Athreya BH. Point prevalence of cardiac abnormalities in children with systemic lupus erythematosus . *J Rheumatol* 2001; **28**: 854–859.
20. Trapani S, Camiciottoli G, Ermini M et al. Pulmonary involvement in juvenile systemic lupus erythematosus: a study on lung function in patients asymptomatic for lung disease . *Lupus* 1998; **7**: 545–550.
21. Gharavi AE. Anticardiolipin syndrome: antiphospholipid syndrome. *Clin Med* 2001; **1**: 14–17.
22. Wilson WA, Gharavi AE, Koike T et al. International consensus statement on preliminary classification criteria for definite antiphospholipid syndrome. *Arthritis Rheum* 1999; **42**: 1309–1311.
23. Buyon JP, Clancy RM. Neonatal lupus: basic research and clinical perspectives. *Rheum Dis Clin North Am* 2005; **31**: 299–231.
24. Tan EM, Cohen AS, Fries JF et al. The 1982 revised criteria for the classification of systemic lupus erythematosus. *Arthritis Rheum* 1982; **25**: 1271–1277.
25. Illei GG, Tackey E, Lapteva L, Lipsky PE. Biomarkers in systemic lupus erythematosus. II. Markers of disease activity. *Arthritis Rheum* 2004; **50**: 2048–2065.
26. Constantin T, Ponyi A, Fekete G. Clinical relevance of anti-phospholipid antibody tests in childhood. *Eur J Pediatr* 2004; **163**: 507.
27. ter Borg EJ, Horst G, Limburg PC et al. C-reactive protein levels during disease exacerbations and infections in systemic lupus erythematosus: a prospective longitudinal study. *J Rheumat* 1990; **17**: 1642–1648.
28. Haq I, Isenberg DA. How does one assess and monitor patients with systemic lupus erythematosus in daily clinical practice? *Best Pract Res Clin Rheumatol* 2002; **16**: 181–194.
29. Brunner HI, Feldman BM, Bombardier C et al. Sensitivity of the systemic lupus erythematosus disease activity index, British Isles lupus assessment group index, and systemic lupus activity measure in the evaluation of clinical change in childhood-onset systemic lupus erythematosus. *Arthritis Rheum* 1999; **42**: 1354–1360.
30. Tucker LB. Controversies and advances in the management of systemic lupus erythematosus in children and adolescents. *Best Pract Res Clin Rheumatol* 2002; **16**: 481–494.
31. The Canadian Hydroxychloroquine Study Group. A randomised study of the effect of withdrawing hydroxychloroquine sulfate in systemic lupus erythematosus. *N Engl J Med* 1991; **324**: 150–154.

32. Ravelli A, Ballardini G, Viola S *et al.* Methotrexate therapy in refractory pediatric onset systemic lupus erythematosus. *J Rheumat* 1998; **25**: 572–575.
33. Buratti S, Szer IS, Spencer CH *et al.* Mycophenolate mofetil treatment of severe renal disease in paediatric onset systemic lupus erythematosus. *J Rheumat* 2001; **28**: 2103–2108.
34. Marks SD, Patey S, Brogan PA *et al.* B lymphocyte depletion therapy in children with refractory systemic lupus erythematosus. *Arthritis Rheum* 2005; **52**: 3168–3174.
35. Wulffraat NM, Sanders EA, Kamphuis SS *et al.* Prolonged remission without treatment after autologous stem cell transplant for refractory childhood systemic lupus erythematosus. *Arthritis Rheum* 2001; **44**: 728–731.
36. Callen JP. Management of 'refractory' skin disease in patients with lupus erythematosus. *Best Pract Res Clin Rheumatol* 2005; **19**: 767–784.
37. Lilleby V, Lien G, Frøslie KF, Haugen M, Flatø B, Rørre Ø. Frequency of osteopenia in children and young adults with childhood-onset systemic lupus erythematosus. *Arthritis Rheum* 2005; **52**: 2051–2059.
38. Cimaz R. Osteoporosis in childhood rheumatic diseases: prevention and therapy. *Best Pract Res Clin Rheumatol* 2002; **16**: 397–409.
39. Lacks S, White P. Morbidity associated with childhood systemic lupus erythematosus. *J Rheumat* 1990; **17**: 941–945.
40. Falaschi F, Ravelli A, Martignoni A *et al.* Nephrotic-range proteinuria, the major risk factor for early atherosclerosis in juvenile-onset systemic lupus erythematosus. *Arthritis Rheum* 2000; **43**: 1405–1409.

Eran Kozer

5

Medication errors in children – first do no harm

One of the first principles we all learned in medical school is *primum non nocere* (first do no harm). As medical knowledge and technology progress, this simple principle should always be kept in mind. We are treating sicker and more complicated patients, using advanced technology and more potent drugs. At the same time, the risk of an error with the potential for severe consequences increases.

Here, the epidemiology of medication errors in paediatrics is reviewed and some risk factors for errors identified. The system approach to errors is described (as opposed to the traditional approach) and strategies suggested to reduce errors.

ADVERSE DRUG EVENT AND MEDICATION ERRORS

There is no consensus on the definitions of medication error and adverse drug event. A common definition for medication error is 'an error in prescribing, dispensing, or administering a medication'. Some definitions require that the result would be that the patient fails to receive the correct drug or the indicated proper drug dosage. This requirement, however, is limited and does not include a wide range of errors that does not reach the patients. Most experts agree that, for the definition of medication error, it is not necessary for the patient to have received one or more doses of the drug or to have been harmed. In this review, this broader definition of medication error will be used. Medication error will include any preventable event that may cause or lead to inappropriate prescribing, dispensing, or administering a medication.

An adverse drug event is an injury resulting from medical intervention related to a drug.[1] It is important to understand that not every medication error will result in an adverse drug event. On the other hand, the same adverse

Eran Kozer MD
Pediatric Emergency Services, Assaf Harofeh Medical Center, Zerifin 70300, Israel
E-mail: erank@asaf.health.gov.il

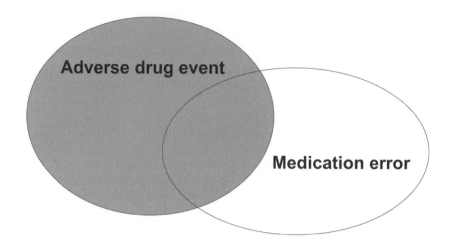

Fig. 1. Medication error and adverse drug event.

drug event (*e.g.* allergic reaction to penicillin) may result from a medication error (if the patient is known to be allergic to the drug) or may be unavoidable if there was no previous history of allergy. Figure 1 illustrates the relationship between adverse drug events and medication errors.

EPIDEMIOLOGY OF MEDICATION ERRORS

Iatrogenic injuries are a significant cause of morbidity and mortality among patients. In 1999, an expert panel of the Institute of Medicine estimated that 44,000–98,000 people in the US die each year as a result of medical errors.[2]

Medication errors are a common cause for iatrogenic adverse events[1,3] and can lead to severe consequences including prolonged hospitalisation, unnecessary diagnostic evaluations, unnecessary treatments and death.[3–5] The cost of medication errors and adverse drug events are extremely high. In the US, medication errors (in hospitalised patients and out-patients) may account for more than 7000 deaths annually.[6] In a report from a teaching hospital in New York, the rate of errors occurring per order written, per admission and per patient-day increased significantly from 1987 to 1995.[7]

Medication errors commonly involve children. Lesar *et al.*[8] compared prescribing errors in different services in a teaching hospital in New York. Error rate per 1000 orders was highest in paediatrics (5.9 in paediatrics, 5.5 in emergency medicine, 4.2 in medicine and obstetrics/gynaecology and 3.6 in surgery). Lesar[9] also found that 69.5% of dosing errors involving calculations occurred in children.

There are number of reasons why medication errors are common in the paediatric population. Many drugs used in paediatrics are off-labelled with no standard dosing.[10] Medication doses must be adjusted for the child's weight or body surface area. The pharmacokinetics of some drugs change according to the child age and this information should be known and incorporated into clinical decisions. Many medications are supplied to the pharmacy in standard dosage forms, usually an adult dose. Such drugs must be diluted or subdivided for administration to children.

TYPES OF ERROR

There are many types of medication errors and no consensus on the classification. The classification can be based on the process of drug administration to distinguish between prescribing errors, dispensing errors and administration errors.[11] Each type can be further divided.[12] Table 1 presents some examples of the different types.

Table 1. Types of medication errors

Error	Example
Prescribing errors	
Wrong drug	Penicillin given to a patient with a known history of allergy to penicillin
	Antibiotic prescribed for simple upper respiratory tract infection
Wrong dose	Tenfold errors
	Total daily dose given as a single dose
	Microgram switched with milligrams
	No adjustment for renal function
Wrong frequency	Giving a potent drug such as methotrexate once daily instead of once weekly
Wrong duration	Prescribing 3-day course of penicillin for streptococcal pharyngitis
Wrong route	Salbutamol for inhalation given as a suspension by mouth
Wrong dosage form	Sustained release preparation crushed and given via a nasogastric tube
Dispensing errors	
Inappropriate delay or failure in supplying a drug	An order sent to pharmacy but did not get to the pharmacist
Wrong drug supplied	Atropine and adrenaline are supplied in 1-ml brown ampoules and stocked in near drawers. The wrong drug is supplied
Failure to identify and remove expired drug from stock	
Error on label of medicine container	
Administration errors	
Wrong drug	Patient received another patient's drug
Wrong preparation of a drug	Cephtriaxone for i.v. administration is dissolved with a solvent used for i.m. injections
Wrong route	Vincristine injected intratracheally instead of i.v.
Wrong rate of administration	Phenytoin given by intravenous push instead of over 30 min
Wrong dose	
Dose delayed or omitted	
Extra dose given	

DOSING ERRORS

In paediatrics, dosing errors are the most common.[13–16] It has been suggested that the reason for the high rate of dosing error is that there are no standard doses, and calculations are needed to prescribe the correct dose for the child's weight. Indeed, even in an ideal setting, a substantial proportion of nurses[17] paediatric residents[18,19] and paediatricians[17] make mistakes when calculating drug doses. The mean score of paediatric residents, in a test of 10 questions on basic calculations, was less than 70%.[18] In an anonymous written test, 7 out of 32 residents committed a 10-fold error.[19] It is not surprising, therefore, that when factors related to medication errors in a general hospital were analysed, the need for dosage calculations was the commonest reason for medication errors in paediatric patients.[12]

TEN-FOLD ERRORS

Ten-fold errors occur when one prescribes or administers a dose which is 10-fold higher or lower than the recommended dose. These errors are a particularly concerning subset of mishaps. They typically involve a calculation (in the majority of cases) or transcription errors, which can be fatal. Such errors can result from not using a zero to the left of a dose less than 1 (*e.g.* .1 rather than 0.1) or from writing a terminal zero to the right of the decimal point (*e.g.* 5.0 rather than 5). Another potential source for a 10-fold error is using the wrong units (*e.g.* milligrams instead of micrograms). Such errors are more likely to occur if units are not specified and when abbreviations are used. Using the letter µ instead of spelling 'micro' may also increase the risk for such an error.

The incidence of 10-fold medication errors in paediatric units varies according to the detection method.[20–22] One study showed that 10-fold errors represent 15% of all medication prescribing errors involving the use of dosage equations in paediatric patients.[9] Since the dose of most drugs given to children is based on their body weight or surface area, there is a need to calculate the dose required. When such calculations are applied to potent drugs and small children, the result is a very small amount of a drug. Indeed, the drugs involved in 10-fold errors are often very potent, given in doses of less than 1 mg/kg, creating a potential source of confusion during the conversion of milligrams to micrograms. In one report,[20] there was a difference between the identity of the drugs for which 10-fold errors were reported and those given commonly to patients suggesting that 10-fold medication errors in children are not a random phenomenon.

AREA OF RISK

There are many factors that can increase the risk for an error. These factors are related to a patient's characteristics, the health professional involved and the setting in which one works.

PATIENTS

Several types of patient are at higher risk for a medication error. Sicker patients with complex medical conditions are more prone to errors.[14] These patients are often treated with multiple medications so the risk for unwanted drug interaction is increased. Compromised renal function is another potential source for errors in critically ill patients. When such patients need urgent care, there is often not enough time for rechecking the doses. The drugs, which are used in such patients, are potent drugs with a narrow therapeutic window and the consequence of an error might be serious.

Studies[11,15,22] have shown that medication errors are more likely to occur in the intensive care setting. In a study by Raju et al.,[23] 15% of patients admitted to the neonatal and paediatric intensive care units were subjected to a medication error; iatrogenic injury due to a medication error was found in 3.1% of the patients. A more recent study[13] reported a higher incidence of errors (28% of the patients) and no difference between the incidence of errors in the neonatal intensive care unit, paediatric intensive care and general paediatric ward. There was a higher risk for a potential adverse drug event in neonates compared to other age groups and a significantly higher rate of potential or preventable adverse drug events in the neonatal intensive care unit compared with other wards.

AMBULATORY CARE AND IN THE HOME

While there is some data on the incidence of medication errors in hospitalised patients, there is very limited data on the incidence of such errors in the ambulatory setting. Data from poison centres and reported cases indicate that therapeutic misadventures, with over-the-counter medications such as acetaminophen, may lead to significant morbidity and even death. Several factors may contribute to such errors. Paediatricians should know that, even when proper instruction are given, only an estimated 30% of caregivers are able to give their child medication correctly.[24] Using an adult preparation in a young child is another common source for errors and may result in a significant overdose.

HEALTH PROFESSIONALS

All health professionals involved in the process of prescribing, administering or dispensing medication commit errors, including prescribers, nurses and pharmacists. Parents and other caregivers also err. In a study by Leape et al.,[25] physicians committed 39% of all detected errors, nurses 38% and pharmacists 12%. This proportion may be different[22,26] when other definitions of error are applied or if different methods of detection are used. Several characteristics of health professionals may increase the risk for an error.

EXPERIENCE

Several studies[8,11,14] found that inexperienced physicians are more likely to err. Wilson et al.[11] reported a 2-fold increase in the rate of medication errors when new physicians started their rotation. Lesar et al.[8] found that first-year residents have higher rates of prescription errors. In a study conducted at the emergency department of a paediatric hospital,[14] the risk of an error was higher when an order was given by a trainee compared with a staff physician.

The finding that trainees made more errors at the beginning of the academic year strengthens the plausibility of the association between level of training and the rate of errors. Contrary to these studies, another study[27] found no difference in rates of error made by attending physicians and residents. Moreover, two studies[18,19] that looked at the basic calculation skills of paediatric residents found no significant correlation between the number of years in residency and errors in calculating drug doses.

The reason why some studies found a large difference between attending physicians and trainees while others did not may be related to whether or not staff physicians actually prescribe medications. In areas such as the emergency department or intensive care units, many orders are given directly by the attending physician while in general wards often the house officer gives the orders and only rarely the attending physician. In such cases, the rate of errors by attending physicians may increase.

TIRED PHYSICIANS MAKE MORE ERRORS

Intuitively, one can assume that long working hours and sleepless nights will increase the risk for medication errors. Yet, a large percentage of physicians deny that fatigue increases their risk to err.[28] Recent studies[29,30] have shown that work load may have a negative effect on a physician's performance. Reducing on-call shifts for interns in the intensive care unit from 30 h to a maximum of 16 h and reducing the weekly working hours from more than 80 h/week to 64 h/week reduced the number of attentional failures by more than half.[30] Such attentional failures may lead to serious errors. Indeed, the same group found that interns who worked on a reduced hours' schedule, made 17% less serious medication errors.[29]

THE SYSTEM APPROACH AND THE PERSON APPROACH

The traditional approach to errors in medicine (including medication errors) focused on unsafe actions by individuals. The assumption behind such an approach was that error is the result of inattention, careless behaviour, negligence and poor motivation. It was believed that the person who made the error is solely responsible for the outcome, which in some cases could be dismal. The person who erred is, therefore, blamed for his or her wrong-doing and disciplinary action may be taken. When such an approach is used, it is not surprising that people cover-up their mistakes and errors become a 'top secret'. The result might be that similar errors happen many times before a change in practice is made.

Contrary to the traditional approach, the system approach view every medical error as a systems failure. The focus is on the system in which one works and not on actions by individuals. When an error occurs, the question is not who made the error but why did it happen and what changes are needed to prevent a recurrence. Examples of such changes could be introducing checkpoints within the process of drug ordering (for example, if a physician ordered a 10-fold higher dose of a drug, the system change may be a requirement to specify the dose per kilogram and setting an upper limit for drug dosage in a computerised ordering system). Re-arranging pharmacy drawers in a way that medications with look-alike packages are kept at maximal distance and actions by regulatory bodies to prevent the occurrence of sound-alike and look-alike drugs in the market are other examples of the system approach for the prevention of medication errors.

STRATEGIES TO REDUCE ERRORS

The effort to reduce errors should involve all participants involved in the complex process of drug prescription.[31] At the national level, professional organisations, drug companies and regulatory bodies should be involved. Regulatory bodies should prevent marketing of look-alike and sound-alike drugs. They can also set rules for the proper use of drugs and limit physicians' working hours.

For in-patients, the hospital administration, physicians, pharmacy services, nursing staff, patients and families should be involved. For out-patients, it should include the treating physician, caregivers and the pharmacy. The following are examples for strategies to reduce medication errors.

COMPUTERISED PHYSICIAN ORDER ENTRY SYSTEMS

Computerised physician order entry systems are based on a computer program that can detect and prevent medication errors. The use of computerised physician order entry systems offers many obvious advantages. There are no handwriting identification problems and less errors associated with similar drug names. The system can be easily linked to drug–drug interaction warnings and decision-support systems.

For decision-support systems the patient's personal information, such as age, weight, allergy to a drug and abnormal renal function, has to be entered into the system. Dosing errors are less likely to occur since the computer calculates the drug dose based on the patient's weight. The order is transferred directly to the pharmacy. The system can also provide an alert when the patient's medical condition requires dose adjustments for specific drugs (*e.g.* the system will alert the physician before prescribing gentamycin if the patient's creatinine is high).

Computerised physician order entry systems significantly reduced medication errors in both adults and paediatric in-patients.[32,33] Medication error rates decreased by 40% in wards that started to use a computerised physician order entry system compared with wards that continued to use hand-written orders.[32] Despite this reduction, there was no change in adverse drug event rate, and the authors' calculations suggest that when using computerised physician order entry systems, 490 patient days are needed to see the benefit of one less medication error. This small effect is probably because medication errors in this study were detected through incident reporting (see below) and the error rate was low.

In a paediatric intensive care unit, implementation of computerised physician order entry systems almost eliminated (99% reduction) prescribing errors.[33] The reported reduction of adverse drug events in the same study was significant but less dramatic (40%).

Since a computerised physician order entry system can also gather data on prescribing habits, it may facilitate research in the field.

Computerised physician order entry systems have several limitations. Such a system will not help in cases where the doses need to be prepared immediately on the ward. Moreover, computerised physician order entry systems are not error proof. Indeed, using a computerised physician order entry system may increase the risk for specific types of medication errors.[34] For example, in a tertiary hospital where a widely used computerised physician order entry system is in place, more than two-thirds of the house staff reported that they were often uncertain about medications and dosages because of difficulty in viewing all the patient's medications on one screen.[33] More than 90% reported that the system was inflexible, generating difficulties in specifying medications or ordering off-formulary medications. One of the major problems of computerised physician order entry systems is the cost. The implementation of computerised physician order entry systems is expensive and they are not available in most hospitals.

The role of computerised physician order entry systems for prescription writing for out-patients

It is not known whether or not existing systems reduce medication errors in out-patients. Recently, a computerised system to calculate the dose of two frequently used drugs (paracetamol and promethazine) for ambulatory and emergency department patients has been evaluated in a children's hospital.[35] It was associated with a significant reduction in error rates. However, even when the computerised system was used, the error rate was more than 12%, unacceptably high.

In adults, physicians often over-ride the alerts generated by the system and a large percentage of the alerts are judged as inappropriate. It is reasonable to assume that the rate of over-riding may be even higher in paediatrics where many drugs are used in an off-label way.[10]

TEMPLATES

Standardised order sheets that include areas for patient weight, old and new allergies, prescriber name, signature, and contact number may be a cheap and easily available alternative to computerised physician order entry systems.[31] In a paediatric emergency department, using a pre-printed order sheet in which the patient's weight, and dose-adjusted weight had to be entered, reduced the number of prescribing errors by half.[36]

ROLE OF PHARMACY AND PHARMACY AUDITING

Several studies have shown the benefit of having a pharmacist as part of the treatment team.[16,37] The pharmacist can review the physician order and detect errors that are not easily identified by physicians, such as drug interactions, wrong solvents and infusion rates. In an adult intensive care unit, the presence of a pharmacist during ward round decreased the rate of adverse drug events due to ordering errors by 66%.[37] Having pharmacy satellites in patient care areas such as the intensive care unit is another effective way to prevent or reduce medication errors.[38] The pharmacist may use computerised systems to review the orders, recheck the calculations and look for potential drug interactions.

USING A STANDARD DOSING SYSTEM

Emergency treatment, for a critically ill child, is an area where the rate of errors may be extremely high.[26] If one assumes that drugs given during extreme conditions have beneficial effects on the outcome, it is important to reduce these errors. The Broselow tape provides standardised, pre-calculated medication doses, dose delivery volumes, and equipment sizes using colour-coded zones based on the child height (which can be measured immediately upon arrival). Shah and his colleges[39] used simulated resuscitation to study medication errors in the paediatric emergency department. Participants were randomised for two different settings of work – using a standard dosing system (Broselow tape) or using traditional dosing references. When compared with the use of traditional dosing references, using the Broselow Paediatric Emergency Tape and colour-coded materials was associated with lower deviation from recommended dose ranges.

In the ambulatory setting, using a colour-coded method may improve caregivers' ability to determine and give the appropriate dose to their child.[40]

EDUCATION

If experienced physicians make fewer errors, it is tempting to assume that better education and training will reduce medication errors. Indeed, medical trainees who attended a tutorial on writing orders scored higher on a written test than those who did not take the tutorial.[41] Even if education reduces the rate of errors in written tests, there is no proof that it has any effect on error prevention. That does not mean that we should abandon education as part of the medical training but one must be aware that the effect on error prevention (if any) is marginal.

TEAM WORK AND OPEN COMMUNICATION

Lack of team work and strict hierarchy, where senior physicians are perceived as those who 'cannot be wrong' and where nurses and junior doctors are afraid to ask the consultants for clarification regarding their orders, may increase the risk for serious errors.[42] Open communication between team members may prevent errors from affecting patients[43] even in the most stressful situations. In a study on medication errors during simulated resuscitations,[26] many of the significant errors (*e.g.* 10-fold errors) were intercepted by a team member.

It is not always simple to build trust between health professionals especially when errors are pointed out; yet, much effort should be devoted to create an environment in which all voices are heard.

Open communication should also be part of the interaction between physicians and their patients. Paediatricians should spend enough time to instruct parents on the proper use of the medication they prescribe and how to use over-the-counter medications. Proper instructions may reduce the number of medication errors by caregivers. Parents and older patients should be encouraged to know which medications they are using and not to hesitate to ask and confirm they are getting the right treatment.

FUTURE DIRECTIONS

Using a hand-held computer containing a drug database may reduce the rate of preventable adverse drug events. This technology, however, has not yet been formally studied.

DETECTING AND IDENTIFYING ERRORS

Detecting and reporting cases of medication errors is a crucial component in developing systems to prevent errors. There are several methods for identifying and monitoring medication errors. Spontaneous voluntary systems, in which health professionals are required to report any medication error and adverse drug event is one crucial measure. An open, non-punitive, approach that encourages voluntary reporting should be preferred. To promote voluntary reporting, confidentiality must be granted. It is also important that such reporting will not be associated with disciplinary or legal actions against those who gave the information. Although it may appear that in such approach accountability is abandoned and patients' safety might be compromised, it is not the case.

VOLUNTARY REPORTING AND ACTIVE SURVEILLANCE

Voluntary reporting may identify a broad range of errors[44] and promote multidisciplinary collaborative efforts to enhance patient safety. The information gathered by such voluntary reports is more important by far than identifying another 'bad apple' and blaming that person for his or her actions. When monitoring medication errors, it is important to identify both errors that reached the patients and those that were intercepted. Identifying near misses (*i.e.* errors identified before reaching the patient) is an opportunity to detect system failures before a catastrophe happens.

Relying on voluntary reporting is not sufficient. Many errors can go undetected unless an active surveillance system is in place.[20,45,46] For example, Cullen *et al.*[45] reported that only 6% of adverse drug events identified by a chart review were reported to a pharmacy hotline. Moreover, a retrospective review of patients' charts, even when done properly, can not detect many types of errors (mainly administration errors). In a study that compared three methods of detecting medication errors,[46] direct observation was more efficient and accurate than reviewing charts and incident reporting.

The difficulty in detecting medication errors is further highlighted by studies[26,47] demonstrating that we do not always administer what we think we give. Parshuram *et al.*[47] analysed 232 morphine infusions prepared for clinical use in paediatric and neonatal intensive care units. The measured morphine concentration was more than 10% different from the ordered concentration in two-thirds of the infusions. In 6% of the infusions, a 2-fold difference was found. These studies,[25,47] showing that, in many cases, there is large discrepancy between the dose ordered and the actual administered dose, are very disturbing. They suggest that the incidence of medication errors reported in the literature (which is based, in most cases, on incident reporting or on chart reviews) may be an underestimate of the true numbers and the problem might be much bigger than it appears.

CONCLUSIONS

Medication errors are common in paediatrics and may account for significant morbidity and mortality. Applying the systems approach towards medication errors will enable hospitals and health organisations to detect and treat the source of many preventable errors before they harm patients. Clinicians and health professionals should adopt strategies that have been shown to reduce errors such as computerised physician order entry systems. Further studies are needed to understand this epidemic better and to develop new preventive measures.

Key points for clinical practice

- Medication errors are common in treating children. Patients at risk include sicker and more complex patients such as those in the neonatal and paediatric intensive care units and those in the emergency department.

- Dosing errors are the most common type of medication errors in children.

- Ten-fold errors are common in paediatrics. The consequence of 10-fold errors may be very serious.

- A medication error that reaches the patient is a system failure. Ask yourself how to change the system in order to prevent the next error.

- Always give parents and other caregivers simple instructions on how to administer medications to their child.

- When prescribing drugs, try to avoid decimal points (use leading zero and avoid trailing zero), spell micrograms and nanograms and avoid abbreviations.

- Encourage teamwork and open communication between health professionals and with the patients and parents.

- Using a standard dosing system for paediatric emergencies and a formatted order sheet may reduce medication errors.

- Using a computerised physician order system reduces the incidence of medication errors.

- A non-punitive approach to medication errors will encourage voluntary reporting of such errors and may help prevent the next mistake.

- Voluntary reporting underestimates the true rate of medication errors. Detection of medication errors can not rely solely on voluntary reports; active surveillance for such errors should be part of any health organisation.

References

1. Bates DW, Cullen DJ, Laird N et al. Incidence of adverse drug events and potential adverse drug events. Implications for prevention. ADE Prevention Study Group. JAMA 1995; **274**: 29–34.

2. Kohn LT. *To err is human: building a safer health system*. Washington, DC: National Academy Press, 2000.

3. Leape LL, Brennan TA, Laird N *et al*. The nature of adverse events in hospitalized patients. Results of the Harvard Medical Practice Study II. *N Engl J Med* 1991; **324**: 377–384.

4. Brennan TA, Leape LL, Laird NM *et al*. Incidence of adverse events and negligence in hospitalized patients. Results of the Harvard Medical Practice Study I. *N Engl J Med* 1991; **324**: 370–376.

5. Koren G, Barzilay Z, Greenwald M. Tenfold errors in administration of drug doses: a neglected iatrogenic disease in pediatrics. *Pediatrics* 1986; **77**: 848–849.

6. Phillips DP, Christenfeld N, Glynn LM. Increase in US medication-error deaths between 1983 and 1993. *Lancet* 1998; **351**: 643–644.

7. Lesar TS, Lomaestro BM, Pohl H. Medication-prescribing errors in a teaching hospital. A 9-year experience. *Arch Intern Med* 1997; **157**: 1569–1576.

8. Lesar TS, Briceland LL, Delcoure K, Parmalee JC, Masta-Gornic V, Pohl H. Medication prescribing errors in a teaching hospital. *JAMA* 1990; **263**: 2329–2334.

9. Lesar TS. Errors in the use of medication dosage equations. *Arch Pediatr Adolesc Med* 1998; **152**: 340–344.

10. Conroy S, Choonara I, Impicciatore P *et al*. Survey of unlicensed and off label drug use in paediatric wards in European countries. European Network for Drug Investigation in Children. *BMJ* 2000; **320**: 79–82.

11. Wilson DG, McArtney RG, Newcombe RG *et al*. Medication errors in paediatric practice: insights from a continuous quality improvement approach. *Eur J Pediatr* 1998; **157**: 769–774.

12. Lesar TS, Briceland L, Stein DS. Factors related to errors in medication prescribing. *JAMA* 1997; **277**: 312–317.

13. Kaushal R, Bates DW, Landrigan C *et al*. Medication errors and adverse drug events in pediatric inpatients. *JAMA* 2001; **285**: 2114–2120.

14. Kozer E, Scolnik D, Macpherson A *et al*. Variables associated with medication errors in pediatric emergency medicine. *Pediatrics* 2002; **110**: 737–742.

15. Vincer MJ, Murray JM, Yuill A, Allen AC, Evans JR, Stinson DA. Drug errors and incidents in a neonatal intensive care unit. A quality assurance activity. *Am J Dis Child* 1989; **143**: 737–740.

16. Folli HL, Poole RL, Benitz WE, Russo JC. Medication error prevention by clinical pharmacists in two children's hospitals. *Pediatrics* 1987; **79**: 718–722.

17. Perlstein PH, Callison C, White M, Barnes B, Edwards NK. Errors in drug computations during newborn intensive care. *Am J Dis Child* 1979; **133**: 376–379.

18. Glover ML, Sussmane JB. Assessing pediatrics residents' mathematical skills for prescribing medication: a need for improved training. *Acad Med* 2002; **77**: 1007–1010.

19. Rowe C, Koren T, Koren G. Errors by paediatric residents in calculating drug doses. *Arch Dis Child* 1998; **79**: 56–58.

20. Kozer E, Scolnik D, Keays T, Shi K, Luk T, Koren G. Large errors in the dosing of medications for children. *N Engl J Med* 2002; **346**: 1175–1176.

21. Lesar TS. Tenfold medication dose prescribing errors. *Ann Pharmacother* 2002; **36**: 1833–1839.

22. Ross LM, Wallace J, Paton JY. Medication errors in a paediatric teaching hospital in the UK: five years operational experience. *Arch Dis Child* 2000; **83**: 492–497.

23. Raju TN, Kecskes S, Thornton JP, Perry M, Feldman S. Medication errors in neonatal and paediatric intensive-care units. *Lancet* 1989; **2**: 374–376.

24. Simon HK, Weinkle DA. Over-the-counter medications. Do parents give what they intend to give? *Arch Pediatr Adolesc Med* 1997; **151**: 654–656.

25. Leape LL, Bates DW, Cullen DJ *et al*. Systems analysis of adverse drug events. ADE Prevention Study Group. *JAMA* 1995; **274**: 35–43.

26. Kozer E, Seto W, Verjee Z *et al*. Prospective observational study on the incidence of medication errors during simulated resuscitation in a paediatric emergency department. *BMJ* 2004; **329**: 1321.

27. West DW, Levine S, Magram G, MacCorkle AH, Thomas P, Upp K. Pediatric medication order error rates related to the mode of order transmission. *Arch Pediatr Adolesc Med*

1994; **148**: 1322–1326.

28. Sexton JB, Thomas EJ, Helmreich RL. Error, stress, and teamwork in medicine and aviation: cross sectional surveys. *BMJ* 2000; **320**: 745–749.

29. Landrigan CP, Rothschild JM, Cronin JW *et al*. Effect of reducing interns' work hours on serious medical errors in intensive care units. *N Engl J Med* 2004; **351**: 1838–1848.

30. Lockley SW, Cronin JW, Evans EE *et al*. Effect of reducing interns' weekly work hours on sleep and attentional failures. *N Engl J Med* 2004; **351**: 1829–1837.

31. Stucky ER. Prevention of medication errors in the pediatric inpatient setting. *Pediatrics* 2003; **112**: 431–436.

32. King WJ, Paice N, Rangrej J, Forestell GJ, Swartz R. The effect of computerized physician order entry on medication errors and adverse drug events in pediatric inpatients. *Pediatrics* 2003; **112**: 506–509.

33. Potts AL, Barr FE, Gregory DF, Wright L, Patel NR. Computerized physician order entry and medication errors in a pediatric critical care unit. *Pediatrics* 2004; **113**: 59–63.

34. Koppel R, Metlay JP, Cohen A *et al*. Role of computerized physician order entry systems in facilitating medication errors. *JAMA* 2005; **293**: 1197–1203.

35. Kirk RC, Li-Meng GD, Packia J, Min KH, Ong BK. Computer calculated dose in paediatric prescribing. *Drug Safety* 2005; **28**: 817–824.

36. Kozer E, Scolnik D ,Macpherson A, Rauchwerger D, Koren G. Using a preprinted order sheet to reduce prescription errors in a pediatric emergency department: a randomized controlled trial. *Pediatrics* 2005; **116**: 1299–1302.

37. Leape LL, Cullen DJ, Clapp MD *et al*. Pharmacist participation on physician rounds and adverse drug events in the intensive care unit. *JAMA* 1999; **282**: 267–270.

38. Bond CA, Raehl CL, Franke T. Medication errors in United States hospitals. *Pharmacotherapy* 2001; **21**: 1023–1036.

39. Shah AN, Frush K, Luo X, Wears RL. Effect of an intervention standardization system on pediatric dosing and equipment size determination: a crossover trial involving simulated resuscitation events. *Arch Pediatr Adolesc Med* 2003; **157**: 229–236.

40. Frush KS, Luo X, Hutchinson P, Higgins JN. Evaluation of a method to reduce over-the-counter medication dosing error. *Arch Pediatr Adolesc Med* 2004; **158**: 620–624.

41. Shaughnessy AF, D'Amico F. Long-term experience with a program to improve prescription-writing skills. *Fam Med* 1994; **26**: 168–171.

42. Dean B, Schachter M, Vincent C, Barber N. Causes of prescribing errors in hospital inpatients: a prospective study. *Lancet* 2002; **359**: 1373–1378.

43. Fortescue EB, Kaushal R, Landrigan CP *et al*. Prioritizing strategies for preventing medication errors and adverse drug events in pediatric inpatients. *Pediatrics* 2003; **111**: 722–729.

44. Suresh G, Horbar JD, Plsek P *et al*. Voluntary anonymous reporting of medical errors for neonatal intensive care. *Pediatrics* 2004; **113**: 1609–1618.

45. Cullen DJ, Bates DW, Small SD, Cooper JB, Nemeskal AR, Leape LL. The incident reporting system does not detect adverse drug events: a problem for quality improvement. *Jt Comm J Qual Improv* 1995; **21**: 541–548.

46. Flynn EA, Barker KN, Pepper GA, Bates DW, Mikeal RL. Comparison of methods for detecting medication errors in 36 hospitals and skilled-nursing facilities. *Am J Health Syst Pharm* 2002; **59**: 436–446.

47. Parshuram CS, Ng GY, Ho TK *et al*. Discrepancies between ordered and delivered concentrations of opiate infusions in critical care. *Crit Care Med* 2003; **31**: 2483–2487.

Malcolm Holliday Aaron Friedman

6

Treating hypovolaemia: avoiding hyponatraemia

Hyponatraemia has been labelled the most common complication of intravenous (i.v.) fluid therapy used for acutely ill children.[1,2] It can cause brain damage or death. Its common cause is giving more free water than can be excreted, thereby diluting body solutes and temporarily expanding cell volume. As brain cell volume increases, brain blood flow becomes restricted, potentially causing brain damage.

Hospital-induced hyponatraemia occurs because hypotonic saline is given to acutely ill children who have a non-osmotic stimulated level of antidiuretic hormone that limits free water excretion. This is often accompanied by an elevated plasma renin activity indicating hypovolaemia.[3] Children presenting to the emergency department who are already hyponatraemic have ingested excess free water, usually associated with hypovolaemia.[4]

In reviewing the literature, we concluded that hypovolaemia is the most common stimulus for non-osmotic antidiuretic hormone release that results in acute hyponatraemia.[5] Although stress, pain, vomiting, and certain drugs also stimulate antidiuretic hormone release, these appear, as judged from clinical experience and changes in urine output, to have shorter periods of action than hypovolaemia.[6,7] Antidiuretic hormone, elevated by hypovolaemia, is suppressed by extracellular fluid expansion with either isotonic saline or Ringer's lactate solution (Table 1) given over a few hours.[8,9] This chapter reviews these relationships, defines the causes and the nature of hypovolaemia and its correction. This correction avoids hyponatraemia.

Malcolm Holliday MD (for correspondence)
Emeritus Professor of Pediatrics, University of California at San Francisco, 1515 Oxford Street, Berkeley, CA 94709, USA
E-mail: mah@itsa.ucsf.edu

Aaron Friedman MD
Professor and Chair of Pediatrics, Brown University and Hasbro Children's Hospital, 593 Eddy Street, Hasbro Children's Hospital, Rm 125, Providence, RI 02903, USA
E-mail: afreidman@lifespan.org

Table 1. Composition of intravenous and oral solutions

Solution	Osmolality (mOsm/l)	Glucose (mmol/l)	Na (meq/l)	Cl (meq/l)	HCO$_3$ (meq/l)	K (meq/l)
Intravenous solutions						
Ringer's lactate	280	–	130	110	25	4
0.9% saline	308	–	154	154	–	–
D$_5$ 0.45% saline	454	300	77	77	–	–
D$_5$ 0.22% saline	377	300	38	38	–	–
Oral solution						
WHO-ORS	330	110	90	80	30	20
Low-Na ORS	270	110	60	50	30	20
Pedialyte	270	140	45	35	30	20

WHO, World Health Organization; ORS, oral rehydration solution.

DEFINING HYPOVOLAEMIA AND ITS CAUSES

The underlying diseases associated with hypovolaemia in acutely ill children include gastroenteritis, pulmonary infections, meningitis, other inflammatory disorders and trauma. Hypovolaemia occurs pre- and post-surgery, particularly post-neurosurgery. In endemic areas, it occurs in patients with malaria and other wasting diseases.

Hypovolaemia is a state in which loss or displacement of extracellular fluid impairs arterial circulation, perfusion of organs and tissues, and lowers central blood volume.[10] The obvious examples are loss of extracellular fluid due to diarrhoea and vomiting, displacement of extracellular fluid into a major burn area, and vasomotor collapse due to sepsis. More subtle forms of extracellular fluid loss and/or displacement that, nonetheless, cause non-osmotic antidiuretic hormone release occur in children who:

1. Drink excess free water when engaged in strenuous sports in hot weather or during an acute illness, or who have cystic fibrosis and are exposed to heat stress.

2. Have meningitis, head injury, or undergo neurosurgery leading to acute cerebral salt wasting.[11]

3. Have renal tubular disease with renal salt wasting and become acutely ill, interrupting replacement intake.

4. Have acute inflammation due to pneumonia, cellulitis and other inflammatory states or sustain trauma and 'third space' losses causing more subtle oedema and dislocations of interstitial fluid.

5. Are fasted and thirsted for long periods in getting to hospital and in waiting to be seen.

6. Experience loss of muscle tone as occurs with anaesthesia, coma or a prolonged passive state.

Table 2. Distribution of extracellular fluid[12]

System	Infant	Adult
Plasma and lymph (ml/kg)	60	55
Muscle and organs (ml/kg)	80	85
Skin and connective tissue (ml/kg)	160	130
Total extracellular fluid (ml/kg)	300	270

While the latter two conditions are well recognised as occurring in patients during surgery and postoperative states, they are often overlooked in children who have been travelling distances to get to an emergency department and have been lying on a trolley waiting to be seen. In these acutely ill children, extracellular fluid is either lost, displaced by inflammation, sequestered thus reducing venous return, or some combination of these. These changes are comparable to the effects of experimental 'quiet standing' described below.

THE INTERPLAY OF ARTERIAL CIRCULATION WITH EXTRACELLULAR FLUID

The interactions of arterial circulation, plasma volume and the two phases of the interstitial fluids (Table 2) and how these react in hypovolaemia are more

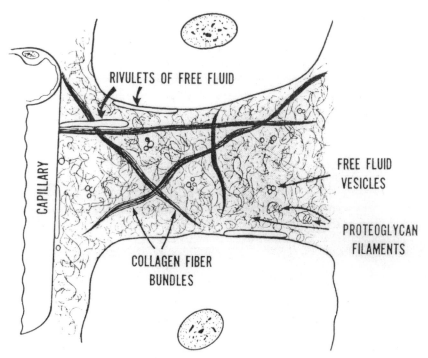

RIVULETS OF FREE FLUID

CAPILLARY

FREE FLUID
VESICLES

PROTEOGLYCAN
FILAMENTS

COLLAGEN FIBER
BUNDLES

Fig. 1. A line drawing of the interstitium indicating the coils of proteoglycans that make interstitial fluid into a gel that is resistant to gravitational stress. The structural rigidity of the collagen fibres maintains the intercapilliary–interstitial space between cells and the negative hydrostatic pressure, P_i, in the interstitium; this assures rapid and efficient exchange of solutes between plasma and cells. From Guyton.[13]

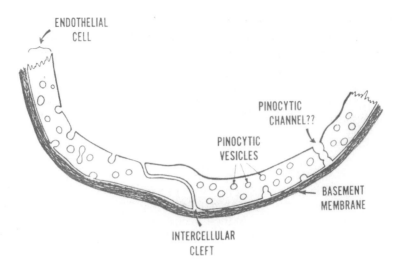

Fig. 2. Structure of the capillary wall. *With permission from* Guyton.[13]

intricate than commonly appreciated.[12] The fluid phase between capillaries and metabolising tissue cells, is a thin gel-like fluid (cell interstitial fluid) that is resistant to gravity and to net change in volume but is a busy pathway for exchange between plasma and tissue cells (Fig. 1). Oxygen and carbon dioxide

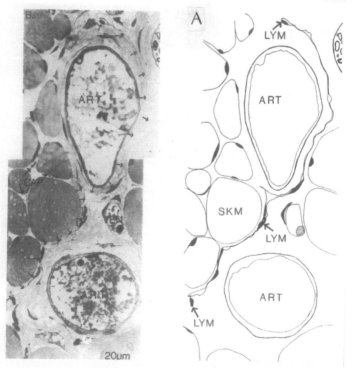

Fig. 3. A photomicrograph and line drawing of skeletal muscle (SKM) showing lymphatics (LYM) and capillaries (CAP) adjacent to arteries (ART) and muscle fibres that will be squeezed to propel lymph and blood forward during exercise, VEN venule. From Holliday.[12]

exchange by diffusion; nutrients and end-products are exchanged by ultrafiltration from plasma into cell interstitial fluid, then taken up into cell fluid by active transport. Plasma ultrafiltrate carrying nutrients passes through capillary epithelium via small intercellular clefts driven by capillary hydrostatic pressure. Plasma albumen filters through larger clefts as a function of cleft diameter and charge that is regulated by factors that also control capillary flow (Fig. 2). A portion of the ultrafiltrate with metabolic end-products is returned to

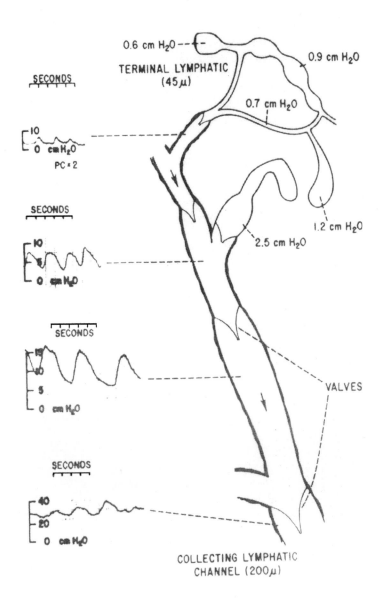

Fig. 4. A line drawing the lymphatics. interstitial fluid and proteins enter the low-pressure terminal lymphatic (upper left) and are propelled forward by pulsating pressures of smooth and skeletal muscle contractions. Valves prevent back flow, P_c hydrostatic capillary pressure. From Holliday.[12]

plasma by net oncotic (Starling) forces; the balance of ultrafiltrate and all the albumen are returned via lymphatics (Fig. 3) propelled by lymphatic smooth muscle and voluntary muscle contraction (Fig. 4) through the lymphatic duct into the vena cava. This entails a brisk exchange of albumen and plasma ultrafiltrate between circulation and interstitial fluid via lymph propelled by muscle tone and activity.

Capillary flow, the oxygen–nutrient delivery system is regulated by oxygen tension; as cell activity increases, oxygen tension drops causing local capillary blood flow to increase. Capillary-cell exchange rates then increase. As the sum of all individual cell metabolic activities changes, so does metabolic rate, capillary blood flow and cardiac output.[12] Dehydration and shock, impairing this sequence, impair cell metabolism.

The second interstitial fluid is a larger collagen-rich interstitial fluid of skin and connective tissue (skin interstitial fluid). It gives structure and elasticity to these areas but has few cells and little metabolic activity (Fig. 5). In contrast to cell interstitial fluid, skin interstitial fluid is a reservoir that decreases to sustain plasma and cell interstitial fluid volume when hypovolaemia develops.[12]

ADAPTATION TO LOSS OR DISPLACEMENT OF EXTRACELLULAR FLUID

With dehydration, plasma volume decreases compromising circulation; skin interstitial fluid also decreases, thereby partially restoring plasma volume, but

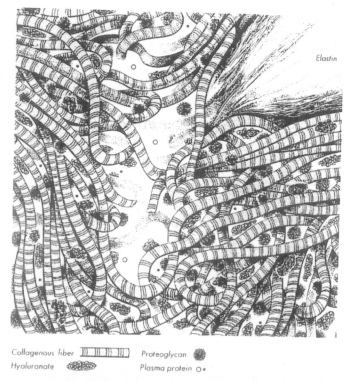

Collagenous fiber   Proteoglycan
Hyaluronate   Plasma protein

Fig. 5. An artist's sketch of skin interstitial fluid (not to scale) illustrating collagen and proteoglycans in relation to free fluid of the interstitium as seen in skin. Note areas of exclusion of large plasma proteins (open circles) where small (filled circles) proteins are present. From Holliday.[12]

causing loss of skin turgor. Cell interstitial fluid and exchange between capillary and cell is preserved. With skin injury, as in burns, the inflammatory response draws plasma volume and skin interstitial fluid to the affected site. Plasma volume, circulating albumin and skin interstitial fluid are reduced. Hypovolaemia from any of these causes stimulates antidiuretic hormone release, activates the renin–angiotensin–aldosterone system, and other factors regulating sodium and/or chloride excretion.

A similar shift occurs with quiet standing and total muscle relaxation of healthy, well-hydrated subjects. In just 15 min of quiet standing, lymph, albumen and venous blood are sequestered, slowing venous return; oedema collects in the dependent limbs and cardiac output is compromised. Substantial skin interstitial fluid, plasma fluid and albumin are displaced from the upper to the dependent extremities causing syncope and hypotension. Once muscle activity or lying down restores lymph flow and albumen to venous circulation, the blood pressure is restored and antidiuretic hormone and renin–angiotensin–aldosterone system levels decline as noted above.[12] A variant is noted when dehydrated subjects with elevated antidiuretic hormone and renin-angiotensin-aldosterone system are immersed in water; central blood volume increases and antidiuretic hormone and renin-angiotensin-aldosterone system decline.[14] These findings illustrate the rather exquisite sensitivity of antidiuretic hormone and renin-angiotensin-aldosterone system to changes in circulation.

EVOLUTION OF TREATMENT FOR DIARRHOEAL DEHYDRATION

Because i.v. fluids were first used to treat cholera and infantile diarrhoeal dehydration and are a common treatment for acutely ill children today, current practices under discussion are, to some extent, an outgrowth of the treatment that evolved for both cholera and infantile diarrhoeal dehydration over the last century.[15] Intravenous isotonic saline was first used in the 19th century for treatment of the severe dehydration of cholera. It was dramatically effective in restoring circulation to patients, even those who were moribund. In some cases, more than 10 l were required: as extracellular fluid was restored, sometimes diarrhoea and dehydration recurred, and extracellular fluid had to be restored again. However, the hundreds of patients in some epidemics exceeded the resources able to deliver this i.v. therapy. Finding an effective oral rehydration solution became a priority.

The use of i.v. isotonic saline for the treatment of the severe dehydration of infantile diarrhoea began in the early 20th century lowering mortality rate from ~80% to ~20% by the 1930s.[15] Darrow et al.,[16] in the 1940s, described a comprehensive treatment regimen based on replacing estimated deficits of sodium, chloride, potassium and water which was combined with maintenance solutions, to replace insensible and urinary water losses. These fluids were given over several days; oral feedings were introduced slowly. Variations on this approach were the guiding principles for textbook treatment plans for the next half century.[15] The effectiveness of this regimen was compromised because the potassium concentration in the i.v. solution slowed the permissible infusion rate and, therefore, the rate of extracellular fluid restoration.

An effective oral rehydration solution was developed in the 1960s for treating cholera. Adding 2% glucose to an oral saline solution (Table 1) stimulated glucose/sodium co-transport increasing not only sodium, but chloride, potassium, and water uptake as well that corrected dehydration and electrolyte disturbances of cholera. Oral rehydration solution proved dramatically effective in the 1963 Bangladesh epidemic dropping mortality to single digits. Intravenous saline was needed initially only for patients with profuse vomiting or in shock.[17]

The same regimen was similarly successful in treating children with diarrhoeal dehydration in areas with limited resources. An aggressive regimen, 100 ml/kg in 6 h, was equally effective in treating children with hyponatraemia, normonatraemia and hypernatraemia, restoring serum sodium to normal in all cases.[18] Initial i.v. solutions were seldom needed. Some reported mortality rates below 1%. Solutions of between 60–90 meq/l of sodium with chloride proved equally effective.[17] In the industrialised world, diarrhoea, when it does occur, often is treated with i.v. saline – sometimes isotonic, sometimes half isotonic – followed by oral rehydration solution. Those treated with half isotonic are prone to become hyponatraemic.[9] The complex i.v. fluid regimen of the 1950s changed into the rapid extracellular fluid expansion, oral rehydration solution regimen of the 1980.

SURGICAL PRACTICE

It has long been established practice in surgical patients to maintain isotonic saline as a 'keep open' line, before, during and after surgery. More isotonic saline is given to maintain or restore effective circulation: offsetting the effects of muscle relaxation, tissue injury (third-space loss) and absent oral intake. Oral feedings are initiated postoperatively as soon as practical, usually bypassing the need for long-term i.v. maintenance therapy. The same regimen is suitable for many acutely ill children with medical problems.

Burn patients with more than 30% skin surface burn have an intense inflammatory response that transfers extracellular fluid, mostly skin interstitial fluid and plasma volume, into the injured site causing burn shock. The standard acute treatment is to give Ringer's lactate solution or isotonic saline at an initial rate of 2 ml/kg/percentage burn surface in the first 4 h, repeating this infusion over the next 18–24 h to establish and maintain an effective arterial circulation as indicated by blood pressure, skin temperature, alertness, and renal and gastrointestinal perfusion. A 30-kg child with 40% burn will receive 2400 ml (80 ml/kg) in the first 4 h to accomplish these goals; a similar amount is scheduled for the next 18–24 h.[19] Moyers and his associates,[20] in 1965, gave 150–260 ml/kg of Ringer's lactate solution but no plasma or albumen; patients responded with good perfusion and normal blood pressure. They were conversing, taking fluid and food and passing suitable urine within 12 h. Subsequent refinements have confirmed the value of this approach. Ringer's lactate solution, in overexpanding extracellular fluid and making up for fluid lost in the burn site, restores circulation and perfusion and salvages dislocated albumen. Extracellular fluid adjusts by excreting the excess sodium chloride and water.

The very high antidiuretic hormone levels noted in patients with burn shock remain well above normal throughout the first 24 h. Yet urine output is normal or high and urine osmolality averages ~700 mOs/l from the first voiding; serum sodium averages > 133 meq/l despite persistence of stress, pain, and continued morphine administration and oral water intake. In other words, an elevated but declining antidiuretic hormone may not so inhibit free water excretion as to cause hyponatraemia.[8]

This finding points to the need for comparing concurrent urine concentration with plasma antidiuretic hormone toward defining the relation between an elevated but declining antidiuretic hormone and the capacity to excrete urine, not maximally concentrated.

MAINTENANCE THERAPY

The maintenance programmes developed by Darrow et al.,[16] by Talbot and colleagues[21] and by Holliday and Segar[22] in the 1950s were approximations of the anticipated insensible and urinary losses of children with diarrhoeal dehydration **once rehydrated** but not yet on oral feedings. These losses scale to a metabolic rate or surface area rather than body weight as growth proceeds. Differences among these programmes were negligible. Updated versions of i.v. maintenance therapy note the case of children with obligatory oliguria or other exceptional problems not noted by to the originators of these earlier programmes.[22]

Over the last quarter century, diarrhoeal dehydration has become less common in the industrialised world; children with the diverse acute illnesses are the ones now being treated in emergency departments. It became common practice to give a new version of original i.v. maintenance, half or quarter isotonic saline often in excess of recommended maintenance to replace physiological losses and would, it was reasoned, replace any subtle sodium chloride or water losses. It was this development that led to the scourge of hyponatraemia and its sometimes dire consequences. The call for using isotonic saline as initial i.v. fluid therapy has greatly reduced the problem.[24] Terming isotonic saline a generic maintenance solution is more problematic.

Isotonic saline itself given as a bolus or as 'maintenance' has its own complications. Either sometimes leads to urinary sodium excretion sufficient to lower serum sodium.[4,7,25] Current physiological studies describing controls over sodium and chloride excretion[26,27] have not yet developed to become dependable guidelines for establishing clinical practices.

CONCLUSIONS

The call that has come to test whether initial i.v. fluid therapy should be isotonic or hypotonic addresses the wrong question. Isotonic saline is usually the preferred initial therapy because hypovolaemia and elevated antidiuretic hormone levels are common but not always apparent. Following initial i.v. treatment, maintenance therapy for infants can be met by oral rehydration solution with sodium concentrations from 30–90 meq/l; for older patients, oral rehydration solution or liquid diets should suffice. It is safer to plan 24-h i.v. maintenance to replace minimum, not generous losses. Generous 24-h i.v. prescription for maintenance water causes hyponatraemia; generous 24-h i.v. prescription for sodium chloride has some unanticipated effects that are noted above. Prudence argues to plan replacing minimum 24-h sodium chloride losses with a hypotonic maintenance solution, reserving isotonic saline at 20–40 ml/kg/over 2–4 h when expansion for hypovolaemia is warranted.

Key points for clinical practice

- Observe respiration, heart beat and skin temperature for signs of hypovolaemia or overload. Obtain history of appetite, thirst and urine output.

- If intravenous therapy is planned, obtain serum electrolytes.

- In the absence of signs of overload give 20–40 ml/kg of isotonic saline or Ringer's lactate solution over a 2–4-h period and monitor urine output (and concentration).

- If further observation or admission is planned following the above intravenous regimen, continue a keep open intravenous isotonic saline. Initiate oral liquids if practical: in infants, use an oral rehydration solution; in children, an oral rehydration solution or clear liquids plus salted crackers. If intravenous maintenance is required, use minimum levels appropriate to the patient's status. Do not give excess salt or water loads.

- If discharging home, initiate oral feedings: in infants, use an oral rehydration solution; in children, an oral rehydration solution or clear liquids plus salted crackers. Caution family about overzealous use of 'clear liquids' free of salt in follow-up and subsequent episodes.

References

1. Shann F, Germer S. Hyponatremia associated with pneumonia or bacterial meningitis. *Arch Dis Child* 1985; **60**: 963–966.
2. Gerigk M, Bald M, Feth F, Rascher W. Clinical settings and vasopressin function in hyponatremic children. *Eur J Paediatr* 1993; **152**: 301–305.
3. Gerigk M, Gnehm HE, Rascher W. Arginine vasopressin and renin in acutely ill children: implications for fluid therapy. *Acta Pediatr* 1996; **85**: 550–553.
4. Hoorn EJ, Geary D, Robb M, Halperin ML, Bohn D. Acute hyponatremia related to intravenous fluid administration in hospitalized children: an observational study. *Pediatrics* 2004; **113**: 1279–1284.
5. Holliday MA, Friedman A, Segar WE, Chesney R, Finberg L. Avoiding hospital-induced hyponatremia: a physiological approach. *J Pediatr* 2004; **145**: 584–587.
6. Friedman AL, Segar WE. Antidiuretic hormone excess. *J Pediatr* 1979; **94**: 521–526.
7. Duke T, Molyneux EM. Intravenous fluids for seriously ill children: time to reconsider. *Lancet* 2003; **362**: 1320–1323.
8. McIntosh N, Michaelis L, Barclay C, Muir M, Stephen R, Sedowofia K. Dissociation of osmoregulation from plasma arginine vasopressin levels following thermal injury in childhood. *Burns* 2000; **26**: 543–547.
9. Neville KA, O'Meara M, Verge CF, Walker JL. Normal saline is better than half normal saline for rehydration of children with gastroenteritis. Pediatric Acad Soc Annual Meeting, Seattle, WA, 2003.
10. Holliday MA. Fluid and nutrition support [Ch. 14A]. In: Holliday MA, Barratt TM, Avner ED (eds) *Pediatric Nephrology*, 3rd edn. Baltimore, MD: Williams and Wilkins, 1993; 287–298.

11. Ganong CA, Kappy MS. Cerebral salt wasting in children. *Am J Dis Child* 1993; **147**: 167–169.
12. Holliday MA. Extracellular fluid and its proteins: dehydration, shock, and recovery. *Pediatr Nephrol* 1999; **13**: 989–995.
13. Guyton AC. Capillary dynamics and exchange of fluid between the blood and interstitisl fluid. In: Guyton AC, Hall JE. (eds) *Medical Physiology*, 6th edn. Philadelphia, PA: WB Saunders, 1996; Chapter 30: Fig.1 = p359, Fig.30.2; Fig.2 = p362, Fig. 30.4.
14. Epstein M, Preston S, Weitzman RE. Isosmotic central blood volume expansion suppresses plasma arginine vasopressin in normal man. *J Clin Endocrinol Metab* 1981; **52**: 256–262.
15. Holliday MA. The evolution of therapy for dehydration: should deficit therapy still be taught? *Pediatrics* 1996; **98**: 171–177.
16. Darrow DC, Pratt EL, Flett J, Gamble AH, Weiss HA. Disturbances of water and electrolytes in infantile diarrhea. *Pediatrics* 1949; **1**: 129–156.
17. Hirschhorn N. The treatment of acute diarrhea in children: an historical and physiological perspective. *Am J Clin Nutr* 1980; **33**: 637–663.
18. Pizarro D, Posada G, Villavicencio N, Mohs E, Levine MM. Oral rehydration in hypernatremic and hyponatremic diarrheal dehydration. *Am J Dis Child* 1983; **137**: 730–734.
19. Puffinbarger NK, Tuggle DI, Smith EI. Rapid isotonic fluid resuscitation in pediatric thermal injury. *J Pediatr Surg* 1994; **29**: 339–341.
20. Moyers CA, Margraf HW, Monafo WW. Burn shock and extravascular sodium deficiency – treatment with Ringer's solution with lactate. *Arch Surg* 1965; **90**: 799–811.
21. Talbot NB, Crawford JD, Butler AM. Homeostatic limits to safe parenteral fluid therapy. *N Engl J Med* 1953; **248**: 1100–1108.
22. Holliday MA, Segar WE. The maintenance need for water in parenteral fluid therapy. *Pediatrics* 1957; **19**: 823–832.
23. Friedman AL. Fluid and electrolyte therapy. In: Berhman RE, Kliegman RM. (eds) *Nelson's Essential Pediatrics*, 4th edn. Philadelphia, PA: WB Saunders, 2002; 671–709.
24. Moritz ML, Ayus JC. Prevention of hospital acquired hyponatremia: a case for using isotonic saline in maintenance fluid therapy. *Pediatrics* 2003; **111**: 227–230.
25. Steele A, Gowrishankar M, Abrahamson S *et al*. Postoperative hyponatremia despite near isotonic saline infusion: a phenomenon of desalination. *Ann Intern Med* 1997; **126**: 823–832.
26. Singer DRJ, Markandu ND, Buckley MG *et al*. Contrasting endocrine responses to acute oral compared with intravenous sodium loading in normal humans. *Am J Physiol* 1998; **274**: F111–F119.
27. Rasmussen MS, Simonsen JA, Sandgaard NCF, Hoilund-Carlsen PF, Bie P. Mechanisms of acute natriuresis in normal humans on low sodium diets. *J Physiol* 2003; **546**: 591–603

Jordan Greenbaum Cindy W. Christian

7

Asphyxiation in children

Asphyxia is derived from the Greek word *asphuxia*, meaning 'a stopping of the pulse'. In modern usage. it refers to 'a lack of oxygen', and describes a wide variety of causes that interfere with oxygen uptake or utilisation, and elimination of carbon dioxide.[1] Causes include neck or chest compression, airway obstruction, exclusion of atmospheric oxygen by an inert gas, and interference with oxygen uptake and metabolism.

Some of the more common types of asphyxia are defined in Table 1.[2] In some cases, asphyxia results from a combination of the conditions described in Table 1. An adult asphyxiating a small child with a pillow, for example, may not only obstruct the external air passages (smother), but also compress the child's neck (strangulation).

Asphyxia may be accidental or inflicted. A soundly sleeping older child, or intoxicated adult may overlay a prone infant, causing asphyxia through facial obstruction and/or chest compression. An adult may intentionally asphyxiate a young child by obstructing the nose and mouth with his or her hand. Clinical or autopsy findings may not allow differentiation between accidental and inflicted asphyxia.

EPIDEMIOLOGY

Suffocation is a relatively common cause of injury death in young children, but infrequent in older children and adolescents. Data from the Centers for Disease

Jordan Greenbaum MD (for correspondence)
Medical Director, Child Protection Center, Children's Healthcare of Atlanta, MOB, Suite 500, 1001
Johnson Ferry Rd, NE Atlanta, GA 30342, USA
E-mail: virginia.greenbaum@choa.org

Cindy W. Christian MD
Associate Professor of Paediatrics, The University of Pennsylvania School of Medicine and
Chair, Child Abuse and Neglect Prevention, Room 2405, The Children.s Hospital of Philadelphia,
34th Street and Civic Center Blvd, Philadelphia, PA 19104, USA. E-mail: christian@email.chop.edu

Table 1 Common types of asphyxia

Suffocation	A general term implying death from oxygen deprivation, including lack of atmospheric oxygen or obstruction of the nose and mouth
Smothering	Deprivation of oxygen by obstruction of the nose and mouth. This may entail an object being pressed over the face, the face being pressed against an object, or an object occluding the mouth (as in a gag), which eventually leads to obstruction of the nasal passages by edema or mucus
Choking	Obstruction of the upper airway by a foreign body
Strangulation	External compression of the neck by hand(s) or ligature
Throttling	External compression of the neck by hand(s)
Traumatic asphyxia	Asphyxia caused by severe chest compression
Hanging	A form of ligature strangulation in which the force of the neck compression derives from the weight of the victim's body (or a portion of the body)
Wedging	A type of mechanical asphyxia in which the face or thorax is compressed, preventing adequate respiration[3]
Overlying	A form of asphyxia in which the body, or portion of the body, of an adult or older child lies atop the victim resulting in airway obstruction, and/or compression of the abdomen/thorax, and/or compression of the neck[3]

Control (CDC; unintentional injury deaths) in 2002[4] indicate that suffocation accounted for 67% (636/946) of unintentional injury deaths in infants less than 1 year of age, and 8.5% (139/1641) of such deaths in children 1–4 years old. In contrast, suffocation accounted for only 3.4% (40/1176) and 1.6% (138/8679) of the unintentional injury deaths in children 5–9 and 10–19 years of age, respectively (Fig. 1).

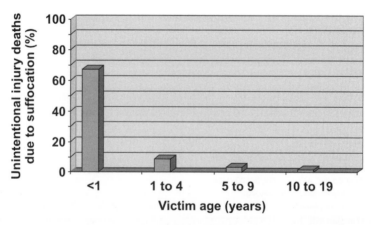

Fig. 1 Unintentional injury deaths related to suffocation by victim age, 2002. Adapted from WISQARS database, Office of Statistics and Programming, National Center for Injury Prevention and Control, Centers for Disease Control.[4]

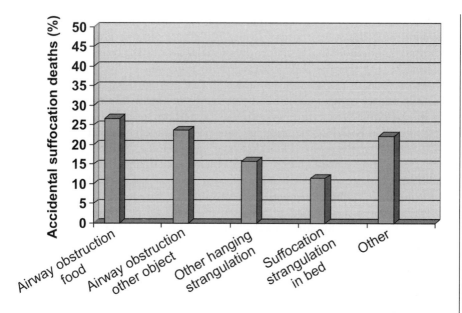

Type of accidental suffocation

Fig. 2 Mechanism of unintentional suffocation deaths in children 1–4 years old, 2002. Adapted from WISQARS database, Office of Statistics and Programming, National Center for Injury Prevention and Control, Centers for Disease Control.[4]

Accidental asphyxia in infants commonly involves entrapment/wedging, obstruction of the nose and mouth by loose bedding, or overlying. In the study by Scheers *et al.*[5] of accidental suffocation and sleep location in infants, entrapment was the most common form of suffocation in infants sleeping in adult beds, accounting for about half the deaths. This typically involved the child becoming trapped between the bed and the wall or the mattress and the head/foot board. For infants sleeping in cribs, the majority of accidental suffocation deaths involved entrapment and soft bedding, while for those sleeping on sofas or chairs the primary causes of asphyxia were entrapment and overlying. The risk of suffocation was 40 times higher for infants sleeping in adult beds than for those sleeping in cribs.

Frequent causes of wedging or neck compression deaths involve defective cribs or mattresses that are too small for the crib. In addition, an infant may become entangled in a low-hanging cradle gym, and a toddler climbing out of the crib may become wedged between that structure and adjacent furniture.[6,7]

Toddlers and pre-school aged infants are also vulnerable to asphyxia from inhalation of food and other foreign objects. Data from the CDC[4] show that aspiration accounted for 50% of the unintentional suffocation deaths for children 1–4 years old in 2002 (Fig. 2).

Accidental neck compression in toddlers and young children occasionally occurs with hanging cords or ropes.[4,6,8] Even school-aged children are vulnerable to accidental hanging from neck compression, often involving outer clothing becoming stuck on a protruding object during play.[8] Adolescents are more likely to engage in suicidal strangulation or incur accidental asphyxial injuries while 'acting out' after punishment, or while playing with ropes and cords.[6] In the 10–19-year-old age group, CDC data showed 60 unintentional neck compression deaths in 2002, compared with 704 suicides using this method of asphyxia. In their study of deaths related to mechanical asphyxia in children under 15 years of age, Nixon et al.[9] found a peak incidence of self-inflicted hanging deaths in boys 8–14 years old. Details of the incidents were not described, but the authors indicated most involved 'play that had gone badly wrong'; in some cases, it involved the child imitating acts depicted in the media. Flobecker et al.[8] also found a distinct group of boys who apparently placed a noose around their necks deliberately, and suffered fatal neck compression. Auto-erotic asphyxia is an unusual practice involving self-induced asphyxia, usually accomplished by some form of neck compression, and designed to heighten the pleasure of sexual activity. It is typically practised by adult males, but it has been reported infrequently in adolescents and can lead to unexpected accidental death.[8–10]

A significant number of intentional injury deaths in young children are due to asphyxia.[11–14] In one study of infant deaths classified as either intentional or 'undetermined intent', 10.2% were due to suffocation or strangulation.[12] Two additional studies of infanticide found that asphyxia accounted for 23–24% of the deaths (Fig. 3).[13,14] While estimates vary considerably, the American Academy of Pediatrics estimates that < 5% of sudden infant death syndrome (SIDS) cases are 'missed' homicides.[5] Given that intentional asphyxia often leaves no evidence at autopsy (see below), the majority of those missed cases likely involve an asphyxial death. There is evidence that historical factors may help to differentiate SIDS deaths from intentional asphyxia.[15] In a study of covert homicide victims, Meadow[15] found that about half of families had a history of multiple child deaths. In addition, 70% of index victims had experienced unexplained illnesses and greater than 50% had been hospitalised during the previous month. In ~50% of cases, Munchausen syndrome by proxy was suspected. In this study, smothering was the most common cause of death,

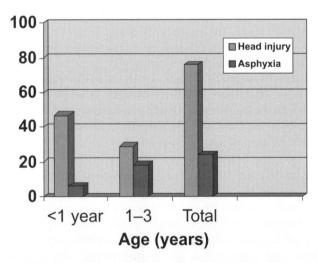

Fig. 3 Cause of death according to age. From de Silva and Oates.[13]

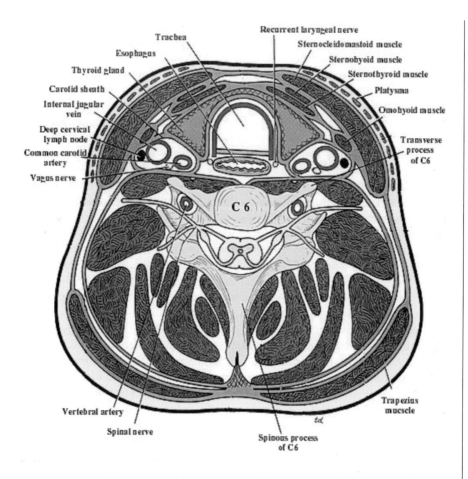

Recurrent laryngeal nerve
Trachea
Sternocleidomastoid muscle
Esophagus
Sternohyoid muscle
Thyroid gland
Sternothyroid muscle
Carotid sheath
Platysma
Internal jugular vein
Omohyoid muscle
Deep cervical lymph node
Transverse process of C6
Common carotid artery
Vagus nerve
C 6
Vertebral artery
Trapezius muscle
Spinal nerve
Spinous process of C6

Fig. 4 Anatomy of the neck. *Adapted from* Snell.[62]

with 19 of the 50 parents who confessed reporting they had smothered the child. Notably, 42 cases had been diagnosed as SIDS at the time of autopsy.

Inflicted asphyxia may be associated with paediatric condition falsification (also referred to as Munchausen syndrome by proxy)[16,17] or with more 'traditional' forms of physical abuse, related to frustration and anger by the caregiver toward the child.[18] The more common methods include smothering,[15,17,18] manual strangulation,[9] or chest compression.[19]

PATHOPHYSIOLOGY OF COMMON CAUSES OF PAEDIATRIC ASPHYXIA

NECK COMPRESSION

There are five possible consequences of external compression of the neck. There may be: (i) isolated venous obstruction; (ii) venous and arterial obstruction; (iii) vascular and airway occlusion; (iv) reflex cardiac arrest; or (v) varying combinations of these changes. The consequence depends on the amount of force used, the distribution and location of the compressing force, movements of victim and compressing object, and arterial/venous pressures at the time of the event. The major vascular structures of the neck to be affected are those supplying the brain: the common carotid arteries and the internal jugular veins (Fig. 4). The carotid arteries are located relatively deep in the tissues of the neck, medial to the internal jugular veins. This relatively deep location, the protection by the overlying sternomastoid muscles and the sturdy, muscular nature of the arterial walls ensure that it is more difficult to occlude blood supply to the brain than it is to obstruct venous return. The large, thin-walled internal jugular veins are relatively close to the surface and more vulnerable to compression. The vertebral arteries are well protected from compression as they tunnel upwards through intervertebral foramina within the transverse processes of the cervical vertebrae and are generally uninvolved in neck compression injury (see Fig. 4). The trachea, with its cartilaginous wall, is more difficult to compress than the nearby vascular structures. This is especially true in older children, in whom the cartilage of the tracheal wall is stiffer than in newborns. Depending on the application of the compressive force, airway occlusion may occur at the level of the pharynx rather than the trachea, as the larynx may be lifted upwards, and the root of the tongue pressed against the soft palate and roof of the mouth. Assuming an even distribution of forces, gradually increasing pressure will typically occlude the jugular veins first, followed by the carotid arteries and then the trachea. The degree of pressure may well change during the asphyxial event, leading to changing degrees of occlusion of the various structures over time.

Isolated and complete obstruction of the internal jugular veins leads to increasing venous congestion, as the drainage of blood from the brain is interrupted while the arterial supply continues. Eventually, the cerebral vascular congestion reduces blood flow and hypoxia/hypercapnia ensue. As there is no obstruction to coronary flow, there is no myocardial ischaemia, as long as respiration continues.

The situation changes when both venous and arterial blood flow are interrupted. Here, there is abrupt cessation of oxygenated blood flow to the brain, as well as blocked venous return. Because the blood supply is drastically reduced (the vertebral arteries continue to deliver blood, but this supply is not sufficient to support the cortex), there is no marked increase in venous pressure, as will occur with isolated venous occlusion. Hypoxia develops more quickly, as does hypercapnia, given the lack of blood flow. In fact, the inability of the brain to obtain oxygen rapidly leads to a cessation of metabolic activity. As long as the airway is open and respirations continue, however, there is no myocardial hypoxia.

If the force of neck compression is great enough to occlude venous and arterial supply, as well as obstruct the airway, there will be minimal blood flow to and from the brain and no marked venous congestion. However, the obstructed airway will lead to reduced oxygen delivery to the myocardium.

At any time during the compressive event, baroreceptors in the carotid sinus, carotid sheath and/or carotid body may be stimulated by the external pressure, initiating a reflex arc that leads to bradycardia and possibly asystole. Afferent impulses from the carotid structures travel to the Xth nucleus in the brainstem via the glossopharyngeal nerve. Efferent signals travel to the heart via the vagus nerve. It is unknown how often this vagal reflex occurs, and if it can lead directly to asystole or must be preceded by bradycardia.[2]

During the course of the compressive episode, conditions may change so that one or more of the above situations arises. There may be continuous or intermittent compression of the vessels and airway; there may be alterations in the location of pressure, as the victim or compressing object moves. There may be partial or complete obstruction of vascular and/or respiratory structures, or asymmetry in the external pressure applied. This variability may have significant effects on clinical presentation, as well as time to unconsciousness and time to death.

ISOLATED AIRWAY OBSTRUCTION

When a child's face is obstructed by bedding or other object, there is an abrupt cessation of oxygen delivery to the blood. The vascular structures of the neck remain patent, so blood flow continues, but there is a gradual decline in the level of oxygen delivered to the brain. Other nutrients continue to be delivered to the neurons, and carbon dioxide is cleared, albeit increasingly less effectively. As hypoxia ensues, anaerobic metabolism causes a marked increase in lactic acid production. The decline in neuronal metabolic activity is slower in this form of asphyxia than that involving total obstruction of all vascular structures.

The mechanism of sudden death or deterioration related to aspiration/ ingestion of foreign bodies varies.[20,21] Typically, asphyxia arises from direct obstruction of the airway (occlusion may occur anywhere from the oropharynx to the major bronchi), but it may also be related to occlusion by submucosal bleeding, inflammation with mucus production, or by external compression of the trachea by a foreign body impacted in the adjacent oesophagus. Theoretically, there may be a role for vagal reflex bradycardia and apnoea related to oesophageal obstruction as a cause of death, but it is difficult to be certain if this actually occurs, and if so, and how often it plays a clinically significant role.

CHEST COMPRESSION

In this type of mechanical asphyxia, an external force crushes or compresses the thorax and prevents adequate respiration. Expansion of the chest wall may be totally prevented, or partially compromised, effecting the time necessary for loss of consciousness and death. Depending on the degree of force, there may or may not be accompanying venous obstruction. In the classic 'traumatic asphyxia', the force is tremendous (typically occurring when a child is run over by a car, trampled by a crowd, or trapped beneath a very heavy object), and often sudden and violent.[22,23] In these cases, the crushing force produces a sudden and dramatic increase in intrathoracic pressure, which is transmitted to the right heart and superior vena cava, and in retrograde fashion, to the veins of the upper body. This results in rupture of venules and capillaries, as well as dilatation and atony of the small vessels with consequent dramatic craniocervical congestion and cyanosis, as well as massive skin and subconjunctival petechiae – the so-called 'masque ecchymotique'.[24] For those who survive, facial changes may persist for hours to many days. There may also be transient changes in mental status, including confusion and lethargy, and visual changes (with or without retinal haemorrhages and exudates).[25,26] It is thought that to incur these pathophysiological and clinical changes, the victim must close the glottis and tense the thoraco-abdominal muscles in a valsalva manoeuvre at the time of the event, perhaps related to a 'fear response'. The closed glottis prevents inspired air from escaping the lungs and decreasing the thoracic pressure.[24] If the compression is brief, there may be no associated hypoxia, despite the dramatic facial and upper body changes.

When a child's chest is compressed during an episode of physical abuse, there is typically no evidence of the masque ecchymotique, likely due to the considerably lower pressures involved (adult squeezing a child's chest or pressing down on the back), and possibly to a lack of glottic closure and significant valsalva. The episode may be sustained, however, leading to significant, if not lethal, hypoxia and anoxia from compromised respiratory efforts.[19]

CLINICAL AND AUTOPSY FINDINGS

The clinical presentation in non-fatal cases, and the autopsy findings in fatal ones, will differ according to the type of mechanical asphyxia.

NECK COMPRESSION

Isolated venous obstruction may lead to showers of petechiae over the skin of the face and postauricular region, the conjunctivae, oral mucosa, the temporalis muscles, and undersurface of the scalp (Figs 5 and 6). The mechanism for these petechiae involves increased vascular pressure, with rupture of small venules.[27] There may be intense facial congestion as well, especially in fatal cases. If pressure applied to the neck is asymmetric, there

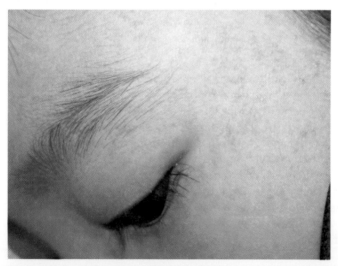

Fig. 5 Facial petechiae and subconjunctival haemorrhage in a young child who was the victim of attempted strangulation.

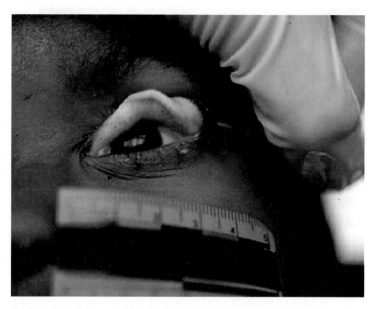

Fig. 6 Scattered subconjunctival petechiae in victim of fatal strangulation.

may be more petechiae and/or facial congestion on one side of the head than the other. Evidence suggests that the appearance of petechiae in cases of hanging is related to the degree of body support present at the time of the hanging event: victims who are partially supported (feet or buttocks on the ground) are more likely to develop petechiae than are those who are completely suspended. This is probably a function of the level of force applied to the neck, with partial body support making isolated venous obstruction more likely (with consequent vascular engorgement and small vessel rupture).[28] The presence or absence of petechiae is not a reliable indicator of the life-threatening status of the event. Harm and Rajs[29] studied homicide victims and survivors of manual strangulation; they found that while petechiae were significantly more common in fatal cases, almost 50% of the survivors with petechiae never lost consciousness. It must be emphasised that the presence of petechiae is a non-specific finding that may be seen in natural deaths, as well as asphyxial episodes, and in benign processes associated with an intense valsalva manoeuvre (intense coughing, for example).

Combined (and complete) arterial and venous obstruction (with or without airway occlusion) leads to 'pale' asphyxia, as there is no marked increase in venous pressure. Clinically, there is no prominent facial congestion or oedema, and no showers of petechiae. The same would be expected in cases of reflex bradycardia and asystole, provided this occurred very early during the course of the neck compression.

In cases of neck compression, there may be external and/or internal injuries to the neck structures.[2,28–31] Abrasions from fingernails (child's or perpetrator's), bruises with or without overlying abrasions from fingerpads (typically the perpetrator's), and abrasions/contusions from a ligature may be seen (Fig. 7). The thumb typically generates more force than other fingers, so

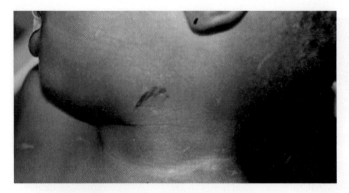

Fig. 7 Abrasions on neck of strangulation victim.

there may be one or two thumb marks in isolation. Clusters of 1–2-cm bruises on one side of the neck, and a single bruise on the other side may correspond to the fingers and thumb of the adult, but caution should be exercised in drawing this type of conclusion, as some fingers may not leave marks (especially over the firm surface of the posterior neck), while other fingers may shift position during the asphyxial episode, yielding more than one bruise. Similarly, the size of the fingerpad bruises and distance between clustered bruises are poor indicators of the size of the adult's hand. Fingernail abrasions on the neck may represent static pressure from nails, in which case the marks may be linear or curvilinear (in either direction), this being influenced by the distortion of the child's skin under pressure, the shape of the nail, orientation of the adult's hands and other factors.[29] Fingernail marks may also reflect movement of the fingers down the skin, in which case the abrasions are typically long, linear or curvilinear, and often parallel.[2] In cases of hanging, there may be abrasions and furrows associated with the ligature (Fig. 8).[6,7]

Internal neck injury often consists of small areas of haemorrhage within the sternomastoid and strap muscles of the neck (Fig. 9). There may be bruising beneath the thyroid capsule. Because of the cartilaginous nature of the hyoid, cricoid and thyroid cartilage, fracture of these structures is not seen in children, but is much more common in older adults, whose structures are heavily calcified.[2,6] Unusually, there may be damage to the carotid arteries, with dissection or perivascular haemorrhage.[32,33] In some cases, there is submucosal haemorrhage of the epiglottis or even the base of the tongue (as the tongue is pushed up against the soft palate).

Internal examination at autopsy may or may not show intrathoracic petechiae, congested, oedematous lungs with focal or wide-spread atelectasis, aspiration of gastric contents (likely representing a non-specific agonal event), and cerebral oedema with uncal grooving.[7] If there is a period of survival, there may be massive cerebral oedema with global softening and necrosis indicative of 'respirator brain', or cystic infarcts with wide-spread encephalomalacia, indicative of severe global hypoxia–anoxia.[34] In a study of adult males dying of asphyxiation, Hadley and Fowler[35] found increased weights of the lungs, liver, kidneys and spleen (but not brain) relative to victims of trauma. However, the range of organ weights was similar in the two groups, significantly limiting the diagnostic value of these findings.

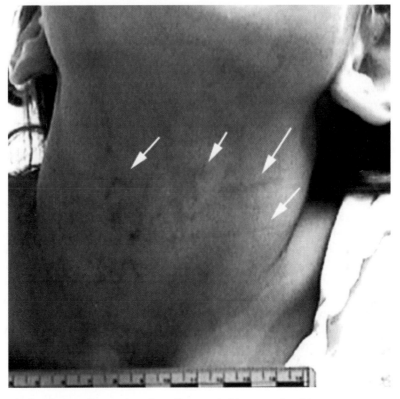

Fig. 8 Neck abrasions and contusions from ligature (white arrowheads).

In a study of lung histology from adult and paediatric cases of fatal asphyxia, Delmonte and Capelozzi[36] obtained a discriminant function of histological variables that adequately classified 85% of cases of strangulation, suffocation, aspiration and drowning. Strangulation victims typically showed lungs with increased alveolar

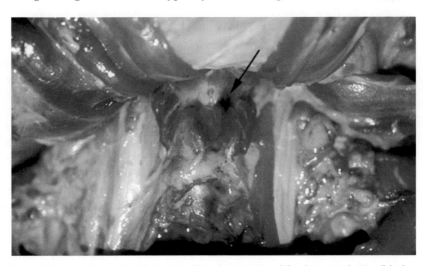

Fig. 9 Small haemorrhage in soft tissues of neck in victim of fatal strangulation (black arrow).

haemorrhage, alveolar collapse and overinsufflation (emphysema), as well as alternating zones of bronchiolar constriction and dilatation. They suggested their semiquantitative method of analysis was potentially useful as a supplementary tool in the evaluation of possible asphyxial deaths.

Survivors of strangulation or hanging incidents may be completely asymptomatic, or they may complain of sore throat, pain with palpation of the larynx, cough, stridor, muffled voice, respiratory distress or mental status changes.[37] They may develop pulmonary oedema,[6,7,38] aspiration pneumonia,[39] laryngeal oedema (sometimes delayed), and signs/symptoms of global hypoxic–ischaemic encephalopathy.[18,40] Cerebral oedema may vary and, in some cases, be quite severe, with typical 'watershed' infarcts and laminar necrosis noted on CT/MRI scans.[18,34] Cerebrovascular haemo-dynamics may demonstrate cortical hyperaemia, as well as dissociative vasoparalysis with failed autoregulation but persistent CO_2 reactivity.[39] Neurological outcome varies in hanging and strangulation cases, ranging from full recovery to severe encephalopathy, persistent vegetative state, and death.[34,39–41] Further, initial presentation and history may not predict outcome. In the study of Hanigan et al.,[39] two adolescent boys were both found hanging about 10 min after last being seen, both required cardiopulmonary resuscitation by the caregiver and had initial Glasgow Coma Scores of 4 and 5. Their initial CT scans were normal. One fully recovered while the other sustained severe and persistent neurological deficits.

ISOLATED AIRWAY OBSTRUCTION

Accidental or intentional smothering often leaves no trace at autopsy, making it difficult to differentiate these causes of death from SIDS. DiMaio[42] found that of 18 fatal suffocation victims up to 2 years of age, only one had petechial haemorrhages, and this child had only a single conjunctival petechiae and a single scleral haemorrhage. In the study by Meadow[15] of covert homicides, 57% of the infants had no bruises, petechiae or oronasal blood at the time of autopsy. In their evaluation of 18 paediatric deaths due to plastic bag suffocation, Perez-Martinez et al.[43] found no external trauma in 15 cases. The remaining 3 cases showed conjunctival petechiae, petechiae of the lip and peri-orbital region , and 'congestion of the eyes'. Four cases showed intrathoracic petechiae. The majority (11/18) showed only non-specific findings of pulmonary congestion and oedema.

There is evidence that asphyxia is more likely than SIDS to be associated with frank oronasal bleeding (as opposed to the serosanguinous fluid so often seen emanating from nose and mouth in SIDS). Krous et al.[44] found only 3% of SIDS victims had frank oronasal blood in the absence of, or before, cardiopulmonary resuscitation. In contrast, oronasal blood was seen in 14% of known accidental suffocation cases. Occasionally, one may see subtle facial or oronasal injuries, such as subconjunctival haemorrhages, or contusions and abrasions to the lips, cheek, gums or nose (Fig. 10). Frenulum lacerations may also occur (Fig. 11). With slightly older victims of homicidal smothering (1.5–7 years), Banaschak et al.[45] found more prominent and numerous cutaneous injuries than are typically seen in young infants. Superficial injuries were seen even in cases in which smothering occurred with a pillow. In some cases, there was

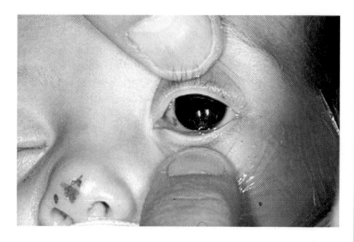

Fig. 10 Nose abrasions and subconjunctival haemorrhage in victim of smothering.

evidence of both smothering and neck compression. The authors made the point that not all facial petechiae are necessarily related to neck compression, but could also be related to venous congestion associated with a severe valsalva manoeuvre made during attempts to cry or scream against an obstructed airway. Clustered petechiae may also represent sites of blunt trauma.

There has been a great deal of interest in the possibility that differences in the amount of intra-alveolar haemorrhage and hemosiderin may help distinguish asphyxial deaths from SIDS.[46–50] While there is some evidence to suggest that asphyxia may be associated with pulmonary haemorrhage, and

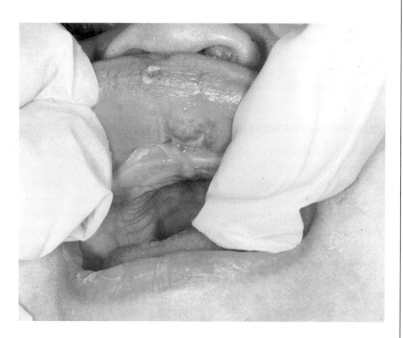

Fig. 11 Healing frenulum laceration and associated contusion in victim of attempted smothering.

repeated asphyxial events associated with increased hemosiderin-laden macrophages within the lungs, not all studies support this theory.[51] Much additional research must be done to further clarify any relationship, and exclude the contribution of potentially confounding factors (young age, for example).[52] It does seem clear, however, that increased pulmonary haemorrhage (or signs of previous haemorrhage) is neither necessary nor sufficient to diagnose asphyxia. In addition, the differential diagnosis for pulmonary haemorrhage is quite large (small amounts of pulmonary haemorrhage are often seen in SIDS), further limiting the utility of this variable in making a diagnosis of asphyxia.

Additional efforts to differentiate types of asphyxia from other causes of death have also focused on pulmonary pathology. Delmonte and Capelozzi[36] showed that relative to cases of drowning, strangulation and aspiration, the lungs in cases of suffocation deaths were characterised by ductal overinsufflation, interstitial oedema and bronchiolar constriction. In a study of 146 children less than 2 years of age, Betz et al.[53] showed that asphyxia/strangulation cases were characterised by the simultaneous presence of conjunctival petechiae and acute pulmonary emphysema (noted in 71% of cases). These changes were not identified concurrently in any of the patients dying of SIDS or other natural causes or trauma.

CHEST COMPRESSION

Chest compression may or may not be forceful enough to lead to severely increased intrathoracic pressure, with resultant intense upper body congestion, plethora and petechiae.[22] In some cases, the child's chest may be compressed only to the point that it cannot be expanded during respiration, thereby incurring significant respiratory compromise. In such cases, there may be little or no internal or external evidence of the asphyxial episode. Kohr[19] reported a case of a 2-year-old who was restrained by an adult who placed her legs (one was casted) on the prone child's back for ~30–40 min. The child died of asphyxia but the only external finding at autopsy was an abrasion on the back. Internally, there were rare intrathoracic petechiae.[19]

OVERLYING AND WEDGING

The exact mechanism of asphyxia in overlying and wedging may vary. When an infant is overlain, he may suffer facial obstruction, with or without chest compression, with or without neck compression. Thus, the clinical presentation may vary according to the mechanism, but in many cases there is little or no external evidence of the event. Occasionally, one may see anterior lividity with sparing over regions subjected to the weight of the adult's body, or even pressure marks from that person's clothing. In a study of overlying deaths, Collins[3] reported superficial injuries in 6 of 11 infants (facial abrasions, a single contusion, a few ocular petechiae; facial petechiae) and one infant with pressure marks over the face. Since wedging may involve face and/or thoracic compression, the mechanism and findings may also vary; however, as in overlying deaths, there are usually few positive findings at autopsy. Of 8 wedging cases, Collins[3] found a chin abrasion in one, and a single contusion (face, cheek) in two children. Two had external petechiae and three children had linear impressions on the body reminiscent of the wedging object. Notably, overlying and wedging victims may or may not have intrathoracic petechiae, a finding very common to SIDS victims.[7]

COMMON QUESTIONS IN INVESTIGATIONS OF ASPHYXIAL CASES

HOW LONG DOES IT TAKE FOR A CHILD TO LOSE CONSCIOUSNESS DURING AN ASPHYXIAL EPISODE?

The time to loss of consciousness is influenced by many factors, including the type of asphyxia experienced (venous compression, venous/arterial compression, airway obstruction, *etc.*), the degree of vascular or airway obstruction (partial versus complete occlusion), the consistency of the obstruction (continuous versus intermittent), and the age and health of the child. Thus, in the absence of an eyewitness, it is not possible to give a definitive answer in any particular case. Southall *et al.*[17] reported two cases of imposed airway obstruction of infants captured on videotape. Both infants struggled violently during the episode, but at least 70 s passed before electroencephalographic changes indicated probable loss of consciousness.

The data of Southall *et al.*[17] reflect the time to unconsciousness for a child who is asphyxiated by isolated upper airway obstruction. As the vascular supply to and from the brain remains intact in this situation (there being no neck compression), the time to loss of consciousness will likely be somewhat delayed, as the brain continues to receive blood (albeit poorly oxygenated) for a period after the obstruction begins. In contrast, if a child sustains severe neck compression in which the carotid artery supply is occluded, the brain will become hypoxic more quickly, and loss of consciousness will likely occur more rapidly. In a study of sudden, complete, cerebral blood flow obstruction in young adult human males (including vertebral artery flow), Rossen *et al.*[54] showed an average time to loss of consciousness of 6.8 s. (This study, and some others performed during this period, employed methods that would be considered inappropriate by today's standards.)

HOW LONG DOES IT TAKE FOR A CHILD TO DIE FROM ASPHYXIA?

For obvious reasons, this cannot be experimentally determined. Some of the most illuminating information we have comes from animal experiments, some of which were performed more than 25 years ago.[55–57]

Ikeda *et al.*[56] studied 'typical' hanging in dogs, analysing vital signs after occlusion of the jugular veins, carotid and vertebral arteries, and trachea. This most closely approximates a severe episode of neck compression in a child (although one would not expect vertebral artery compromise in this situation). The authors identified four distinct stages of response: (i) a dyspnoea stage beginning just after occlusion and lasting 1–1.5 min; (ii) an initial apnoea stage following the dyspnoea and lasting 0.5–1 min; (iii) a stage of terminal respiration during which breathing was sporadic and abrupt; followed by (iv) a secondary apnoea and circulatory collapse. The heart rate initially increased after occlusion, and remained fairly regular until circulatory collapse; blood pressure rose abruptly at the onset, but then gradually declined after the dyspnoea stage. The entire time course of respiration and circulation ranged from 4–6 min.

In their discussion of the pathophysiology in 'typical hanging', Ikeda et al.[56] compared these results with those of Suzuki et al.,[63] who studied isolated airway occlusion in dogs. In the latter experiments, the same sequence of four stages occurred, but the dyspnoea stage lasted about twice as long, and the initial apnoea was also prolonged. The terminal respiration stage was shorter, so that the total time course was similar to the dogs that experienced both vascular and airway occlusion (4–6 min).

DOES A LACK OF SIGNS OR SYMPTOMS IMPLY THE ASPHYXIAL EVENT WAS MINOR?

When a child is brought to the emergency department with a history of attempted strangulation, there is often no external evidence of trauma and the child may appear asymptomatic. There may be several reasons for this. The asphyxial episode may have been brief and/or mild, causing no residual signs or symptoms. In an effort to protect the perpetrator, the child may not disclose existing symptoms. Signs may be present but misinterpreted (for example, a hoarse voice interpreted as a consequence of screaming during an argument).[58] As noted above, asphyxial events (even fatal ones) may leave no external signs of trauma. Superficial injuries may be overlooked or misinterpreted. Signs and symptoms may be delayed, only developing after the child has left the emergency department. Many of these problems are reported in adult victims of intimate partner violence.[58] In short, there are many reasons for a lack of obvious traumatic injury in cases of asphyxia, and lack of trauma should not be interpreted as necessarily meaning the episode was insignificant. Certainly, fatal asphyxial events are not insignificant, and even brief, non-fatal episodes of smothering or neck compression may be extremely frightening to the child. They may also be painful (as the child struggles to get free), and uncomfortable (if the child experiences air hunger, for example).[59–61]

PREVENTION

Arguably, the best way to prevent accidental asphyxia in infants and children is to educate caretakers on appropriate cribs and sleep conditions, on the need to keep cords well away from toddlers, and on the need for close supervision of young, curious children. The Consumer Product Safety Commission is active in its efforts to improve the quality and design of cribs, and to prohibit the sale of pacifiers with attached cords.[6] Continued research and advocacy by paediatricians is needed to help shed light on the safety hazards surrounding accidental asphyxia in children, and to prompt legislative change that will mandate safer conditions.

Prevention of intentional asphyxia is difficult, not only because it is hard to predict which children will be at risk, but also because it is often impossible to detect attempted smothering or neck/chest compression, making it challenging to intervene before a subsequent lethal episode. Knowledge of risk factors associated with smothering infanticide,[15] an awareness of possible signs and symptoms of asphyxia, and general screening for child abuse risk factors may prevent some cases. Additionally, medical practitioners should keep asphyxia in the differential diagnosis whenever evaluating a child with unexplained loss of consciousness, seizure, cyanosis, etc., especially if the child has subtle facial or oronasal trauma.

Key points for clinical practice

- Asphyxia in children may be accidental of inflicted. Suffocation accounts for the majority of unintentional injury deaths in infants less than 1 year of age.

- The risk of accidental asphyxia is greatly increased when infants sleep in defective or poorly maintained cribs, or sleep in adult beds.

- Asphyxia accounts for ~25% of infanticide cases. While autopsy is frequently negative, certain historical factors or subtle physical findings may alert the medical practitioner to possible abuse.

- Asphyxia from neck compression may involve isolated venous obstruction, combined venous and arterial occlusion, both vascular and airway obstruction or reflex vagal response. Multiple conditions may occur during the course of an asphyxial event.

- When associated with massive forces, chest compression may cause 'mask ecchymotique', but in many cases the force is considerably less and physical findings are minimal.

- Prolonged chest compression with a moderate weight can cause delayed death from incomplete but significant respiratory compromise.

- Facial and mucosal petechiae are relatively common in cases of neck and/or chest compression, but are not necessary or specific for asphyxia.

- Older victims of smothering may have multiple superficial facial/oral injuries, even when smothered by a soft pillow. This may be related to their ability to struggle harder than infants.

- Research is inconclusive about the possible relationship between asphyxia and significant pulmonary haemorrhage, and increased pulmonary hemosiderin. However, pulmonary haemorrhage is neither necessary nor sufficient to diagnose asphyxia.

- Time to loss of consciousness depends on multiple factors. Evidence suggests unconsciousness occurs more quickly with vascular obstruction (as in hanging or strangulation), than with isolated airway obstruction (as in smothering). Very limited data on infants suggest the time to unconsciousness may be greater than 60 s during a smothering episode.

- Animal studies of asphyxia show four stages of physiological response, including a dyspnoea stage, initial period of apnoea, a terminal respiration stage, followed by circulatory collapse. The time to death averaged 4–6 min.

- For many reasons, inflicted or accidental asphyxia may cause no signs or symptoms, but this does not mean the event was a trivial one. Fatal cases of asphyxia often leave no external injuries. Children may experience tremendous fright, anxiety and discomfort during an asphyxial episode, even a brief one.

(continued on next page)

> ## Key points for clinical practice *(continued)*
>
> - Education of caretakers regarding safe sleep practices and a safe home environment may be the best prevention of unintentional asphyxia. Screening for risk factors of abuse, and keeping the possibility of intentional asphyxia in mind may allow prevention or early detection of inflicted asphyxia.

References

1. Spitz WU. Asphyxia. In: Spitz WU. (ed) *Medicolegal Investigation of Death: Guidelines for the Application of Pathology to Crime Investigation*, 3rd edn. Springfield: Charles Thomas, 1993; 444.
2. Saukko P, Knight B. Suffocation and 'asphyxia'. In: Knight B. (ed) *Knight's Forensic Pathology*, 3rd edn. London: Arnold, 2004; 352–394.
3. Collins KA. Death by overlaying and wedging: a 15-year retrospective study. *Am J Forensic Med Pathol* 2001; **22**: 155–159.
4. Office of Statistics and Programming. *WISQARS database: National Center for Injury Prevention and Control*. Atlanta, GA: Centers for Disease Control, 2002.
5. Scheers NJ, Rutherford GW, Kemp JS. Where should infants sleep? A comparison of risk for suffocation of infants sleeping in cribs, adult beds, and other sleeping locations. *Pediatrics* 2003; **112**: 883–889.
6. Feldman KW, Simms RJ. Strangulation in childhood: epidemiology and clinical course. *Pediatrics* 1980; **65**: 1079–1085.
7. Moore L, Byard RW. Pathological findings in hanging and wedging deaths in infants and young children. *Am J Forensic Med Pathol* 1993; **14**: 296–302.
8. Flobecker P, Ottosson J, Johansson L, Hietala MA, Gezelius C, Eriksson A. Accidental deaths from asphyxia. A 10-year retrospective study from Sweden. *Am J Forensic Med Pathol* 1993; **14**: 74–79.
9. Nixon JW, Kemp AM, Levene S, Sibert JR. Suffocation, choking, and strangulation in childhood in England and Wales: epidemiology and prevention. *Arch Dis Child* 1995; **72**: 6–10.
10. Byard RW, Hucker SJ, Hazelwood RR. A comparison of typical death scene features in cases of fatal male and autoerotic asphyxia with a review of the literature. *Forensic Sci Int* 1990; **48**: 113–121.
11. Vanamo T, Kauppi A, Karkola K, Merikanto J, Rasanen E. Intra-familial child homicide in Finland 1970–1994: incidence, causes of death and demographic characteristics. *Forensic Sci Int* 2001; **117**: 199–204.
12. Overpeck MD, Brenner RA, Trumble AC, Trifiletti LB, Berendes HW. Risk factors for infant homicide in the United States. *N Engl J Med* 1998; **339**: 1211–1216.
13. de Silva S, Oates RK. Child homicide – the extreme of child abuse. *Med J Aust* 1993; **158**: 300–301.
14. Brewster AL, Nelson JP, Hymel KP *et al.* Victim, perpetrator, family, and incident characteristics of 32 infant maltreatment deaths in the United States Air Force. *Child Abuse Negl* 1998; **22**: 91–101.
15. Meadow R. Unnatural sudden infant death. *Arch Dis Child* 1999; **80**: 7–14.
16. Meadow R. Suffocation, recurrent apnea, and sudden infant death. *J Pediatr* 1990; **117**: 351–357.
17. Southall DP, Stebbens VA, Rees SV, Lang MH, Warner JO, Shinebourne EA. Apnoeic episodes induced by smothering: two cases identified by covert video surveillance. *BMJ Clin Res Edn* 1987; **294**: 1637–1641.
18. McIntosh BJ, Shanks DE, Whitworth JM. Child abuse by suffocation presenting as hypoxic–ischemic encephalopathy. Report of a patient. *Clin Pediatr (Phila)* 1994; **33**: 561–563.
19. Kohr RM. Inflicted compressional asphyxia of a child. *J Forensic Sci* 2003; **48**: 1148–1150.

20. Byard RW. Mechanisms of unexpected death in infants and young children following foreign body ingestion. *J Forensic Sci* 1996; **41**: 438–441.
21. Byard RW. Accidental childhood death and the role of the pathologist. *Pediatr Dev Pathol* 2000; **3**: 405–418.
22. Byard RW, Hanson KA, James RA. Fatal unintentional traumatic asphyxia in childhood. *J Paediatr Child Health* 2003; **39**: 31–32.
23. Campbell-Hewson G, Egleston CV, Cope AR. Traumatic asphyxia in children. *J Accid Emerg Med* 1997; **14**: 47–49.
24. Nunn CR, Bass JG, Nastanski F, Morris Jr JA. Traumatic asphyxia syndrome. *Tenn Med* 1997; **90**: 144–146.
25. Gorenstein L, Blair GK, Shandling B. The prognosis of traumatic asphyxia in childhood. *J Pediatr Surg* 1986; **21**: 753–756.
26. Ravin JG, Meyer RF. Fluorescein angiographic findings in a case of traumatic asphyxia. *Am J Ophthalmol* 1973; **75**: 643–647.
27. Ely SF, Hirsch CS. Asphyxial deaths and petechiae: a review. *J Forensic Sci* 2000; **45**: 1274–1277.
28. Luke JL, Reay DT, Eisele JW, Bonnell HJ. Correlation of circumstances with pathological findings in asphyxial deaths by hanging: a prospective study of 61 cases from Seattle, WA. *J Forensic Sci* 1985; **30**: 1140–1147.
29. Harm T, Rajs J. Types of injuries and interrelated conditions of victims and assailants in attempted and homicidal strangulation. *Forensic Sci Int* 1981; **18**: 101–123.
30. Camps FE, Hunt AC. Pressure on the neck. *J Forensic Med* 1959; **6**: 116–135.
31. Taff ML, Boglioli LR. Strangulation. A conceptual approach for courtroom presentation. *Am J Forensic Med Pathol* 1989; **10**: 216–220.
32. Clarot F, Vaz E, Papin F, Proust B. Fatal and non-fatal bilateral delayed carotid artery dissection after manual strangulation. *Forensic Sci Int* 2005; **149**: 143–150.
33. Malek AM, Higashida RT, Halbach VV *et al.* Patient presentation, angiographic features, and treatment of strangulation-induced bilateral dissection of the cervical internal carotid artery. Report of three cases. *J Neurosurg* 2000; **92**: 481–487.
34. Simpson RK, Goodman JC, Rouah E *et al.* Late neuropathological consequences of strangulation. *Resuscitation* 1987; **15**: 171–185.
35. Hadley JA, Fowler DR. Organ weight effects of drowning and asphyxiation on the lungs, liver, brain, heart, kidneys, and spleen. *Forensic Sci Int* 2003; **137**: 239–246.
36. Delmonte C, Capelozzi VL. Morphologic determinants of asphyxia in lungs: a semiquantitative study in forensic autopsies. *Am J Forensic Med Pathol* 2001; **22**: 139–149.
37. Ernoehazy WJ, Ernoehazy WS. Hanging injuries and strangulation: E-medicine; 2001.
38. Rubin DM, McMillan CO, Helfaer MA, Christian CW. Pulmonary edema associated with child abuse: case reports and review of the literature. *Pediatrics* 2001; **108**: 769–775.
39. Hanigan WC, Aldag J, Sabo RA, Rose J, Aaland M. Strangulation injuries in children. Part 2. Cerebrovascular hemodynamics. *J Trauma* 1996; **40**: 73–77.
40. Sabo RA, Hanigan WC, Flessner K, Rose J, Aaland M. Strangulation injuries in children. Part 1. Clinical analysis. *J Trauma* 1996; **40**: 68–72.
41. Pradeep KG, Kanthaswamy V. Survival in hanging. *Am J Forensic Med Pathol* 1993; **14**: 80–81.
42. DiMaio VJ. Homicidal asphyxia. *Am J Forensic Med Pathol* 2000; **21**: 1–4.
43. Perez Martinez AL, Chui P, Cameron JM. Plastic bag suffocation. *Med Sci Law* 1993; **33**: 71–75.
44. Krous HF, Nadeau JM, Byard RW, Blackbourne BD. Oronasal blood in sudden infant death. *Am J Forensic Med Pathol* 2001; **22**: 346–351.
45. Banaschak S, Schmidt P, Madea B. Smothering of children older than 1 year of age-diagnostic significance of morphological findings. *Forensic Sci Int* 2003; **134**: 163–168.
46. Becroft DM, Lockett BK. Intra-alveolar pulmonary siderophages in sudden infant death: a marker for previous imposed suffocation. *Pathology (Phila)* 1997; **29**: 60–63.
47. Berry PJ. Intra-alveolar haemorrhage in sudden infant death syndrome: a cause for concern? *J Clin Pathol* 1999; **52**: 553–554.
48. Hanzlick R, Delaney K. Pulmonary hemosiderin in deceased infants: baseline data for further study of infant mortality. *Am J Forensic Med Pathol* 2000; **21**: 319–322.
49. Schluckebier DA, Cool CD, Henry TE, Martin A, Wahe JW. Pulmonary siderophages and unexpected infant death. *Am J Forensic Med Pathol* 2002; **23**: 360–363.

50. Yukawa N, Carter N, Rutty G, Green MA. Intra-alveolar haemorrhage in sudden infant death syndrome: a cause for concern? *J Clin Pathol* 1999; **52**: 581–587.
51. Jackson CM, Gilliland MG. Frequency of pulmonary hemosiderosis in Eastern North Carolina. *Am J Forensic Med Pathol* 2000; **21**: 36–38.
52. Forbes A, Acland P. What is the significance of haemosiderin in the lungs of deceased infants? *Med Sci Law* 2004; **44**: 348–352.
53. Betz P, Hausmann R, Eisenmenger W. A contribution to a possible differentiation between SIDS and asphyxiation. *Forensic Sci Int* 1998; **91**: 147–152.
54. Rossen R, Kabat H, Anderson JP. Acute arrest of cerebral circulation in man. *Arch Neurol Psychiatry* 1943; **50**: 510–528.
55. Godfrey S. Respiratory and cardiovascular changes during asphyxia and resuscitation of foetal and newborn rabbits. *Q J Exp Physiol Cogn Med Sci* 1968; **53**: 97–118.
56. Ikeda N, Harada A, Suzuki T. The course of respiration and circulation in death due to typical hanging. *Int J Legal Med* 1992; **104**: 313–315.
57. Swann HG, Brucer M. The cardiorespiratory and biochemical events during rapid anoxic death; obstructive asphyxia. *Tex Rep Biol Med*. 1949; **7**: 593–603.
58. McClane GE, Strack GB, Hawley D. A review of 300 attempted strangulation cases Part II: clinical evaluation of the surviving victim. *J Emerg Med* 2001; **21**: 311–315.
59. Guz A. Brain, breathing and breathlessness. *Respir Physiol* 1997; **109**: 197–204.
60. McQuillen EN, McQuillen JB. Pain and suffering. and unconsciousness. *Am J Forensic Med Pathol* 1994; **15**: 174–179.
61. Moosavi SH, Golestanian E, Binks AP, Lansing RW, Brown R, Banzett RB. Hypoxic and hypercapnic drives to breathe generate equivalent levels of air hunger in humans. *J Appl Physiol* 2003; **94**: 141–154.
62. Snell RS. *Clinical Anatomy for Medical Students*, 2nd edn. Boston: Little, Brown & Company; 1981.
63. Suzuki T, Ikeda N, Umetsu K, Sashimura S. The course of respiration in death caused by obstructive asphyxia [German]. *Z Rechtsmed* 1986; **96**: 105–109.

Prakesh S. Shah Max Perlman

8

Birth asphyxia and multi-organ dysfunction

Dysfunction of various organs other than brain is observed following birth asphyxia. Multi-organ dysfunction is one of the criteria for the clinical diagnosis of neonatal asphyxia.[1-5] The detection of 'multi-organ dysfunction' or multisystem dysfunction (for simplicity, we use the term multi-organ dysfunction to cover both) is also important for management of infants in the postnatal period. The pathophysiological basis for multi-organ dysfunction, namely the 'diving reflex', is interesting due to the quantitative and qualitative variations in the activation of this reflex among fetuses when exposed to asphyxia of similar severity.

In this chapter, we: (i) summarise current knowledge of the pathophysiology of multi-organ dysfunction; (ii) delineate the post-asphyxial dysfunctions and rare permanent injuries of each organ as observed pathologically and clinically; (iii) explore the relationships between multi-organ dysfunction and long-term outcome; and (iv) provide suggestions for optimal timing of assessment of organ functions for infants with asphyxia.

PATHOPHYSIOLOGY

To understand the pathophysiological mechanisms of multi-organ dysfunction, the effects of asphyxia on the blood flow of organs have been studied. These effects in

Prakesh S. Shah MBBS MD DCH(London) MRCP(UK) MRCPCH(UK) FRCPC MSc (for correspondence)
Assistant Professor and Consultant Neonatologist, Department of Paediatrics, and Department of
Health Policy, Management and Evaluation, University of Toronto, Room 775A, Mount Sinai
Hospital, 600 University Avenue, Toronto, Ontario M5G 1X5, Canada
E-mail: pshah@mtsinai.on.ca

Max Perlman MB FRCP FRCPC
Professor Emeritus, Department of Paediatrics, University of Toronto and Honorary Consultant
Neonatologist, Division of Neonatology, The Hospital for Sick Children, 555 University Avenue,
Toronto, Ontario M5G 1X8, Canada
E-mail: max.perlman@sympatico.ca

Table 1 Effect on blood flow to various organs following different mechanisms of hypoxia–ischaemia in animals[6]

Mechanism of asphyxia	Maternal hypoxaemia	Graded reduction of umbilical BF	Repeated reduction of uterine BF	Graded reduction of uterine BF	Arrest of uterine BF	Reduction in fetal blood volume by 15%
Brain	I	I	I	I	D*	I
Heart	I	I	I	I	I	D*
Adrenal	I	I	I	I	I	I
Liver	O	D	D	I*	D	I*
Renal	D	I*	D	D	D	D
Carcass	D	I*	D	D	D	D
Lungs	D	D	I*	D	D	D
Gut	D	I*	D	D	D	D

BF, blood flow; I, increased; D, decreased; O, no change; *refers to the atypical responses.

different animals and using various mechanistic models of asphyxia are summarised in Table 1.

The 'diving reflex' is pivotal to understanding these effects. In response to significant stress, blood from the skin and splanchnic area (kidneys, liver and intestine) is diverted to the heart, adrenals and brain, so-called 'centralisation' of cardiac output.[6–8]

However, in various models of asphyxia, responses have not been observed to follow this pattern consistently (Table 1). Although generally adhering to the above 'centralisation' pattern, organ blood flows have atypical responses in some models. Blood flow to the brain unexpectedly decreased in the 'arrest of uterine blood flow' model. In the 'reduction in fetal blood volume' model, in distinction to the typical 'diving reflex', cardiac blood flow was reduced and hepatic blood flow was increased. An unexpected increase in blood flow to 'non-essential' organs occurred in the 'graded reduction of umbilical blood flow' model.

Similar local protective responses have been observed within the central nervous system. Regional cerebral blood flow increases or decreases according to the metabolic rate, energy requirements and oxygen consumption within particular areas. Regions having high oxygen consumption such as brainstem have greater fractional extraction of oxygen, use more alternative fuels and have a marked increase in blood flow prior to the development of dysfunctional changes. Viability is preferentially preserved in these areas, vital for life.[6] However, with a progressive asphyxial insult or during an agonal heart rate pattern, cardiovascular collapse ensues.[9] Blood pressure, combined ventricular output and blood flow to all organs decrease significantly. This collapse is considered to precipitate brain injury.[10] Thus, the impact of asphyxial injury on non-essential organs is likely to occur in the early stages of the asphyxial insult, and if the insult is prolonged, again in the terminal stages.

CLINICOPATHOLOGICAL CORRELATES OF POST-ASPHYXIAL MULTI-ORGAN DYSFUNCTION IN HUMANS

The time-honoured pathophysiological definition of asphyxia is hypoxia, hypercapnia and a mixed respiratory and metabolic acidosis.[1] The metabolic acidosis occurs due to anaerobic metabolism. The clinical criteria for birth or neonatal asphyxia in the past included multi-organ dysfunction as a prerequisite,[1,2,4,5] but more recently multi-organ dysfunction has been categorised as a 'suggestive' and 'non-specific' criterion for an 'acute intrapartum hypoxic event sufficient to cause cerebral palsy'.[3]

There is marked variability in several aspects of ascertainment of multi-organ dysfunction in published studies. These variations include: (i) what constitutes multi-organ dysfunction (how many organs – usually investigators have included at least one organ other than brain); (ii) which organs to be included in multi-organ dysfunction (central nervous, cardiovascular and respiratory systems and kidneys are most consistent); (iii) what criteria define a particular organ dysfunction; (iv) what is the precise timing for assessment of particular organ dysfunction; (v) what investigations are necessary to identify the presence of multi-organ dysfunction; and (vi) which patients are at risk of multi-organ dysfunction and need to be investigated?

Based on pathophysiological findings in experimental fetal and neonatal animals, it is assumed that human neonates with clinically detectable cardiac dysfunction and hypoxic ischaemic encephalopathy resulting from birth asphyxia, and even more, those who will prove to have permanent brain injury, activated the 'diving reflex' for protection. From clinical and pathological perspectives, asphyxial insults cause a spectrum of effects on various organs (including brain) from no effect, through transient dysfunction ('insult'), to permanent impact ('injury'). 'Activation' (stimulation of organ such as marrow) of certain organ/system may also occur in response to birth asphyxia. Data on human neonates, the approximate definitions used, the populations studied and the incidences of dysfunctions of various organs are summarised in Tables 2 and 3.

Pathological findings and clinical aspects of various organ dysfunctions following birth asphyxia are summarised below.

RENAL

In infants who die of asphyxia, acute tubular necrosis is the most common autopsy finding.[20] Renal hypoperfusion results in variable duration of oliguria or anuria, usually followed by polyuria. Oliguria leads to fluid retention accompanied by postnatal weight gain during first few days after birth (instead of the normal postnatal weight loss) and hyponatraemia. Haematuria and proteinuria are usually present. Elevated serum creatinine, blood urea nitrogen, and urinary of β_2-microglobulin levels[11–19] and, at times, myoglobinuria[21] have been observed following renal involvement. A variety of criteria for defining asphyxial renal dysfunction exist in the literature. Differences in the definitions together with the variation in severity of illness of the populations studied explain the wide variation in the reported incidence of post-asphyxial renal dysfunction (15–95%). Renal dysfunction is usually suspected when oliguria lasts for 24 h or more. Blood urea and serum creatinine concentrations during the first 24 h after birth reflect maternal values rather than neonatal renal function; thus, to determine dysfunction, measurements should be delayed for 24 h. A rise in creatinine concentration is a more likely indicator of renal dysfunction.[22] During the period of oliguria,

Table 2 Definitions of organ dysfunctions used in studies of multi-organ dysfunction in birth asphyxia*

Study	Hankins et al.[11]	Korst et al.[12]	Low et al.[13]	Martin-Ancel et al.[14]	Perlman et al.[15]	Shah et al.[16]	Shankaran et al.[17]	Tack et al.[18]
CNS	HIE	Permanent neurological injury on follow-up	Encephalopathy	HIE	Encephalopathy or USG evidence of haemorrhage or echodensity	Moderate-to severe HIE	Seizures, abnormal USG, CT scan or EEG	Seizures or abnormal imaging
Renal	Creatinine >108 or oliguria or persistent haematuria or proteinuria	Creatinine >110 or oliguria or serum Na <130 for > 3 days	Haematuria, creatinine >100, oliguria	Oliguria for >24 h; urea >7; creatinine > 110 for >48 h	Oliguria or β_2-microglobulin in the first void or urea >7 or creatinine >90	Oliguria >24 h and creatinine >100 or oliguria >36 h or creatinine >125	Acute tubular necrosis or renal failure	Oliguria, urea >7, creatinine >110
Cardiac	Need for pressors >2 h after birth, elevated CK-MB	Use of pressors >3 days, persistent fetal circulation, abnormal ECG, cardiac failure	Heart rate, blood pressure and ECG changes	Murmur or ECG suggestive of transient ischaemia or signs of cardiac failure	ECG or echocardiogram findings >2 SD deviant from normal	Need for pressor > 24 h or ECG evidence of transient ischaemia	Hypotension cardiomegaly, cardiac dysfunction or sinus bradycardia	Abnormal ECG or echocardiogram
Hepatic	AST, ALT or LDH >1.5 times upper normal limit	AST or AST >100 during first week	NR	NR	NR	AST or ALT >100 during the first week	NR	NR
Pulmonary	NR	Ventilatory support for >24 h	Need for oxygen, need for transient or prolonged ventilation	Need for FiO₂ >0.4 for >4 h; need for mechanical ventilation	Need for intubation >48 h or persistent pulmonary hypertension	Need for assisted ventilation with FiO₂ >0.4 for the first 4 h	Meconium aspiration, air leaks, persistent fetal circulation	Persistent pulmonary hypertension
Gut	NR	Necrotising enterocolitis	NR	Bleeding, necrotising enterocolitis	Necrotising enterocolitis	NR	NR	Necrotising enterocolitis
Hemato-logical	Platelet <150, or NRBC >26	DIC or platelet <150	NR	NR	NR	NR	Thrombo-cytopaenia, DIC	NR

HIE, hypoxic ischaemic encephalopathy; NR, not reported; ECG, electrocardiogram; DIC, disseminated intravascular coagulation; NRBC, nucleated red blood cell. Units of measurement: creatinine mmol/l, urea mmol/l, Na meq/l, AST IU/L, ALT IU/L, platelets x10⁹/l and NRBC per 100 white blood cells.
*Sexson et al.[19] did not report individual organ criteria.

Table 3 Incidence of multi-organ dysfunction reported in various studies

Study	Hankins et al.[11]	Korst et al.[12]	Low et al.[13]	Martin-Ancel et al.[14]	Perlman et al.[15]	Sexson et al.[19]	Shah et al.[16]	Shankaran et al.[17]	Tack et al.[18]
Population studied	Intrapartum asphyxia	Children with post-asphyxial CNS injury	Metabolic acidosis	Asphyxia	Asphyxia	Apgar < 5 at 5 min	Moderate-to-severe post-asphyxial HIE	Perinatal asphyxia	Perinatal asphyxia
Total number of patients	46	47	59	72	35	59	130	28	60
Number of patients with HIE	32	47	36	52	13	N/R	130	19	25
Renal	72%	17%	24%	42%	57%	15%	70%	54%	95%
Cardiac	78%	26%	61%	29%	28%	34%	62%	50%	44%
Hepatic	80%	23%	NR	NR	NR	20%	85%	NR	NR
Pulmonary	NR	55%	47%	26%	29%	39%	86%	86%	5%
Gut	NR	0%	NR	29%	0%	20%	NR	NR	2%
Hematological	54%	23%	NR	NR	NR	NR	NR	36%	NR
Metabolic*	NR	NR	NR	NR	NR	NR	NR	46%	56%
No multi-organ dysfunction	NR	36%	22%	18%	57%	47%	0%	25%	NR

*S Na < 130 or S Ca < 7 mg/l or glucose < 2.3.
HIE, hypoxic ischaemic encephalopathy; NR, not reported.

careful monitoring of fluid and electrolytes is indicated. Post-asphyxial acute renal failure is mostly transient.[23] Rarely, survivors develop chronic renal failure requiring renal replacement therapy and even renal transplantation.

CARDIOVASCULAR SYSTEM

Necrosis of papillary muscles, subendocardial necrosis or haemorrhage, and congestion and petechiae were noted at autopsy in infants who died of asphyxia.[20] Papillary muscles are supplied by end-arteries, and thus are vulnerable to ischaemia and hypoxia.[24] Myocardial hypoperfusion, acidosis and responses from sympathetic nervous system and peripheral vascular receptors lead to hypotension and poor perfusion to other organs. In addition to systemic hypotension requiring inotropic support, the clinical effects of transient myocardial ischaemia include electrocardiographic changes, cardiac murmur due to valvular incompetence, and ventricular or congestive heart failure.[24,25] Again, investigators have used various definitions to ascertain cardiac dysfunction depending upon access to diagnostic modalities. Myocardial ischaemia is evaluated by electrocardiography, echocardiography and elevated levels of cardiac enzymes (creatinine kinase-MB fraction or troponin T).[26–28] The incidence of cardiovascular involvement is reported between 26–78%.[11–19] The timing of evolution of cardiac changes is within hours or minutes of birth as evident by clinical picture of haemodynamic instability. Both electrocardiographic and echocardiographic changes are most evident during the first 24 h, but T-wave changes and the rise of creatine kinase-MB can be delayed beyond 24 h.[29] Ascertainment of the degree and the type of cardiovascular system involvement have important roles in the management of infant. Severe refractory hypotension can be lethal in neonatal period. Apart from rare cases of long-term myocardial damage, cardiovascular injury is usually reversible.

HEPATIC

Hepatic pathology varies from congestion through fatty changes to massive ischaemic necrosis.[20] Hepatic changes are thought to be less marked than changes in other organs, perhaps because of the multiple sources of blood supply to liver (umbilical, portal venous and hepatic arterial). While the fetal umbilical–portal venous circulation still continues, blood is diverted away from the liver, especially the right lobe, via the ductus venosus, which causes hepatic cellular hypoxia/ischaemia. The increased permeability of the liver cell membranes to cytoplasmic enzymes causes a rise in serum levels of the transaminases and lactate dehydrogenase.[30] Apart from rare instances of cholestasis, no overt clinical manifestations are ascribed to asphyxial liver insults.[31] Significantly deranged liver function can lead to reduced synthesis of coagulation factors. This may aggravate the co-existing consumptive coagulopathy due to disseminated intravascular coagulation that at times accompanies asphyxia. Liver dysfunction as indicated by elevated aminotransferase levels is reported for 20–85% of cases.[11,12,16,19] Knowledge of the timing of onset and the time-course of serum enzyme concentration is limited.[28] The mean aspartate aminotransferase (AST) and alanine aminotransferase (ALT) levels increased significantly during the first 72 h after birth in asphyxiated newborns, remained elevated between day 5 and day 10, and returned to normal levels between day 20 and day 30. Our impressions are that AST levels peak at about 18–24 h post-insult followed by a fairly rapid fall to normal values, whereas ALT levels peak at about 30–36 h post-insult, followed by a slower fall to normal values. No long-term hepatic complications have been reported in the literature.

LUNGS

Hypoxaemic or hypovolaemic lung insults can result in delayed pulmonary adaptation to extra-uterine life; for example, delayed clearance of lung fluid, secondary inactivation of surfactant, delayed fall in pulmonary vascular resistance leading to persistence of pulmonary hypertension, and haemorrhagic pulmonary oedema. Impaired control of breathing results in apnoea and hypoventilation. Prolonged intubation and ventilation may be needed for depressed brainstem responses, and for the pulmonary complications of asphyxia including the meconium aspiration syndrome. Certain pathological mechanisms of meconium aspiration syndrome, however, are distinct from the effects of birth asphyxia. In cases of severe respiratory failure, aggressive ventilation and occasionally nitric oxide inhalation may be needed. Definitions of respiratory involvement vary greatly, as do reported incidence rates (between 5–86%).[12–19] Post-asphyxial pulmonary hypertension can cause a protracted course of respiratory failure, and rarely death. Long-term adverse effects on the lungs have not been reported.

GASTROINTESTINAL SYSTEM

Paralytic ileus is common after birth asphyxia, presenting with increased residual gastric volumes or feeding intolerance.[32] Akinbi et al.[33] reported reversal or absence of anterograde superior mesenteric artery blood flow in severely asphyxiated neonates. Necrotising enterocolitis and gastric or intestinal perforation are uncommon complications. Enteral feeding of infants with birth asphyxia should be delayed until clinical signs of ileus have resolved to allow time for restoration of gastrointestinal blood flow and recovery of the structural integrity of the gastrointestinal tract. The frequency of gastrointestinal involvement has been reported between 0–29%.[12,14,15,18,19] Provided that damage to the gut wall is not extensive, recovery is usually complete and there are no long-term sequelae.

HAEMATOLOGICAL

Haematological changes following birth asphyxia have been studied mainly from the perspective of identifying the time of the asphyxial insult. Most haematological changes represent 'activation' by an asphyxial insult rather than dysfunction of haematopoietic tissue. Lymphocytosis and elevated nucleated red blood cell counts are described within about an hour of the asphyxial episode, with return to normal values over the next several hours in most patients.[34,35] Platelet counts tend to be normal at birth and fall during the first day or two after the insult, taking 5–7 days to recover. The changes in nucleated red blood cells and platelets are attributed to the marked stimulation of erythroid cells by erythropoietin and a resultant decreased number of immature megakaryocytes leading to diminished thrombocytopoiesis. These marrow responses are transient. The clinical significance of these findings is minimal, except for severe thrombocytopaenia as a manifestation of disseminated intravascular coagulation, requiring platelet transfusion.

METABOLIC

Hypoglycaemia, hypocalcaemia, hyponatraemia, the syndrome of inappropriate antidiuretic hormone secretion,[17,18] and hyperammonaemia[36] are reported metabolic complications of asphyxia. These complications are probably more prevalent than reported. Not all studies have considered these as part of multi-organ dysfunction as each of these complications can result from multiple factors operating in various organs. Additionally, definitions of these complications vary. Importantly, these complications have obvious implications for diagnosis and therapy.

Finally, it is important to recognise that most of the data reported in the various studies (Tables 1 and 2) were collected without standardised timing of assessment of multi-organ dysfunction. The incidence of organ dysfunctions was reported in a recently completed multicentre trial of selective brain cooling for post-asphyxial hypoxic ischaemic encephalopathy patients. The timing of data collection was prespecified. Renal dysfunction was present in 70%, hypotension in 52%, elevated liver enzymes in 53%, thrombocytopaenia in 22%, coagulopathy in 14%, hyponatraemia in 39%, hypoglycaemia in 17% and hypocalcaemia in 43% of the patients who met the inclusion criteria for the trial and were randomised to the control group[37] (we elected to present data only from control group as some of the complications in the treatment groups could be attributed to hypothermia). These frequencies are within the ranges of those previously reported. Thus, variable involvement of organs following asphyxia supports the notion that the diving reflex is inconsistently activated in the asphyxiated human fetus, as in experimental animals.[6]

MULTI-ORGAN DYSFUNCTION AND LONG-TERM OUTCOMES

LONG-TERM OUTCOMES

A few studies of associations between multi-organ dysfunction and long-term outcomes have been published. Perlman et al.[38] evaluated the relationship between renal injury and short- and long-term neurological outcomes in a cohort that included preterm as well as term infants. All six patients with persistent oliguria for > 36 h developed hypoxic ischaemic encephalopathy and all had abnormal brain imaging. Of the six, one patient died, two had spastic quadriplegia, two had spastic diplegia and one was normal. Of 8 patients with transient oliguria for < 24 h, two patients developed hypoxic ischaemic encephalopathy and one developed a left hemiplegia. Of the 22 patients with normal urine output, two developed hypoxic ischaemic encephalopathy and four had abnormal brain imaging; only one patient had developmental delay at follow-up examination. The authors concluded that the duration of neonatal oliguria was a sensitive predictor of long-term neurological outcomes.

Moller *et al.*[27] reported elevated levels of creatinine, creatine kinase and troponin T in asphyxiated infants compared to controls. Troponin T levels were significantly higher in asphyxiated infants with heart failure; however, none of these parameters helped to differentiate infants with neurological sequelae from infants without such sequelae.

Saili *et al.*[39] reported a 60% mortality rate among asphyxiated neonates with liver dysfunction compared to 9% mortality among those with normal liver function, as measured by transaminases and alkaline phosphatase.

We observed no differences in the incidence of different organ dysfunctions in neonates with moderate-to-severe post-asphyxial hypoxic ischaemic encephalopathy who had severe adverse outcome (neurodevelopmental deficit or death) and those free of adverse outcome.[16] The kidneys, cardiovascular system, lungs and liver were involved in 60%, 58%, 86% and 88%, respectively, among patients free of severe adverse outcomes, and 70%, 62%, 86% and 85%, respectively, among patients with adverse outcomes. Analysis of the relationship between the number of organs involved (other than brain) and long-term outcomes showed no significant differences between patients with adverse outcome and those free of adverse outcomes. Every one of our patients (*n* = 130) who had all four organs assessed had at least one organ dysfunction in addition to brain dysfunction. This highlights the importance of assessment of all organs to ascertain whether multi-organ dysfunction is present or not.

On the other hand, Phelan *et al.*[40] reviewed children who developed brain injury due to asphyxial insult during intrapartum period and found that multi-organ dysfunction was absent in 14 of 47 patients, questioning the inclusion of multi-organ dysfunction as an essential criterion for the definition of 'neonatal asphyxia'; however, the eligibility criterion was survival for 6 days and the development of cerebral palsy, and the criteria for renal and cardiovascular dysfunction were rather strict.

LONG-TERM INDIVIDUAL ORGAN OUTCOMES

Most of the effects of asphyxia on organs other than the brain are transient and survivors appear to have no sequelae. However, occasional cases of chronic renal failure, acute myocardial infarction, mitral or tricuspid valve incompetence, acute hepatic insufficiency, and necrotising enterocolitis have been observed. Myocardial infarction and massive hepatic necrosis are usually lethal in the neonatal period. Barberi *et al.*[26] reported severe EKG changes, depressed left ventricular function and creatine kinase-MB levels of > 154 IU/l as prognostic markers for poor short-term survival due to extensive myocardial damage. Primhak *et al.*,[28] however, reported that creatine kinase-MB levels lacked specificity for myocardial injury. Other severe organ specific disabilities in survivors can lead to significant permanent disability.

TIMING OF ASSESSMENT OF VARIOUS ORGAN/SYSTEM DYSFUNCTION

As pointed out above, the optimal timing of laboratory and other investigations of organ dysfunction has not been established. No clearly defined algorithms are available for a clinician to follow. We attempt here to suggest the best estimates for timing of each organ function assessment following birth of an asphyxiated infant, based on the available literature and experience.

RENAL

Fluid and electrolyte balance should be monitored for the first 72 h and longer if needed. Urine testing for blood and protein is suggested from birth. Serum creatinine and electrolyte concentrations are suggested at about 24 h of age. These may be repeated every 12–24 h until levels approach normal values.

CARDIOVASCULAR

Blood pressure, perfusion and heart rate should be monitored until values are normal and stable without treatment. The optimal timing for the electrocardiogram is 24 h of age[29] and for creatine kinase-MB measurement 27 h.[28] Echocardiographic evaluation is indicated in patients with persistent hypotension, an unexplained persistent murmur and in patients with electrocardiographic evidence of myocardial ischaemia.

LIVER

Estimation of ALT and AST should be performed at 24 h of age and repeated again at 12-h intervals until levels approach normal. Normal levels at 24 h and 36 h of age require no further action. Further testing of liver synthetic function (serum albumin and coagulation factors) is indicated in patients with significantly elevated AST and ALT and/or bleeding tendency.

LUNGS

Evidence of pulmonary dysfunction is derived from the standard patient ventilation records, blood gas measurements and chest radiographs. The most likely timing of dysfunction is in the hours after birth. No additional investigations are necessary to assess pulmonary dysfunction.

HAEMATOLOGICAL MEASUREMENTS

Performance of a full blood count as early as possible including a manual differential count is indicated to screen for the presence of anaemia, thrombocytopaenia, lymphocytosis and an elevated nucleated red blood cell count. Blood counts are repeated as clinically indicated (*e.g.* more frequently in cases of haemorrhagic shock and if thrombocytopaenia is detected) until normalisation. Assessment of coagulation function is needed for patients with bleeding tendency.

METABOLIC

Blood sugar should be estimated at the earliest possible time until the untreated infant is euglycaemic and stable. Serum calcium measurement is suggested at 24 h and repeated as necessary.

THE FUTURE

In most publications, infants with 'asphyxia' have been the subject of study, defined by various criteria. Investigators have also analysed the relationship between multi-organ dysfunction and metabolic acidosis,[13] multi-organ dysfunction and depression at birth with or without neonatal hypoxic ischaemic encephalopathy,[11,14,15,17,18] multi-organ dysfunction and moderate-to-severe post-intrapartum asphyxial hypoxic ischaemic encephalopathy,[16] and multi-organ dysfunction and cerebral palsy attributed to intrapartum asphyxia.[12,40] Each analysis has contributed to the understanding of the mechanisms of the diving reflex and asphyxial brain injury. The clinically most important patients in which to study multi-organ dysfunction are those who can be defined to have had 'intrapartum asphyxia'. A significant proportion of infants develop post-asphyxial hypoxic ischaemic encephalopathy. It is important to know organ dysfunction in infants who do not develop hypoxic ischaemic encephalopathy because these infants may have invoked a strong protective reflex at the cost of peripheral organ dysfunction to spare the brain. On the other hand, it is equally important to know multi-organ dysfunction in patients with hypoxic ischaemic encephalopathy for postnatal management. The information regarding multi-organ dysfunction may also contribute to understanding of the severity of insult and prognosis.

To further our understanding of the role of the diving reflex and the factors that affect the reflex in the protection of the fetal brain from hypoxic ischaemic injury, more prospective studies are needed. Future research should start with the development, in an international context, of the various criteria that can be used conventionally to define multi-organ dysfunction at appropriate post-insult times. Accurate obstetric data should be collected simultaneously to determine the aetiology and mechanisms of the asphyxia. Studies should include infants with asphyxial insults and these infants should be followed up to determine their long-term neurodevelopmental outcome. This will help to understand relationship between multi-organ dysfunction and neurological outcome.

CONCLUSIONS

Post-asphyxial multi-organ dysfunction is considered to reflect an efficient 'diving reflex' mechanism, preserving cerebral circulation at the expense of blood flow to other, non-essential organs. However, activation of the diving reflex varies, both in experimental animals and probably in humans. The criteria for defining individual organ dysfunction, the optimal timing for testing, and the organs and specific dysfunctions to include in the definition of multi-organ dysfunction have not been standardised. This has resulted in wide variation in the reported incidence of each organ involved and of multi-organ dysfunction. Based on the information available, with reservations arising from the observed variability of definitions and criteria, no clear relationship has been established between the degree and severity of multi-organ dysfunction and long-term outcome. Most organ dysfunction is reversible in survivors and does not reflect permanent injury; however, rare cases of long-term organ morbidity are observed. Further research to standardise the assessment of multi-organ dysfunction and to understand its role in long-term outcome is needed.

Key points for clinical practice

- Multi-organ dysfunction is considered an important, but not absolute, prerequisite for the diagnosis of severe potentially brain-damaging birth asphyxia.

- Animal experiments reveal that in most models of fetal asphyxia, blood flow is diverted from non-essential to essential organs (brain, heart and adrenals), a protective mechanism known as 'diving reflex'.

- Different mechanisms of asphyxia have been shown to produce variable changes in the blood flow to organs in animals and probably this is applicable to humans.

- The spectrum of effects of birth asphyxia on organs (together with brain) includes no effects, activation of organ/system (bone marrow), transient impairment, or permanent injury; the later being rare for all organs other than brain.

- Renal involvement results in anuria or oliguria of variable duration, weight gain, hyponatraemia, haematuria, or elevated serum creatinine concentration. Urine output needs to be monitored from birth until it normalises. Creatinine needs to be checked at age 24 h and 48 h and subsequently if required until normalisation.

- Cardiovascular involvement is manifested as systemic hypotension requiring inotropic support, electrocardiographic findings of transient myocardial ischaemia, ventricular or congestive failure, or cardiac murmur due to valvular incompetence. Blood pressure needs monitoring from birth until normalisation. An electro-cardiogram needs to be performed at 24 h of age. Echocardiogram (when required) and serum creatine kinase-MB estimation (after 24 h) are suggested if indicated clinically.

- Hepatic involvement results in elevated levels of transaminases. Aminotransferase alanine aminotransferase levels need to be measured at 24 h, 36 h and 48 h, and if required they should be repeated until normalisation.

- Pulmonary involvement results in need for assisted respiratory support and oxygen for delayed adaptation (ranging from mild respiratory distress to evolution of persistent pulmonary hypertension of newborn). Monitoring of respiratory status is needed from birth until normalisation without artificial support.

- Haematological involvement (activation) results in elevated nucleated red blood cell count, lymphocytosis and thrombocyto-paenia. A complete blood count is suggested at birth and needs to be repeated as necessary. Coagulation function assessment is indicated if there is bleeding tendency or marked liver dysfunction.

- Metabolic involvement results in hypoglycaemia, hypocalcaemia, or hyponatraemia. Estimation of glucose is suggested at the earliest possible time after stabilisation and repeated until it is normal without additional nutritional support. Serum calcium and electrolytes need to be measured at 24 h and repeated as required.

Key points for clinical practice (*continued*)

- Correlations between individual organ dysfunction, its severity, or the number of dysfunctional organs and long-term outcome are not established.
- The suggested timings of assessment of multi-organ dysfunction are for guideline purposes and may need to be modified according to clinical status of the infant and future research.

References

1. Anon. Policy statement: Task force on cerebral palsy and neonatal asphyxia (part 1). *J Soc Obstet Gynecol Can* 1996; **18**: 1267–1279.
2. ACOG Committee Opinion. Inappropriate uses of the terms fetal distress and birth asphyxia. *Int J Gynecol Obstet* 1998; **61**: 309–310.
3. American College of Obstetricians and Gynecologists' Task Force on Neonatal Encephalopathy and Cerebral Palsy. *Neonatal encephalopathy and cerebral palsy: defining the pathogenesis and pathophysiology.* Washington, DC: The American College of Obstetricians and Gynecologists, 2003; 1–85.
4. Australian and New Zealand Perinatal Societies. The origin of cerebral palsy: a consensus statement. *Med J Aust* 1995; **162**: 85–90.
5. MacLennan A. A template for defining a causal relation between acute intrapartum events and cerebral palsy: international consensus statement. *BMJ* 1999; **319**: 1054–1059.
6. Jensen A, Garnier Y, Berger R. Dynamics of fetal circulatory responses to hypoxia and asphyxia. *Eur J Obstet Gynecol Reprod Biol* 1999; **84**: 155–172.
7. Bocking AD, Gagnon R, White SE, Homan J, Milne KM, Richardson BS. Circulatory responses to prolonged hypoxemia in fetal sheep. *Am J Obstet Gynecol* 1988; **159**: 1418–1424.
8. Peeters LL, Sheldon RE, Jones MD, Makowski EL, Meschia G. Blood flow to fetal organs as a function of arterial oxygen content. *Am J Obstet Gynecol* 1979; **135**: 637–646.
9. Yaffe H, Parer JT, Block BS, Llanos AJ. Cardiorespiratory responses to graded reductions of uterine blood flow in the sheep fetus. *J Dev Physiol* 1987; **9**: 325–336.
10. Block BS, Schlafer DH, Wentworth RA, Kreitzer LA, Nathanielsz PW. Intrauterine asphyxia and the breakdown of physiologic circulatory compensation in fetal sheep. *Am J Obstet Gynecol* 1990; **162**: 1325–1331.
11. Hankins GD, Koen S, Gei AF, Lopez SM, Van Hook JW, Anderson GD. Neonatal organ system injury in acute birth asphyxia sufficient to result in neonatal encephalopathy. *Obstet Gynecol* 2002; **99**: 688–691.
12. Korst LM, Phelan JP, Wang YM, Martin GI, Ahn MO. Acute fetal asphyxia and permanent brain injury: a retrospective analysis of current indicators. *J Matern Fetal Med* 1999; **8**: 101–106.
13. Low JA, Panagiotopoulos C, Derrick EJ. Newborn complications after intrapartum asphyxia with metabolic acidosis in the term fetus. *Am J Obstet Gynecol* 1994; **170**: 1081–1087.
14. Martin-Ancel A, Garcia-Alix A, Gaya F, Cabanas F, Burgueros M, Quero J. Multiple organ involvement in perinatal asphyxia. *J Pediatr* 1995; **127**: 786–793.
15. Perlman JM, Tack ED, Martin T, Shackelford G, Amon E. Acute systemic organ injury in term infants after asphyxia. *Am J Dis Child* 1989; **143**: 617–620.
16. Shah P, Riphagen S, Beyene J, Perlman M. Multiorgan dysfunction in infants with post-asphyxial hypoxic-ischaemic encephalopathy. *Arch Dis Child Fetal Neonatal Ed* 2004; **89**: F152–F155.
17. Shankaran S, Woldt E, Koepke T, Bedard MP, Nandyal R. Acute neonatal morbidity and longterm central nervous system sequelae of perinatal asphyxia in term infants. *Early Hum Dev* 1991; **25**: 135–148.
18. Tack E, Perlman JM, Hausel C, Griften M. Systemic manifestations of perinatal asphyxia in the newborn. *Pediatr Res* 1986; **20**: 362A.

19. Sexson WR, Sexson SB, Rawson JE, Brann AW. The multisystem involvement of the asphyxiated newborn. *Pediatr Res* 1976; **10**: 432.
20. Barnett CP, Perlman M, Ekert PG. Clinicopathological correlations in postasphyxial organ damage: a donor organ perspective. *Pediatrics* 1997; **99**: 797–799.
21. Kojima T, Kobayashi T, Matsuzaki S, Iwase S, Kobayashi Y. Effects of perinatal asphyxia and myoglobinuria on development of acute, neonatal renal failure. *Arch Dis Child* 1985; **60**: 908–912.
22. Roberts DS, Haycock GB, Dalton RN *et al*. Prediction of acute renal failure after birth asphyxia. *Arch Dis Child* 1990; **65**: 1021–1028.
23. Stapleton FB, Jones DP, Green RS. Acute renal failure in neonates: incidence, etiology and outcome. *Pediatr Nephrol* 1987; **1**: 314–320.
24. Donnelly WH. Ischemic myocardial necrosis and papillary muscle dysfunction in infants and children. *Am J Cardiovasc Pathol* 1987; **1**: 173–188.
25. Bucciarelli RL, Nelson RM, Egan EA, Eitzman DV, Gessner IH. Transient tricuspid insufficiency of the newborn: a form of myocardial dysfunction in stressed newborns. *Pediatrics* 1977; **59**: 330–337.
26. Barberi I, Calabro MP, Cordaro S *et al*. Myocardial ischaemia in neonates with perinatal asphyxia. Electrocardiographic, echocardiographic and enzymatic correlations. *Eur J Pediatr* 1999; **158**: 742–747.
27. Moller JC, Thielsen B, Schaible TF *et al*. Value of myocardial hypoxia markers (creatine kinase and its MB-fraction, troponin-T, QT-intervals) and serum creatinine for the retrospective diagnosis of perinatal asphyxia. *Biol Neonate* 1998; **73**: 367–374.
28. Primhak RA, Jedeikin R, Ellis G *et al*. Myocardial ischaemia in asphyxia neonatorum. Electrocardiographic, enzymatic and histological correlations. *Acta Paediatr Scand* 1985; **74**: 595–600.
29. Jedeikin R, Primhak A, Shennan AT, Swyer PR, Rowe RD. Serial electrocardiographic changes in healthy and stressed neonates. *Arch Dis Child* 1983; **58**: 605–611.
30. Zanardo V, Bondio M, Perini G, Temporin GF. Serum glutamicoxaloacetic transaminase and glutamicpyruvic transaminase activity in premature and fullterm asphyxiated newborns. *Biol Neonate* 1985; **47**: 61–69.
31. Herzog D, Chessex P, Martin S, Alvarez F. Transient cholestasis in newborn infants with perinatal asphyxia. *Can J Gastroenterol* 2003; **17**: 179–182.
32. Berseth CL, McCoy HH. Birth asphyxia alters neonatal intestinal motility in term neonates. *Pediatrics* 1992; **90**: 669–673.
33. Akinbi H, Abbasi S, Hilpert PL, Bhutani VK. Gastrointestinal and renal blood flow velocity profile in neonates with birth asphyxia. *J Pediatr* 1994; **125**: 625–627.
34. Hermansen MC. Nucleated red blood cells in the fetus and newborn. *Arch Dis Child Fetal Neonatal Ed* 2001; **84**: F211–F215.
35. Naeye RL, Shaffer ML. Postnatal laboratory timers of antenatal hypoxemic-ischemic brain damage. *J Perinatol* 2005; **25**: 664–668.
36. Giacoia GP, Padilla-Lugo A. Severe transient neonatal hyperammonemia. *Am J Perinatol* 1986; **3**: 249–254.
37. Gluckman PD, Wyatt JS, Azzopardi D *et al*. Selective head cooling with mild systemic hypothermia after neonatal encephalopathy: multicentre randomised trial. *Lancet* 2005; **365**: 663–670.
38. Perlman JM, Tack ED. Renal injury in the asphyxiated newborn infant: relationship to neurologic outcome. *J Pediatr* 1988; **113**: 875–879.
39. Saili A, Sarna MS, Gathwala G, Kumari S, Dutta AK. Liver dysfunction in severe birth asphyxia. *Indian Pediatr* 1990; **27**: 1291–1294.
40. Phelan JP, Ahn MO, Korst L, Martin GI, Wang YM. Intrapartum fetal asphyxial brain injury with absent multiorgan system dysfunction. *J Matern Fetal Med* 1998; **7**: 19–22.

Laura E. Mitchell Richard H. Finnell
Alexander S. Whitehead

9

Aetiology and prevention of spina bifida

Spina bifida is a relatively common, serious malformation of the neural tube. There are several known causes of spina bifida, which account for a relatively small proportion of affected individuals. In the majority of cases, the aetiology of this condition is unknown. Research conducted in the 1990s and early 2000s has provided the opportunity for the primary prevention of spina bifida as well as new tools for identifying the determinants of this condition.

EMBRYOLOGY

The spinal cord and brain arise from the embryonic neural plate, which is transformed into the neural tube through a complex set of molecular and cellular events. The process of neural tube formation can be divided into two phases – primary and secondary neurulation.[1]

PRIMARY NEURULATION

The brain and most of the spinal cord are formed by primary neurulation, which involves shaping, folding and midline fusion of the neural plate. The

Laura E. Mitchell PhD (for correspondence)
Associate Professor, Texas A & M University System Health Science Center, Institute of Biosciences and Technology, Center for Environmental and Genetic Medicine, 2121 W. Holcombe Blvd, Houston, TX 77030, USA
E-mail: lmitchell@ibt.tamhsc.edu

Richard H. Finnell PhD
Regents Professor, Texas A & M University System Health Science Center, Institute of Biosciences and Technology, and Director of Center for Environmental and Genetic Medicine, 2121 W. Holcombe Blvd, Houston TX 77030, USA

Alexander S. Whitehead DPhil
Professor, Department of Pharmacology and Center for Pharmacogenetics, University of Pennsylvania School of Medicine, Philadelphia, PA 19104, USA

portion of the neural tube formed by primary neurulation extends posteriorly to the region of the first to fifth sacral vertebrae (the exact location is not known) and is subsequently covered by surface ectoderm. Primary neurulation is completed by approximately 27 days post-conception.

SECONDARY NEURULATION

Following the completion of primary neurulation, the most caudal portions of the spinal cord are formed by secondary neurulation. This process does not involve the neural plate. Rather, the condensation and epithelialisation of mesenchymal cells forms the secondary neural tube, the lumen of which is contiguous with the primary neural tube.

NEURULATION DEFECTS

Congenital defects arising from primary and secondary neurulation can be distinguished by the absence or presence, respectively, of skin covering the defect. Hence, defects of primary neurulation are thought to include meningomyelocele (commonly referred to as spina bifida), in which a portion of the spinal cord and its covering membranes are exposed to the body surface. The lethal conditions, anencephaly, in which the brain tissue is exposed to the surface, and craniorachischisis, in which the brain and a large segment of the spinal cord are exposed to the surface, are also thought to result from defects in the process of primary neurulation. Skin-covered defects involving the neural tube may result from defects of secondary neurulation (for sacral level defects), or post-neurulation events. Such conditions include encephalocele, in which intracranial contents are herniated through a skull defect, and a wide variety of skin-covered defects of the lower spine, including sacral agensis, spina bifida occulta and lipomeningocele.[2]

The aetiologies of neural tube defects that are exposed to the body surface or 'open' and those that are skin covered or 'closed' are generally believed to differ, because of the different embryological processes that underlie these conditions. However, families including individuals with open and individuals with closed defects have been reported,[3] and there is evidence that maternal folic acid status may influence the risk of encephaloceles as well as anencephaly and spina bifida.[4] Hence, it is possible that there may be some overlap in the factors that give rise to open and closed defects of the neural tube.

CLASSIFICATION

Spina bifida cases are often divided into three subgroups – syndromic, multiple and isolated. The syndromic subgroup includes individuals with spina bifida who also have an identified syndrome of known (e.g. chromosomal or single-gene) or unknown origin, or who were exposed to a known teratogenic agent. The multiple subgroup includes individuals with spina bifida who have additional, major malformations but who do not have an identified malformation syndrome. The isolated subgroup includes individuals who have spina bifida and no other major malformations. These sub-groupings are not perfect (e.g. the multiple group may include individuals with unrecognised chromosomal anomalies), but can be beneficial for both clinical and research purposes.

SYNDROMIC

The subgroup of syndromic spina bifida cases is aetiologically heterogeneous, and may include individuals with chromosomal anomalies, single gene (*i.e.* Mendelian) disorders, known teratogenic exposures (*e.g.* valproic acid) and recognisable patterns of malformations for which the underlying aetiology is unknown.

Chromosomal anomalies

The most frequent chromosomal anomaly observed in individuals with spina bifida is trisomy 18. However, several other autosomal trisomies have been reported in individuals with spina bifida, including trisomy 21 and trisomy 13. Smaller chromosomal anomalies (*e.g.* insertions and deletions), including deletion of chromosome 22q11, which is associated with the velocardiofacial syndrome, have also been reported to occur in association with spina bifida.[5]

Single gene disorders

The subgroup of syndromic spina bifida cases also includes individuals with single gene disorders (*e.g.* Waardenburg syndrome).[5] However, since single gene disorders are individually rare, it is often unclear whether the occurrence of spina bifida in individuals with such disorders represents a chance finding or whether spina bifida is truly a part of the underlying disease phenotype.

Teratogenic exposures

Spina bifida may occur as part of the constellation of defects associated with the teratogenic effects of maternal, pre-gestational diabetes or maternal use of valproic acid and/or carbamazepine.[6]

MULTIPLE

The subgroup that includes individuals with spina bifida who have other major malformations that do not form part of a recognised syndrome is perhaps the least well defined. This subgroup is likely to include individuals with unrecognised syndromes or undocumented teratogenic exposures who, if correctly classified, would be included in the syndromic subgroup. The multiples subgroup may also include individuals that share aetiological factors with the subgroup of isolated cases. However, the extent to which the multiple and isolated subgroups overlap is not known.

ISOLATED

The vast majority of live-born infants with spina bifida do not have an underlying syndrome, or even additional, non-secondary malformations. This subgroup has been the focus of extensive epidemiological and genetic investigations (reviewed below).

Clinically, the distinction between the syndromic, multiple and isolated forms of spina bifida is important for establishing prognosis, determining recurrence risks and evaluating options for prenatal diagnosis in subsequent pregnancies. These distinctions are also important for studies aimed at determining aetiology, since they help to define relatively homogeneous subgroups of patients. The determination as to which subgroup a patient belongs requires a thorough evaluation by a medical geneticist or dysmorphologist, as well as the collection of detailed family and pregnancy histories. Additional testing (*e.g.* cytogenetic analysis, genetic mutation analysis) may also be indicated. Moreover, since features of some syndromes may not be immediately diagnosed (*e.g.* learning disabilities and velopharyngeal dysfunction in the 22q11.2 deletion syndrome), patients should periodically be re-evaluated for the presence of an underlying syndrome.

EPIDEMIOLOGY

The epidemiology of spina bifida has been extensively studied for several decades, and much is known about the distribution of this condition as a function of 'person, place and time'. In addition, a large number of potential risk factors have been investigated, but surprisingly few have been established as, or are strongly suspected to be risk factors for this condition.

PREVALENCE

Although spina bifida is one of the most common, serious malformations, it can be difficult to make specific statements about the prevalence of this condition. This difficulty is due to the fact that the prevalence of spina bifida varies quite extensively across populations, regions and time. In many regions, estimation of the prevalence of spina bifida is also complicated by prenatal diagnosis and termination of affected fetuses. For some populations and population subgroups, accurate, contemporary estimates of the prevalence of spina bifida can be obtained from an existing birth defect registry. For example, based on data from the Texas Birth Defects Registry (Texas Department of State Health Services, Birth Defects Epidemiology and Surveillance Branch) the prevalence of spina bifida in Texas, 1999–2001, is estimated to be 3.8 per 10,000 births (3.4 per 10,000 in non-Hispanic whites, 3.4 per 10,000 in African-Americans and 4.2 per 10,000 in Hispanics) <http://soupfin.tdh.state.tx.us/defectc.htm>.

RISK FACTORS

Established and suspected risk factors for spina bifida include individual characteristics of mother and child, nutritional factors and exogenous exposures. Given that primary neurulation is completed by day 27 post-conception, these risk factors must be present prior to this time in order to influence the risk of spina bifida.

Maternal race

Maternal race and ethnicity are related to the risk of having a child with spina bifida. For example, in the US, the risk of having a child with spina bifida appears to be highest in Hispanic women, intermediate in non-Hispanic Whites and lowest in Blacks and Asians.[7]

Maternal diabetes

Maternal pre-gestational diabetes is a strong risk factor for spina bifida and other malformations. Among diabetic women, the risk of having a child with a malformation is increased by 2–10-fold, relative to non-diabetic women, and appears to be related to the level of periconceptional glycaemic control.[8] There is also evidence that women who develop gestational diabetes are at increased risk for having a child with spina bifida,[9] but this association is not as firmly established as that between pre-gestational diabetes and spina bifida.

Maternal obesity

The risk of having a child with spina bifida is also related to the level of maternal obesity. Among women with the highest body mass indices, usually defined as > 29 kg/m^2, the risk of having a child with spina bifida is increased by approximately 3-fold, relative to women with lower body mass indices.[9]

Maternal hyperthermia

There is relatively strong evidence that elevated maternal body temperature due to febrile illness or external heat sources (*e.g.* sauna, hot tub, electric blanket) is associated with a modest increase (about 2-fold) in the risk of having a child with spina bifida or anencephaly.[10]

Infant sex

Spina bifida is more frequent in female than in male infants.

Folic acid and other vitamins

An association between maternal intake of folate and folic acid and the risk of spina bifida has been firmly established. Inadequate maternal intake of folate/folic acid is associated with a 2–8-fold increase in the risk of having a child with spina bifida or anencephaly. In addition, mandatory folic acid fortification of the food supplies has been associated with declines in the population prevalence of these conditions in several countries.[11,12]. Maternal vitamin B_{12} status[13] and other aspects of the maternal diet (*e.g.* glycaemic index, consumption of fumonisins, dieting behaviours) have also been associated with the risk of spina bifida, but require additional research in order to verify the reported associations.

Medications

Maternal use of valproic acid and/or carbamazipine for the treatment of seizures or other conditions (bipolar disease, migraine, chronic pain) is associated with a 10–20-fold increase in the risk of having a child with spina bifida, relative to the general population.[14,15]

Exogenous exposures

There is considerable interest in the relationship between spina bifida risk and exposures that occur in the workplace and living environment. However, such exposures have not been firmly linked with the risk of this condition.

The risk factors outlined above are not particularly new. They have been known or suspected to influence the risk of spina bifida for years if not decades. More recently, two additional risk factors have been suggested: (i) maternal autoantibodies that bind to the folate receptor and may, therefore, block the cellular uptake of folate;[16] and (ii) *in vitro* fertilisation.[17] However, the evidence relating these two factors to spina bifida is preliminary and remains to be confirmed.

GENETICS

As for many conditions, the strongest risk factor for having a child with spina bifida is a positive family history. It is well established that spina bifida and anencephaly aggregate within families and, further, that these conditions co-segregate within the same family. Families that include individuals with spina bifida and individuals with closed neural tube defects have also been reported. However, such families are rare, relative to those that include only spina bifida or both spina bifida and anencephaly.

INHERITANCE

The risk for spina bifida and/or anencephaly in the siblings of affected individuals ranges from 3–5%, and increased risks have also been reported for mono- and dizygotic twins, and second and third degree relatives.[18–21] The observed familial aggregation pattern for spina bifida and anencephaly is inconsistent with single gene (*i.e.* Mendelian) inheritance, and the observed risks are too high to be solely attributable to familial clustering of environmental risk factors. Hence, the familial recurrence patterns for spina bifida are widely believed to provide a classic example of multifactorial threshold inheritance, in which liability to a trait is determined by multiple factors each with a relatively small effect, and disease status (affected/unaffected) is determined relative to a threshold liability value. In contemporary terminology, spina bifida is regarded to be a complex trait determined by the effects of multiple genetic and non-genetic factors that, individually, have only a small effect on risk.

Genetic risk factors

The involvement of genetic factors in the aetiology of spina bifida has long been suspected, because this condition aggregates within families. However, few studies aimed at identifying specific genes or regions of the genome associated with the risk of spina bifida were conducted until the 1990s. Prior to this time, linkage analysis was the primary tool for identifying regions of the genome that were linked to disease risk. However, linkage analyses require data from families with two or more affected individuals, and such families are rare for spina bifida. Fortunately, the Human Genome Project[22] has provided genetic information and tools that can be used to identify and evaluate potential genetic risk factors for spina bifida. Specifically, the identification of a large number of genetic variants throughout the genome provides the opportunity to undertake association studies that, unlike linkage analyses, do not require data from families with multiple affected members.

CANDIDATE GENE STUDIES

The majority of studies that have been conducted to identify genetic risk factors for spina bifida have taken a 'candidate gene' approach. A candidate gene is a gene that is suspected to be involved in the aetiology of a given condition (*e.g.* spina bifida). A gene may be a candidate because it is involved in processes that are related to the condition (*e.g.* a gene involved in cholesterol metabolism and cardiovascular disease), or it is located in a region of the genome that is associated with the condition (*e.g.* a gene located in the 22q11.2 chromosome region and congenital heart defects), or it is associated with a similar condition in an animal model system.

Many of the reported candidate gene studies for spina bifida have focused on genes that are involved in the transport and metabolism of folate. These studies have been motivated by the known, spina bifida-protective, effect of maternal periconceptional use of folate. The hypothesis underlying these studies is that functional variation within folate-related genes influences folate requirements during embryonic development (*i.e.* individuals with variants that are associated with inefficient transport or metabolism of folate have higher folate requirements and are, therefore, at increased risk of spina bifida). The 'individuals' of interest may be the mothers, the embryos or both, which significantly complicates studies of these candidate genes, because both mothers and their affected offspring must be studied.

Studies of folate-related candidate genes have identified several specific genes that may be related to the risk of spina bifida. However, for most of these genes, the association with spina bifida is weak and/or has been difficult to replicate in independent studies. The strongest evidence is for an association between spina bifida and the folate-related gene methylenetetrahydrofolate reductase (MTHFR) variant C677T (*i.e.* at nucleotide position 677 of the MTHFR gene the nucleotide may include either the base cytosine or the base thymine).[23] However, even for this variant, there are studies that have failed to find an association with spina bifida. Moreover, among studies that have found an association, there is conflicting evidence regarding the importance of the maternal and embryonic genotypes.

Other categories of candidate genes, including genes that may be related to obesity, genes involved in the metabolism of potentially teratogenic agents, and genes that are related to spina bifida in animal models have also been evaluated for an association with spina bifida. As described above, the association between spina bifida and most candidate genes has been weak and/or has been difficult to replicate in independent studies.[24] Consequently, at this time, there are no genetic variants that can be used to determine the risk of spina bifida in an individual pregnancy or embryo.

LINKAGE STUDIES

In addition to candidate gene studies, a whole genome-wide linkage screen has also been conducted for neural tube defects. In contrast to candidate gene studies, a genome-wide linkage screen does not focus on a specific gene, but rather surveys the entire genome for regions that are associated with the condition of interest. Such studies require information (*i.e.* disease status and DNA) from families that include two or more individuals who are affected with the condition of interest and are, therefore, extremely difficult to undertake for conditions such as spina bifida. Indeed, the single reported linkage screen for neural tube defects is based on data from only 44 families, identified by collaborators from 14 institutions.[25] Despite the relatively small sample size, this study identified several regions of the genome that may harbour genes related to spina bifida (and other neural tube defects). Future studies will narrow down the regions of interest and evaluate specific candidate genes within these regions.

Although studies of potential genetic risk factors for spina bifida have not yet provided compelling evidence for specific genetic risk factors, such studies are in their infancy. New information regarding the composition of the human genome and new tools for evaluating this information are emerging at a rapid pace and provide the opportunity to refine approaches for studying the genetic contribution to spina bifida. Hence, the prospects of identifying genes, or combinations of genes that influence the development of spina bifida remain high.

HEALTH IMPACT

MORBIDITY

Spina bifida, even when it occurs as an isolated condition, impacts on multiple body systems. Individuals with spina bifida typically have some degree of lower limb weakness and paralysis. The extent to which lower limb function will be compromised can generally be predicted by the anatomical level of the bony defect, as determined by radiology. However, function may be better or worse than predicted based on the anatomical level.[26] In addition, individuals with spina bifida often have additional malformations of the central nervous system. Hydrocephalus is common and related to the level of the spinal lesion, with shunting required more often in those with thoracic level defects than in those with lower lesions.[26] Chiari II malformations are also common, and are clinically significant in approximately one-third of patients.[27]

Individuals with spina bifida are also at increased risk for neurological (*e.g.* tethered cord) orthopaedic (*e.g.* scoliosis), and urological (*e.g.* ureteric reflux) complications.[28] Individuals with spina bifida generally have normal intelligence levels. However, specific cognitive and language difficulties are quite common.[29]

Because individuals with spina bifida have a range of health issues, care is often best provided by a multidisciplinary team that specialises in the evaluation and treatment of individuals with spina bifida. The patient's primary care physician should work with this team to monitor health status (*e.g.* shunt functioning, weight) and provide routine care (*e.g.* immunisations) and support.

SURVIVAL

The survival rate for infants born with spina bifida is relatively high and continues to increase due to advances in medical treatment. For example, among infants born in Atlanta, Georgia (US) between 1979 and 1994, survival to 1 year was 87% and survival to 17 years was 78%.[30] Shunt status (shunted versus unshunted with clinically insignificant hydrocephalus) does not appear to influence survival through childhood.[30,31] However, survival is markedly lower in individuals with unshunted hydrocephalus or additional birth defects.[31]

PREVENTION

Spina bifida is one of the few birth defects for which there are multiple levels of prevention. Secondary prevention, through prenatal diagnosis and elective termination of affected pregnancies was introduced in the 1970s.[32] Maternal serum α-fetoprotein evaluation and routine ultrasound are used to screen pregnancies for spina bifida, and both amniocentesis (for amniotic fluid α-fetoprotein, acetylcholinesterase and possibly chromosomal analyses) and high-level ultrasound can be used to diagnose this condition. Moreover, *in utero* treatment of spina bifida, a procedure that is currently being evaluated as part of a randomised clinical trial, may provide the opportunity to prevent or reduce some of the complications associated with spina bifida.[33]

The primary prevention of a large proportion of spina bifida cases can be achieved by ensuring that all women of reproductive potential consume adequate levels of folate or folic acid. Randomised clinical trials indicate that up to 70% of all cases of spina bifida can be prevented through the use of supplements containing folic acid prior to and through the first trimester of pregnancy.[34,35] However, public health efforts and policies to increase the use of such supplements, which have been implemented in several countries, have been largely unsuccessful in reducing the prevalence of spina bifida and other neural tube defects.[36–38] In contrast, mandatory folic acid fortification of the food supply, which has now been implemented in several countries (*e.g.* Canada, Chile, US) has consistently been associated with a subsequent decline in the prevalence of spina bifida and other neural tube defects.[11,12]

COUNSELLING

Appropriate genetic and reproductive counselling for individuals and families concerned about their risk of having a child affected with spina bifida requires a thorough evaluation of family, maternal health and pregnancy histories. When there is a family history of spina bifida or other neural tube defect (open or closed), recurrence risks and reproductive options will depend on the underlying cause of the condition in the affected relative(s). For example, recurrence risks and potential prevention strategies will differ for a woman who has had a child with spina bifida in association with trisomy 18, and a woman who took valproic acid early in gestation and subsequently gave birth to a child with spina bifida. When the affected relative(s) appears to have isolated spina bifida with no identifiable, underlying cause, empirical recurrence risks based on historical data are typically provided. However, the data upon which most of these estimates are based are quite old, and the extent to which they reflect recurrence risks in contemporary populations (*e.g.* populations in which mandatory folic acid fortification of the food supply has been implemented) is not known.

In the vast majority of cases, there are no tests that can be performed prior to conception to establish a woman's (couple's) risk of having a child with spina bifida. Evaluation of maternal folate status and/or genotyping for the MTHFR C677T variant is not recommended, since such tests have low predictive value.[39]

In general, maternal use of supplements containing folic acid prior to and during pregnancy is recommended for all women of reproductive potential.

This recommendation is likely to be made, even within populations that have implemented a mandatory folic acid food fortification program because such programmes do not ensure that individual women will consume adequate amounts of folic acid. It remains unclear whether folic acid supplementation reduces the risk of spina bifida in the offspring of women with pregestational diabetes, women taking valproic acid, or women who have had a child with spina bifida despite taking folic acid during pregnancy.

Prenatal screening and diagnosis, through a combination of maternal serum α-fetoprotein evaluation, ultrasound and amniocentesis, should continue to be considered for all pregnancies, since folic acid supplementation and fortification are unlikely to prevent all cases of spina bifida.

Key points for clinical practice

- Spina bifida is an open neural tube defect that results from a disruption in primary neurulation.

- Open neural tube defects, such as spina bifida, and closed neural tube defects result from different embryological processes and are thought to have different aetiologies. However, open and closed defects can occur in the same family.

- Spina bifida can occur as part of syndromes resulting from chromosomal abnormalities, single gene disorders or teratogenic exposures (syndromic). Spina bifida may also occur in association with other anomalies that do not form a recognised syndrome (multiple) or it may occur as an isolated defect (isolated).

- Evaluation by a clinical geneticist and/or dysmorphologist, and possibly additional testing, is required to determine to which subgroup (*i.e.* syndromic, multiple or isolated) a patient belongs. Since some syndromic features may not be immediately diagnosed, periodic re-evaluations may be necessary.

- The subgroup to which a patient belongs has important implications for prognosis, recurrence and counselling.

- Established risk factors for spina bifida include family history, race/ethnicity, sex, maternal pre-gestational diabetes, maternal use of valproic acid and/or carbamazipine, and maternal folic acid intake.

- Additional factors that may influence the risk of spina bifida include gestational diabetes, maternal obesity and maternal hyperthermia.

- The relatives of an individual with spina bifida are at increased risk (relative to the general population) of having a child with spina bifida or anencephaly.

- The Human Genome Project has provided new tools for studying the genetic contribution to spina bifida. However, at this time, there are no genetic tests that can be used to determine the risk of spina bifida in an individual pregnancy or embryo.

> ## Key points for clinical practice *(continued)*
>
> - A substantial proportion of spina bifida cases can be prevented by adequate maternal intake of folic acid prior to and through the first trimester or pregnancy.
>
> - Prenatal screening and/or diagnosis of spina bifida should be offered to all pregnant women.

References

1. Copp AJ, Green NDE, Murdoch JN. The genetic basis of mammalian neurulation. *Nat Rev Genet* 2003; **4**: 784–793.
2. Lemire RJ. Neural tube defects. *JAMA* 1988; **259**: 558–562.
3. Sebold CD, Melvin EC, Siegel D *et al.* Recurrence risks for neural tube defects in siblings of patients with lipomyelomeningocele. *Genet Med* 2005; **7**: 64–67.
4. Castilla EE, Orioli IM, Lopez-Camelo JS, da Graca Dutra M, Nazer-Herrera J. Preliminary data on changes in neural tube defect prevalence rates after folic acid fortification in South America. *Am J Med Genet* 2003; **123A**: 123–128.
5. Lynch SA. Non-multifactorial neural tube defects. *Am J Med* 2005; **135C**: 69–76.
6. Mitchell LE, Adzick NS, Melchionne J, Pasquariello PS, Sutton LN, Whitehead AS. Spina bifida. *Lancet* 2004; **364**: 1885–1895.
7. Feuchtbaum LB, Currier RJ, Riggle S, Roberson M, Lorey FW, Cunningham GC. Neural tube defect prevalence in California (1990-1994): eliciting patterns by type of defect and maternal race/ethnicity. *Genet Test* 1999; **3**: 265–272.
8. McLeod L, Ray JG. Prevention and detection of diabetic embryopathy. *Community Genet* 2002; **5**: 33–39.
9. Anderson JL, Waller DK, Canfield MA, Shaw GM, Watkins ML, Werler MM. Maternal obesity, gestational diabetes, and central nervous system birth defects. *Epidemiology* 2005; **16**: 87–92.
10. Moretti ME, Bar-Oz B, Fried S, Koren G. Maternal hyperthermia and the risk for neural tube defects in offspring. *Epidemiology* 2005; **16**: 216–219.
11. Lopez-Camelo JS, Orioli IM, da Graca Dutra M *et al.* Reduction of birth prevalence rates of neural tube defects after folic acid fortification in Chile. *Am J Med Genet* 2005; **135B**: 120–125.
12. Williams LJ, Rasmussen SA, Flores A, Kirby RS, Edmonds LD. Decline in the prevalence of spina bifida and anencephaly by race/ethnicity 1995–2002. *Pediatrics* 2005; **116**: 580–586.
13. Ray JG, Blom HJ. Vitamin B_{12} insufficiency and the risk of fetal neural tube defects. *Q J Med* 2003; **96**: 289–295.
14. Lammer EJ, Sever LE, Oakley GP. Teratogen update: valproic acid. *Teratology* 1987; **35**: 465–473.
15. Matalon S, Schechtman S, Goldzweig G, Ornoy A. The teratogenic effect of carbamazepine: a meta-analysis of 1255 exposures. *Reprod Toxicol* 2002; **16**: 9–17.
16. Rothenberg SP, da Costa MP, Sequeira JM *et al.* Autoantibodies against folate receptors in women with a pregnancy complicated by neural tube defects. *N Engl J Med* 2004; **350**: 134–142.
17. Kallen B, Finnstrom O, Nygren KG, Olausson PO. *In vitro* fertilization (IVF) in Sweden: risk for congenital malformations after different IVF methods. *Birth Defects Res A Clin Mol Teratol* 2005; **73**: 162–169.
18. Carter CO, Evans K. Spina bifida and anencephaly in greater London. *J Med Genet* 1973; **10**: 209–234.
19. Hunter AGW. Neural tube defects in eastern Ontario and western Quebec: demographic and family data. *Am J Med Genet* 1984; **19**: 45–63.
20. Janerich DT, Piper J. Shifting genetic patterns in anencephaly and spina bifida. *J Med Genet* 1978; **15**: 101–105.

21. Zackai EH, Spielman RS, Mellman WJ *et al*. The risk of neural tube defects to first cousins of affected individuals. In: Crandall BF, Brazier MAB. (eds) *The Prevention of Neural Tube Defects: the Role of Alpha-fetoprotein*. New York: Academic Press, 1978; 99–100.
22. Collins FS, Morgan M, Patrinos A. The human genome project: lessons from large-scale biology. *Science* 2003; **300**: 286–290.
23. Botto LD, Yang Q. 5,10-Methylenetetrahydrofolate reductase gene variants and congenital anomalies: a HuGE review. *Am J Epidemiol* 2000; **151**: 862–877.
24. Mitchell LE. Epidemiology of neural tube defects. *Am J Med Genet* 2005; **135C**: 88–94.
25. Rampersaud E, Bassuk AG, Enterline DS *et al*. Whole genome-wide linkage screen for neural tube defects reveals regions of interest on chromosomes 7 and 10. *J Med Genet* 2005; **42**: 940–996.
26. Rintoul NE, Sutton LN, Hubbard AM *et al*. A new look at myelomeningoceles: functional level, vertebral level, shunting and the implications for fetal intervention. *Pediatrics* 2002; **109**: 409–413.
27. Just M, Schwarz M, Ludwig B, Ermert J, Thelen M. Cerebral and spinal MR-findings in patients with post repair myelomeningocele. *Pediatr Radiol* 1990; **20**: 262–266.
28. Bowman RM, McLone DG, Grant JA, Tomita T, Jacobsen JS. Spina bifida outcome: a 25-year prospective. *Pediatr Neurosurg* 2001; **34**: 114–120.
29. Vachha B, Adams R. Language differences in young children with myelomeningocele and shunted hydrocephalus. *Pediatr Neurosurg* 2003; **39**: 184–189.
30. Wong LC, Paulozzi LJ. Survival of infants with spina bifida: a population study, 1979-1994. *Paediatr Perinat Epidemiol* 2001; **15**: 374–378.
31. Davis BE, Daley CM, Shurtleff DB *et al*. Long-term survival of individuals with myelomeningocele. *Pediatr Neurosci* 2005; **41**: 186–191.
32. Evans MI, O'Brien JE, Dvorin E, Harrison H, Bui T-H. Second-trimester biochemical screening. *Clin Perinatol* 2001; **28**: 289–301.
33. Moise KJ. Maternal-fetal surgery for spina bifida: on the brink of a new era? *Am J Obstet Gynecol* 2003; **189**: 311.
34. MRC. Prevention of neural tube defects. *Lancet* 1991; **338**: 131–137.
35. Czeizel A, Dudas I. Prevention of the first occurrence of neural tube defects by periconceptional vitamin supplementation. *N Engl J Med* 1992; **327**: 1832–1835.
36. Ray JG, Singh G, Burrows RF. Evidence for suboptimal use of periconceptional folic acid supplements globally. *Br J Obstet Gynaecol* 2004; **111**: 399–408.
37. Botto LD, Lisi A, Robert-Gnansia E *et al*. International retrospective cohort study of neural tube defects in relation to folic acid recommendations: are the recommendations working? *BMJ* 2005 [doi: 10.1136/bmj.38336.664352.52 (published 18 Feb 2005)].
38. Busby A, Abramsky L, Dolk H, Armstrong B, a Eurocat Folic Acid Working Group. Preventing neural tube defects in Europe: population based study. *BMJ* 2005; **330**: 574–575.
39. Finnell RH, Shaw GM, Lammer EJ, Volcik KA. Does prenatal screening for 5,10-methylenetetrahydrofolate reductase (MTHFR) mutations in high-risk neural tube defect pregnancies make sense? *Genet Test* 2002; **6**: 47–52.

Neil Murray Irene Roberts

10

Neonatal transfusion of blood products

In the past 15 years, there have been rapid changes in neonatal medicine. The vast majority of mothers delivering preterm neonates are now given antenatal corticosteroids and most of the ensuing very preterm neonates (< 28 weeks' gestational age) are given prophylactic surfactant.[1] As a result, there has been a very considerable reduction in the severity of initial lung disease suffered by these neonates and, in parallel, a considerably reduced necessity for critical neonatal care.[1] The overall consequence of this is a reduced requirement for ventilatory support, both in terms of degree and duration, and, therefore, a reduced requirement for frequent clinical investigations requiring repeated blood tests. This has markedly reduced phlebotomy losses for these patients and, in many cases, has all but removed the primary indication for red cell transfusion, *i.e.* replacement of blood loss 'to the laboratory'.

These changes, coupled with increased awareness of the risks of transfused blood products,[2,3] is stimulating a far more critical approach to neonatal transfusion medicine amongst neonatologists. For many, the transfusion question has changed from 'shall we correct this abnormal blood index by transfusion of a blood product because we can?' to 'is there a reasonable likelihood that transfusion of this blood product will stabilise or improve the neonate's clinical condition, without short-term, or particularly important in neonates, long-term adverse consequences?' In this context, many neonatologists are frustrated that, despite extensive research in neonatal

Neil Murray MD MRCP (for correspondence)
Senior Lecturer and Consultant in Neonatal Medicine, Department of Paediatrics, Imperial College London, 5th Floor, Ham House, Hammersmith Campus, Du Cane Road, London W12 0NN, UK
E-mail: neil.murray@imperial.ac.uk

Irene Roberts
Professor of Paediatric Haematology and Honorary Consultant Paediatric Haematologist, Department of Haematology, Commonwealth Building, Hammersmith Campus Imperial College, Du Cane Road, London W12 0NN, UK
E-mail: irene.roberts@imperial.ac.uk

transfusion medicine, most studies have assessed outcome measures (*i.e.* short-term reduction of recurrent apnoea following red cell transfusion) that are likely to be of limited importance to overall neonatal outcome. In addition, very few studies have looked at long-term consequences of multiple blood product, and donor, exposure in very preterm neonates graduating from neonatal intensive care. Taking these points into consideration, and the fact that it is often difficult to appreciate any immediate clinical benefit from blood product use in neonates,[4] transfusion practice in neonates is becoming increasingly conservative. However, it should be remembered that the evidence-base for this change is perhaps just as weak as that supporting previous liberal transfusion strategies. With these points in mind, this paper will present a critical review of contemporary transfusion medicine in neonates, paying particular attention to current research and how this informs modern neonatal practice. Areas where further research is clearly required to inform and improve practice will also be explored.

RED BLOOD CELLS

CLINICAL STUDIES

Restrictive versus liberal red blood cell transfusion
Packed red blood cells (RBCs) remain the commonest blood product administered to sick neonates. For the reasons outlined above, protocols for their use in neonates are becoming increasingly restrictive. Recent studies reflect this change in neonatal transfusion practice with a reduction in the number of units and total volume of transfused RBCs and, more importantly, a reduction in donor exposure.[5–8] Until recently, there had been few reports of restrictive RBC transfusion being associated with adverse effects in preterm neonates.[9] However, Bell *et al.*[10] have recently reported the results of a large, prospective, multicentre trial comparing short-term outcomes in preterm neonates maintained with restrictive and liberal RBC transfusion protocols. They found a positive association between restrictive RBC transfusion practice and the combined outcomes of the severest grade of intraventricular haemorrhage and periventricular leukomalacia. Although the methodology and conclusions of this study can be criticised because of low numbers with these important complications,[11] this association potentially has great importance to neonatal medicine as these are the cerebral lesions most closely associated with future neurodevelopment problems. Perhaps re-assuringly, this association has not been found in another large study of RBC transfusion practice in neonates looking at similar outcomes reported recently by Heddle and colleagues in abstract form.[12]

High threshold red blood cell transfusion strategy
Whereas a number of studies have reported data on preterm neonates maintained with restrictive RBC transfusion protocols, there is less evidence looking at the converse situation, *i.e.* does maintaining a high haemoglobin level improve outcome in preterm neonates? In a study primarily looking at the effect of maintaining a haematocrit > 40% in preterm neonates in an attempt to reduce retinopathy of prematurity, Brooks *et al.*[13] also reported no reduction in other important neonatal complications (intraventricular haemorrhage, chronic lung disease and necrotising enterocolitis) as secondary

outcome measures. This study only assessed preterm neonates greater than 28 days of age (*i.e.* outside the intensive care period). However, the fact that a 'low' haemoglobin or haematocrit by itself, unaccompanied by clinical symptoms, is often the sole trigger factor for transfusion in sick neonates (see below),[14] suggests that clinical situations where haemoglobin-limited oxygen unloading capacity to the tissues are reached is rare, even during intensive care.

RESEARCH STUDIES

Instead of relying on clinical observations and trials to refine RBC transfusion practice in neonates, an alternative strategy is to develop more reliable laboratory or bedside (near patient) tests for 'clinical anaemia' or reduced tissue oxygenation in these patients. This has not proved an easy task in the past but improved and increasingly sophisticated modern investigation techniques may prove clinically useful in the future.

Capillary whole blood lactate

The determination of lactate concentration is now possible by near-patient testing methods and has been assessed as an indicator of tissue oxygenation and/or the need for RBC transfusion in preterm neonates.[15–17] However, during intensive care periods, whole blood lactate levels are highly variable reflecting variations in tissue perfusion rather than haemoglobin-limited oxygen unloading capacity to the tissues. In stable neonates, lactate levels have been shown to decrease following RBC transfusions given for 'symptomatic' anaemia.[15–17] However, even in stable preterm neonates, lactate levels show considerable variation during a 24-h period[15] and pretransfusion lactate levels do not correlate with pretransfusion haemoglobin or haematocrit.[15] Whereas peripheral blood lactate levels are increasingly used by neonatologists in the overall assessment of tissue perfusion and oxygenation in sick neonates, they cannot be used on their own as a reliable indicator of the need for RBC transfusion.

Peripheral fractional oxygen extraction

Peripheral fractional oxygen extraction is currently a technique available only as a research tool in neonatal medicine. However, it may provide a future method of assessing the adequacy of oxygen delivery to the tissues in neonates and, thereby, a surrogate indicator of 'clinical anaemia'. Recently, Wardle *et al.*[14] measured peripheral fractional oxygen extraction by near-infrared spectroscopy in 74 neonates < 1500 g undergoing standard neonatal care. A peripheral fractional oxygen extraction of > 0.47 was taken as a cut-off point of potentially inadequate tissue oxygen delivery and inadequate tissue oxygenation. In 37 neonates, this was used as their sole RBC transfusion trigger with the remaining 37 neonates receiving RBC transfusion guided by a conventional haemoglobin- and clinical status-based protocol. The study demonstrated a trend towards fewer RBC transfusions in the fractional oxygen extraction group, but this was not statistically significant. However, neonates in the fractional oxygen extraction group had lower median haemoglobin during the study, and time to first transfusion from study entry was also longer. No difference in major neonatal complications was seen between the two groups. However, two-thirds of transfusions given in the fractional oxygen extraction group were given 'out of protocol' because of clinical concerns about low haemoglobin or symptoms and not because of high fractional oxygen extraction. Because of these methodological difficulties, this method of assessing trigger thresholds for RBC transfusion in preterm neonates deserves further assessment as sticking closely to high fractional oxygen extraction as a transfusion trigger may prove to be a practical method to reduce RBC transfusions and donor exposure in sick neonates further, without jeopardising outcome. As the equipment required for near-infrared spectroscopy becomes smaller, this may well be a practical possibility in neonatal medicine in the future.

In-line blood gas and chemistry monitoring

Recently, Widness *et al.*[18] reported the results of a randomised, controlled trial comparing RBC transfusion requirements in extremely low birth weight neonates requiring intensive care, whose blood gas and limited blood chemistry values were monitored by near-patient testing in-line methods (with return of analysed blood to the patient) versus standard laboratory-based measurements (and consequent blood loss). There was a trend towards lower RBC transfusion requirements in the in-line monitoring group without any differences in neonatal mortality or morbidity between groups. Again, if such monitoring can be safely, and cost-effectively, introduced into neonatal intensive care units, this may be a method to reduce RBC transfusions and donor exposure in sick neonates further. However, such a method is only applicable to critically ill neonates with in-dwelling arterial catheters, a situation becoming increasing rare in most neonates for the reasons outlined above.

Clearly, none of the above studies definitely answers the question of when an individual sick neonate should be given a RBC transfusion and this will always rely to a certain extent on clinical judgement. Given this, perhaps the most important message from all of these studies is the continued paucity of data available on important neonatal outcomes associated with one of the commonest therapies administered to preterm neonates. They also highlight the need for further, well-designed, research studies, assessing clinically relevant short- and long-term outcomes, to define the optimal use of RBC transfusions in sick neonates. Indeed, this process will continue to be important as the patient populations, their clinical problems, and the therapies offered to ameliorate these clinical problems continue to evolve rapidly within neonatal medicine.

GUIDELINES FOR RED BLOOD CELL TRANSFUSION

Product

The British Committee for Standards in Haematology (BCSH) Transfusion Task Force (19,20) recommends that:

1. Components for transfusion *in utero* or to children under 1 year of age must be prepared from donors who have given at least one donation within the previous 2 years which was negative for all mandatory microbiological markers.

Table 1 Suggested trigger thresholds for red blood cell transfusion in neonates

Assisted ventilation			CPAP		Breathing spontaneously	
<28 days		≥28 days	<28 days	≥28 days	FiO$_2$ >0.21	Well in air
FiO$_2$ ≥0.3	FiO$_2$ <0.3					
Hb <12 g/dl	Hb <11 g/dl	Hb <10 g/dl	Hb <10 g/dl	Hb <8 g/dl	Hb <8 g/dl	Hb <7 g/dl
or	or	or	or	or	or	or
PCV <0.40	PCV <0.35	PCV <0.30	PCV <0.30	PCV <0.25	PCV <0.25	PCV <0.20

Hb, haemoglobin; PCV, packed cell volume.

2. Dedicating aliquots from a single donation to allow sequential transfusions from the same donor for neonates/small children who are likely to be repeatedly transfused is considered good practice.

3. Components transfused in the first year of life should be cytomegalovirus seronegative (since November 2001 all cellular blood products in the UK have been leukocyte-depleted prior to hospital issue and are widely regarded as cytomegalovirus-safe; nevertheless, in the absence of controlled trials, the BCSH continues to recommend cytomegalovirus-negative products for infants).

Triggers for red blood cell transfusion

Several studies now show that appropriate transfusion guidelines reduce transfusion number and donor exposure.[5,6,21] Suggested RBC transfusion triggers for preterm neonates are presented in Table 1. However, it must be stressed that these trigger levels are only guidelines and some neonates will have no clinical compromise at these haemoglobin/haematocrit levels and, therefore, **will not automatically require RBC transfusion**.

FRESH FROZEN PLASMA

Previously, the liberal administration of fresh frozen plasma to neonates was a common phenomenon justified by a wide variety of poorly-defined clinical indications (Table 2).[22] However, there is now accumulating evidence from a number of studies in neonates, and in adults (summarised by Stanworth et al.[23])

Table 2 Traditional indications for fresh frozen plasma use in neonates

- Treatment of proven or suspected disseminated intravascular coagulation
- Prevention of intraventricular haemorrhage
- Blood volume replacement
- Adjuvant therapy during sepsis (addition of opsonising factors)
- During episodes of thrombocytopenia
- To 'correct' prolonged indices of coagulation (unaccompanied by clinical signs of bleeding or other laboratory findings consistent with disseminated intravascular coagulation, e.g. thrombocytopenia or red cell fragmentation).

to show that (with the exception of treatment of disseminated intravascular coagulation) the use of fresh frozen plasma is not appropriate in these clinical situations. As a result, fresh frozen plasma administration to neonates has now dramatically reduced and this probably represents the greatest evidence-based improvement in neonatal transfusion medicine in recent years.

LIMITATIONS OF USE

Prevention of intraventricular haemorrhage
The large study conducted by the Northern Neonatal Network, reported in 1996,[24] clearly shows that prophylactic fresh frozen plasma administered to preterm neonates at birth does not prevent intraventricular haemorrhage or improve outcome at 2 years of life.

Volume replacement
Fresh frozen plasma is not superior to other colloid or crystalloid solutions as a volume replacement solution in standard neonatal practice.[25,26]

Sepsis
Few studies that have assessed the efficacy of fresh frozen plasma during neonatal sepsis. Krediet et al.[27] looked at rises in immunoglobulin G levels and increases in opsonising activity against coagulase negative *Staphylococcus* in preterm neonates given fresh frozen plasma during clinical episodes of sepsis. They found variable changes in both parameters and no influence on outcome.

During neonatal thrombocytopenia
Disseminated intravascular coagulation is associated with about 10% of episodes of neonatal thrombocytopenia.[28,29] Therefore, administration of fresh frozen plasma to non-bleeding thrombocytopenic neonates is not indicated unless there is good laboratory evidence of concurrent disseminated intravascular coagulation.

Prolonged indices of coagulation
Normal values for indices of coagulation have now been defined for both term and preterm neonates.[30,31] However, as with many neonatal 'normal ranges', these studies have not assessed neonates below 30 weeks' gestational age. Unfortunately, these are the very patients who tend to have the highest incidence of haemorrhage, thrombocytopenia, clinical instability and prolonged indices of coagulation compared to more mature preterm neonates or adults. In addition, many extremely preterm newborns transiently exhibit prolonged indices of coagulation which are not accompanied by clinical bleeding and that spontaneously improve over the first days of life. As above, attempting to 'correct' these indices with fresh frozen plasma is not associated with improved outcome.[24] This may well reflect the fact that fresh frozen plasma infusion in preterm neonates has a variable and unpredictable effect on markers of activation of coagulation (*i.e.* thrombin formation),[32] and the response to fresh frozen plasma may not be accurately reflected in changes in standard indices of coagulation (*e.g.* prothrombin time and activated partial thromboplastin time).[32] Clearly, these data show that further research studies

are indicated to define the normal coagulation indices of the immature neonatal population now receiving intensive care, and how such indices can be manipulated to promote or inhibit coagulation in an attempt to improve outcome.

GUIDELINES FOR FRESH FROZEN PLASMA TRANSFUSION

Until such studies are able to refine practice, fresh frozen plasma is recommended in neonates for vitamin K-dependent bleeding, inherited deficiencies of coagulation factors (+ the specific factors), and proven disseminated intravascular coagulation. The largest volume appropriate to the cardiovascular status of the neonate should be administered. For guidance on fresh frozen plasma products suitable for neonates and the new steps being taken to ensure a pathogen-free product for this age group, the reader is referred to the BCSH web site.[20]

PLATELETS

THROMBOCYTOPENIA AS A CLINICAL PROBLEM IN NEONATES

Thrombocytopenia (platelets $<150 \times 10^9/l$) is common in sick neonates occurring in ~25% of neonates admitted to neonatal intensive care units.[28] Episodes of severe thrombocytopenia (platelets $< 50 \times 10^9/l$) are less common, but still occur in 5% of neonatal intensive care unit patients.[28,29] Half of these severely affected neonates receive platelet transfusions[29] prompted by the fact that previous studies suggest that neonatal thrombocytopenia is a risk factor for haemorrhage (particularly intraventricular haemorrhage),[28,29,33] mortality,[28,29,33,34] and adverse neurodevelopmental outcome.[35,36]. However, to date, there has been no neonatal trial that demonstrates reduced haemorrhage or improved outcome in neonates with non-immune-mediated thrombocytopenia treated with platelet transfusions. In the only randomised controlled trial addressing this, reported in 1993, Andrew et al.[37] found no benefit in terms of haemorrhage when maintaining a normal platelet count by platelet transfusion in preterm neonates compared to appropriate controls with moderate thrombocytopenia (platelets $50–150 \times 10^9/l$).

HAEMORRHAGE IN SICK NEONATES WITH THROMBOCYTOPENIA

The vast majority of neonatal platelet transfusions are given in an attempt to prevent major haemorrhage and its potential sequelae rather than as treatment for active bleeding. The commonest form of major haemorrhage in sick neonates, particularly preterm neonates, is intraventricular haemorrhage and most neonates who develop this do so perinatally (within the first 72 h of life). Although, as above, a number of studies have suggested that abnormal haemostasis contributes to the development of intraventricular haemorrhage, others suggest that haemostatic abnormalities are only a minor antecedent of intraventricular haemorrhage development.[38] Other forms of major, life-threatening, neonatal haemorrhage (e.g. pulmonary or intra-abdominal haemorrhage) are more related to clinical condition at the time of bleeding but even these usually occur early in the neonatal course, during intensive care periods. However, with the exception of perinatal asphyxia, the conditions precipitating the majority of episodes of severe thrombocytopenia (*e.g.* late-onset sepsis and necrotising enterocolitis) usually develop well after the first few days of life (Table 2).[29] Interestingly, neonates with these complications rarely have major haemorrhage, even when severely thrombocytopenic, raising the question of whether there is a real, rather than perceived, risk of bleeding in neonates with platelet counts <50 x 10^9/l.

STUDIES OF CONTEMPORARY PLATELET TRANSFUSION PRACTICE IN NEONATES

To investigate these associations further, four recent publications[29,39–41] have retrospectively documented platelet transfusion practice and short-term outcome in a number of neonatal intensive care units in the US, UK and Mexico. Despite the geographical differences, the findings of these studies are remarkably similar and largely confirm previous clinical observations:

1. The majority of platelet transfusions are given as prophylaxis to non-bleeding neonates with platelet counts < 50 x 10^9/l and most commonly in those with counts < 30 x 10^9/l. However, a wide variety of platelet count triggers for transfusion are used within, and between, these centres (range, platelets 30–100 x 10^9/l), depending on the clinical circumstances of the individual neonate.

2. Very few neonates who receive prophylactic platelet transfusions develop major haemorrhage during their period of thrombocytopenia.

3. More than half of neonates given platelet transfusions receive more that one transfusion, with a significant proportion receiving more than four trans-fusions (roughly doubling the donor exposure for the neonatal period).

4. Thrombocytopenic neonates who receive platelets are up to 10 times more likely to die than neonates who do not receive platelet transfusion. (However, the severity of the clinical conditions causing the thrombocytopenia is stressed as the major factor leading to mortality.)

DEVELOPING GUIDELINES FOR PLATELET TRANSFUSION

These data clearly suggest that many neonates receive platelet transfusions when their overall risk of major haemorrhage is low, possibly very low. They also suggest that this is a further area where carefully designed and conducted clinical research trials could significantly improve transfusion practice for neonates (and these are in development in some centres – personal communication). In the absence of these, we have used the natural history of haemorrhage in sick neonates, coupled with these recent clinical reports, to develop guidelines for platelet transfusion in different groups of sick neonates directed by their degree of prematurity, post-natal age, and incidence of concurrent complications (Table 3). Thus, we believe that prophylactic platelet transfusions are not required for stable neonates until the platelet count falls below 30 x 10^9/l (Table 3). (Indeed, many patients may not be at significant risk of haemorrhage until the platelet count falls much lower.) A higher trigger

Table 3 Suggested trigger thresholds for platelet transfusion in neonates

Platelet count (x 10^9/l)	Non-bleeding neonate (or minor bleeding, e.g. via ETT, NGT)	Major bleeding (e.g. frank pulmonary or renal)	Autoimmune or NAITP (proven or suspected)
< 30	**Consider transfusion in all patients**	**Transfuse**	**Transfuse** (using HPA-compatible platelets)
30–49	Do not transfuse if clinically stable **Consider transfusion if:** • < 1000 g and <1 week of age • clinically unstable (e.g. fluctuating blood pressure) • concurrent coagulopathy • requires surgery or exchange transfusion	**Transfuse**	**Transfuse** (using HPA-compatible platelets if minor of major bleeding present)
50–99	Do not transfuse	**Transfuse**	**Transfuse** (using HPA-compatible platelets only if major bleeding present)
> 99	Do not transfuse	Do not transfuse	Do not transfuse

ETT, endotracheal tube; NGT, nasogastric tube; NAITP, neonatal alloimmune thrombocytopenia; HPA, human platelet antigen.

level (platelets < 50 x 10^9/l) should only be used for patients with the greatest risk of haemorrhage, especially extremely low birth weight neonates (<1000 g) in the first week of life with significant clinical instability (*e.g.* fluctuating ventilation requirements or blood pressure).

Neonates with suspected or proven allo- and auto-immune thrombocytopenia require specialised treatment protocols (see below and Table 3).

Dose and product
No trial evidence is currently available regarding the optimal volume (dose) of platelets to administer or when to administer further transfusions. Larger volumes (20 ml/kg) appear to result in larger and more sustained rises in platelet count compared to smaller volumes (10 ml/kg) (personal observations). However, there is no guarantee that simply maintaining a higher count for longer consistently improves haemostasis and in a small number of neonates whose thrombocytopenia is the result of severe platelet consumption (*i.e.* in necrotising enterocolitis), no platelet increment may be apparent even following repeated platelet transfusions. The value of such repeated therapy during necrotising enterocolitis may, therefore, be questionable given the paucity of trial evidence. Indeed, there is evidence from one small study that repeated platelet transfusion in thrombocytopenic neonates with necrotising enterocolitis may actually worsen overall outcome.[42]

For specific guidance on appropriate platelet products the reader is referred to the BCSH web site.[20]

HUMAN ALBUMIN SOLUTION

Human albumin solution is currently used as a primary blood volume expanding solution for sick newborns. However, human albumin solution is not superior to other colloid or crystalloid solutions as a volume replacement solution in standard neonatal practice.[43] Concentrated human albumin solution solutions (20%) are sometimes administered to hypoalbuminaemic neonates with clinically significant peripheral oedema in an attempt to correct the hypoalbuminaemia, improve circulating oncotic pressure, ameliorate oedema and hasten clinical improvement. Although this may occasionally be of benefit in critically ill neonates, there is no convincing evidence to support this practice as part of the standard care of neonatal intensive care unit patients.[44] As the underlying cause of the hypoalbuminaemia is usually inadequate nutritional support, optimising nutrition is the preferred option. Together, these data suggest that there is no valid indication for the use of human albumin solution in standard neonatal practice and concentrated albumin solutions should only be administered to neonates receiving critical care in tertiary neonatal centres.

NORMAL HUMAN IMMUNOGLOBULIN

IMMUNE-MEDIATED THROMBOCYTOPENIA

Normal human immunoglobulin is standard therapy for both allo- and autoimmune neonatal thrombocytopenia and is generally administered to neonates in both clinical situations at platelet counts below $30 \times 10^9/l$. (Platelet transfusion may also be necessary depending on the clinical condition of the neonate; Table 3.) Platelet counts will usually rise promptly following normal human immunoglobulin at a dose of 1 g/kg on 2 consecutive days (in single or divided doses). Further courses may be required in refractory or relapsing cases.

NEONATAL SEPSIS

There have now been a considerable number of trials assessing the value of normal human immunoglobulin as both prophylaxis and adjuvant therapy for neonatal sepsis. The most recent Cochrane Reviews of the accrued evidence continue to suggest that prophylactic normal human immunoglobulin does not cause a clinically significant reduction in neonatal sepsis or improve outcome;[45] but, normal human immunoglobulin may be beneficial where given in conjunction with antibiotic therapy for neonatal sepsis.[46] An international multicentre trial (INIS) is currently underway to address this question further. When administered during sepsis, the standard recommended dose is 500 mg/kg as a single dose.

IMMUNE-MEDIATED ANAEMIA/HYPERBILIRUBINAEMIA

Recently, a number of studies have looked at administration of normal human immunoglobulin to neonates with alloimmune haemolysis to reduce the need for exchange transfusion. Systematic reviews of these studies[47,48] show a trend towards reduced rates of exchange transfusion. However, the number of studies and infants included is small and further well-designed studies are needed before normal human immunoglobulin can be fully recommended for the treatment of neonatal alloimmune haemolysis.

EXCHANGE/DILUTIONAL EXCHANGE TRANSFUSION

EXCHANGE TRANSFUSION

As severe rhesus haemolytic disease of the newborn becomes increasingly rare due to a combination of maternal anti-rhesus D therapy and intra-uterine transfusion of affected fetuses, neonatal exchange transfusion is also becoming an increasingly rare procedure in neonatal medicine. In haemolytic disease of the newborn, when anaemia and heart failure are the most pressing clinical problems, a single blood volume exchange transfusion (80–100 ml/kg) may be sufficient to ameliorate these problems. However, in the treatment of severe haemolytic disease of the newborn, the aim is to remove both the antibody coated red cells (to reduce further haemolysis and bilirubin production) and the bilirubin already in the circulation. In this situation, a double blood volume exchange transfusion (160–200 ml/kg) is recommended and is estimated to remove 90% of the initial red cells and 50% of the available intravascular bilirubin.[19,20] In the majority of cases in the UK, plasma reduced blood with a haematocrit of 0.50–0.60 is used for exchange transfusion to manage both severe anaemia and hyperbilirubinaemia.[19,20]

In view of the decreasing general experience of the practice of exchange transfusion (especially amongst neonatal trainees), all neonatal units must adopt and maintain appropriate written practice guidelines for this procedure.

DILUTIONAL EXCHANGE

Partial/dilutional exchange transfusion is frequently undertaken in order to reduce whole blood viscosity in the 1–5% of neonates born with polycythaemia (packed cell volume > 0.65).[49,50] It is known that whole blood viscosity rises exponentially when packed cell volume exceeds 0.65–0.70 and this may lead to reduced blood flow and oxygenation of organs and tissues. However, even at a packed cell volume > 0.70, only a minority of neonates exhibit clinical symptoms potentially related to hyperviscosity (jitteriness, hypoglycaemia, poor peripheral perfusion)[49,50] and very few have major symptoms (*e.g.* seizures) likely to lead to long-term sequelae. Performing a dilutional exchange on all neonates with a free flowing venous packed cell volume of > 0.70 is one method of ensuring therapy for all neonates at risk of the major complications of hyperviscosity. However, this entails performing this procedure on a large number of asymptomatic neonates when it is likely that only neonates with hyperviscosity and major symptoms of circulatory compromise or persistent hypoglycaemia are actually at risk of an adverse neurological outcome.[51] Indeed, a recent systematic review by Dempsey *et al.*[52] emphasised the lack of evidence for long-term benefit of dilutional exchange transfusion in unselected neonates with polycythaemia.

Progress to resolve this clinical dilemma could be made by further studies measuring whole blood viscosity in polycythaemic neonates and performing dilutional exchange only on those with proven hyperviscosity. As numbers in individual units would be small, this would clearly require a multicentre study coupled to careful neurodevelopmental follow-up – a costly and time-consuming undertaking. Perhaps a more practical solution is to perform dilutional exchange transfusion only in neonates with a packed cell volume > 0.65–0.70 who have symptoms which suggest a possible adverse outcome (principally neurological symptoms, *i.e.* fits, excessive jitteriness, neurological signs, refractory hypoglycaemia). Asymptomatic neonates should be observed only and those with minor symptoms (*i.e.* poor peripheral perfusion or borderline hypoglycaemia) can be treated by standard therapies until polycythaemia/hyperviscosity resolve spontaneously. In addition, it should be remembered in the assessment and treatment of such neonates that umbilical venous catheterisation and dilutional exchange probably increase the risk of necrotising enterocolitis[52,53] and may lead to thrombotic and hepatic complications. In the few cases where dilutional exchange is clinically indicated, a one-third whole blood volume exchange (80 ml/kg) is usually performed. There is no justification for using other than normal saline as the exchange fluid.[54]

Key points for clinical practice

- Many, previously widely accepted neonatal transfusion practices are changing as the clinical problems and transfusion requirements of extremely preterm neonates change in the antenatal steroid, surfactant, nasal CPAP era.

- In view of their longevity, graduates of neonatal intensive care are particularly at risk of any potential long-term effects of transfusion therapy (*e.g.* chronic hepatitis C infection and its sequelae and vCJD).

- Adhering to increasingly restrictive red blood cell transfusion protocols significantly reduces transfusion requirements and donor exposure without obviously prejudicing neonatal outcome.

- The use of fresh frozen plasma in neonates should be strictly confined to those suffering from a proven coagulopathy or specific clotting factor deficiency.

- Current liberal platelet transfusion guidelines result in many neonates receiving unnecessary platelet transfusions. There is a pressing need for further studies to define evidence-based thresholds for platelet transfusion in neonates.

- There is no role for the use of human albumin solution in either standard care or special care neonatal nurseries. Human albumin solution solutions should only be administered to neonatal patients in specialised neonatal units under the direction of specialised neonatal staff.

Key points for clinical practice (continued)

- Normal human immunoglobulin is rapidly effective in raising the platelet count in most cases of auto- and allo-immune thrombocytopenia. Its potential role as a positive adjuvant therapy during neonatal sepsis and haemolytic disease of the newborn is still to be defined.

- Exchange transfusion is now a rare event in most neonatal units. In view of this, all neonatal units must adopt and maintain appropriate written practice guidelines for this procedure in order to prevent both delays and mistakes in the treatment of the few neonates who urgently require this therapy.

- Very few neonates are likely to show long-term benefit from partial/dilutional exchange transfusion. The majority of immediate symptoms attributed to neonatal polycythaemia/ hyperviscosity can be managed by standard neonatal therapies.

- In order to maintain best practice, neonatal units must construct, adhere closely to, and regularly audit and review guidelines for the administration of all blood products to sick neonates.

- Neonatologists should continue to recognise that very little is actually known about the significant short- and long-term effects of blood product use in neonates. This should continue to stimulate the design and conduct of high-quality, randomised, controlled trials of blood product use in neonates in order to define and refine the best evidence-based practice.

References

1. Hintz SR, Poole WK, Wright LL *et al.*, NICHD Neonatal Research Network. Changes in mortality and morbidities among infants born at less than 25 weeks during the post-surfactant era. *Arch Dis Child Fetal Neonatal Edn* 2005; **90**: F128–F133.
2. Stainsby D, Russell J, Cohen H, Lilleyman J. Reducing adverse events in blood transfusion. *Br J Haematol* 2005; **131**: 8–12.
3. Busch MP, Kleinman SH, Nemo GJ. Current and emerging infectious risks of blood transfusions. *JAMA* 2003; **289**: 959–962.
4. Leipala JA, Boldt T, Fellman V. Haemodynamic effects of erythrocyte transfusion in preterm infants. *Eur J Pediatr* 2004; **163**: 390–394.
5. Miyashiro AM, Santos N, Guinsburg R *et al*. Strict red blood cell transfusion guideline reduces the need for transfusions in very-low-birthweight infants in the first 4 weeks of life: a multicentre trial. *Vox Sang* 2005; **88**: 107–113.
6. Franz AR, Pohlandt F. Red blood cell transfusions in very and extremely low birthweight infants under restrictive transfusion guidelines: is exogenous erythropoietin necessary? *Arch Dis Child Fetal Neonatal Edn* 2001; **84**: F96–F100.
7. Maier RF, Sonntag J, Walka MM *et al*. Changing practices of red blood cell transfusions in infants with birth weights less than 1000 g. *J Pediatr* 2000; **136**: 220–224.
8. Widness JA, Seward VJ, Kromer IJ *et al*. Changing patterns of red blood cell transfusion in very low birth weight infants. *J Pediatr* 1996; **129**: 680–687.
9. Alkalay AL, Galvis S, Ferry DA, Simmons CF, Krueger Jr RC. Hemodynamic changes in anemic premature infants: are we allowing the hematocrits to fall too low? *Pediatrics* 2003; **112**: 838–845.

10. Bell EF, Strauss RG, Widness JA *et al*. Randomized trial of liberal versus restrictive guidelines for red blood cell transfusion in preterm infants. *Pediatrics* 2005; **115**: 1685–1691.

11. Murray N, Roberts I, Stanworth S. Red blood cell transfusion in neonates. *Pediatrics* 2005; **116**: 1609.

12. Heddle NM, Whyte R, Asztalos E, Roberts R, Blajchman M. Identifying the optimal red cell transfusion threshold for extremely low birth weight infants: The premature in need of transfusion (PINT) study. *Transfusion* 2004; **44 (Suppl)**: p1A.

13. Brooks SE, Marcus DM, Gillis D *et al*. The effect of blood transfusion protocol on retinopathy of prematurity: a prospective, randomized study. *Pediatrics* 1999; **104**: 514–518.

14. Wardle SP, Garr R, Yoxall CW, Weindling AM. A pilot randomised controlled trial of peripheral fractional oxygen extraction to guide blood transfusions in preterm infants. *Arch Dis Child Fetal Neonatal Edn* 2002; **86**: F22–F27.

15. Frey B, Losa M. The value of capillary whole blood lactate for blood transfusion requirements in anaemia of prematurity. *Intensive Care Med* 2001; **27**: 222–227.

16. Moller JC, Schwarz U, Schaible TF *et al*. Do cardiac output and serum lactate levels indicate blood transfusion requirements in anemia of prematurity? *Intensive Care Med* 1996; **22**: 472–476.

17. Izraeli S, Ben-Sira L, Harell D *et al*. Lactic acid as a predictor for erythrocyte transfusion in healthy preterm infants with anemia of prematurity. *J Pediatr* 1993; **122**: 629–631.

18. Widness JA, Madan A, Grindeanu LA, Zimmerman MB, Wong DK, Stevenson DK. Reduction in red blood cell transfusions among preterm infants: results of a randomized trial with an in-line blood gas and chemistry monitor. *Pediatrics* 2005; **115**: 1299–1306.

19. Gibson BE, Todd A, Roberts I *et al*., British Committee for Standards in Haematology Transfusion Task Force: Writing group. Transfusion guidelines for neonates and older children. *Br J Haematol* 2004; **124**: 433–453.

20. British Committee for Standards in Haematology Transfusion Task Force. <www.bcshguidelines.com>.

21. Alagappan A, Shattuck KE, Malloy MH. Impact of transfusion guidelines on neonatal transfusions. *J Perinatol* 1998; **18**: 92–97.

22. Strauss RG, Levy GJ, Sotelo-Avila C *et al*. National survey of neonatal transfusion practices: II. Blood component therapy. *Pediatrics* 1993; **91**: 530–536.

23. Stanworth SJ, Brunskill SJ, Hyde CJ, McClelland DB, Murphy MF. Is fresh frozen plasma clinically effective? A systematic review of randomized controlled trials. *Br J Haematol* 2004; **126**: 139–152.

24. Northern Neonatal Nursing Initiative Trial Group. Randomised trial of prophylactic early fresh-frozen plasma or gelatin or glucose in preterm babies: outcome at 2 years. *Lancet* 1996; **348**: 229–232.

25. Emery EF, Greenough A, Gamsu HR. Randomised controlled trial of colloid infusions in hypotensive preterm infants. *Arch Dis Child* 1992; **67**: 1185–1188.

26. Supapannachart S, Siripoonya P, Boonwattanasoontorn W, Kanjanavanit S. Neonatal polycythemia: effects of partial exchange transfusion using fresh frozen plasma, Haemaccel and normal saline. *J Med Assoc Thai* 1999; **82** *(Suppl 1)*: S82–S86.

27. Krediet TG, Beurskens FJ, van Dijk H *et al*. Antibody responses and opsonic activity in sera of preterm neonates with coagulase-negative staphylococcal septicemia and the effect of the administration of fresh frozen plasma. *Pediatr Res* 1998; **43**: 645–651.

28. Castle V, Andrew M, Kelton J *et al*. Frequency and mechanism of neonatal thrombocytopenia. *J Pediatr* 1986; **108**: 749–755.

29. Murray NA, Howarth LJ, McCloy MP *et al*. Platelet transfusion in the management of severe thrombocytopenia in neonatal intensive care unit patients. *Transfusion Med* 2002; **12**: 35–41.

30. Andrew M, Paes B, Milner R *et al*. Development of the human coagulation system in the full-term infant. *Blood* 1987; **70**: 165–172.

31. Andrew M, Paes B, Milner R *et al*. Development of the human coagulation system in the healthy premature infant. *Blood* 1988; **72**: 1651–1657.

32. Hyytiainen S, Syrjala M, Fellman V, Heikinheimo M, Petaja J. Fresh frozen plasma reduces thrombin formation in newborn infants. *J Thromb Haemost* 2003; **1**: 1189–1194.

33. Kahn DJ, Richardson DK, Billett HH. Association of thrombocytopenia and delivery method with intraventricular hemorrhage among very-low-birth-weight infants. *Am J Obstet Gynecol* 2002; **186**: 109–116.

34. Murray NA, Roberts IAG. Circulating megakaryocytes and their progenitors in early thrombocytopenia in preterm neonates. *Pediatr Res* 1996; **40**: 112–119.

35. Jhawar BS, Ranger A, Steven DA, Del Maestro RF. A follow-up study of infants with intracranial hemorrhage at full-term. *Can J Neurol Sci* 2005; **32**: 332-9.

36. Andrew M, Castle V, Saigal S, Carter C, Kelton JG. Clinical impact of neonatal thrombocytopenia. *J Pediatr* 1987; **110**: 457–464.

37. Andrew M, Vegh P, Caco C *et al.* A randomized, controlled trial of platelet transfusions in thrombocytopenic premature infants. *J Pediatr* 1993; **123**: 285–291.

38. Lupton BA, Hill A, Whitfield MF, Carter CJ, Wadsworth LD, Roland EH. Reduced platelet count as a risk factor for intraventricular hemorrhage. *Am J Dis Child* 1988; **142**: 1222–1224.

39. Kahn DJ, Richardson DK, Billett HH. Inter-NICU variation in rates and management of thrombocytopenia among very low birth-weight infants. *J Perinatol* 2003; **23**: 312–316.

40. Garcia MG, Duenas E, Sola MC *et al.* Epidemiologic and outcome studies of patients who received platelet transfusions in the neonatal intensive care unit. *J Perinatol* 2001; **21**: 415–420.

41. Del Vecchio A, Sola MC, Theriaque DW *et al.* Platelet transfusions in the neonatal intensive care unit: factors predicting which patients will require multiple transfusions. *Transfusion* 2001; **41**: 803–808.

42. Kenton AB, Hegemier S, Smith EO *et al.* Platelet transfusions in infants with necrotizing enterocolitis do not lower mortality but may increase morbidity. *J Perinatol* 2005; **25**: 173–177.

43. So KW, Fok TF, Ng PC *et al.* Randomised controlled trial of colloid or crystalloid in hypotensive preterm infants. *Arch Dis Child Fetal Neonatal Edn* 1997; **76**: F43–F46.

44. Greenough A, Emery E, Hird MF, Gamsu HR. Randomised controlled trial of albumin infusion in ill preterm infants. *Eur J Pediatr* 1993; **152**: 157–159.

45. Ohlsson A, Lacy JB. Intravenous immunoglobulin for preventing infection in preterm and/or low-birth-weight infants. Cochrane Database Syst Rev. 2004; (1): CD000361.

46. Ohlsson A, Lacy JB. Intravenous immunoglobulin for suspected or subsequently proven infection in neonates. Cochrane Database Syst Rev. 2004; (1): CD001239.

47. Alcock GS, Liley H: Immunoglobulin infusion for isoimmune haemolytic jaundice in neonates. Cochrane database Syst Rev 3: CD003313, 2002.

48. Gottstein R, Cooke RW. Systematic review of intravenous immunoglobulin in haemolytic disease of the newborn. *Arch Dis Child Fetal Neonatal Edn* 2003; **88**: F6–F10.

49. Rothenberg T. Partial plasma exchange transfusion in polycythaemic neonates. *Arch Dis Child* 2002; **86**: 60–62.

50. Merchant RH, Phadke SD, Sakhalkar VS *et al.* Hematocrit and whole blood viscosity in newborns: analysis of 100 cases. *Indian Pediatr* 1992; **29**: 555–561.

51. Drew JH, Guaran RL, Cichello M, Hobbs JB. Neonatal whole blood hyperviscosity: the important factor influencing later neurologic function is the viscosity and not the polycythemia. *Clin Hemorheol Microcirc* 1997; **17**: 67–72.

52. Dempsey EM, Barrington K. Short and long term outcomes following partial exchange transfusion in the polycythaemic newborn: a systematic review. *Arch Dis Child Fetal Neonatal Edn* 2006; **91**: F2–F6.

53. Supapannachart S, Siripoonya P, Boonwattanasoontorn W, Kanjanavanit S. Neonatal polycythemia: effects of partial exchange transfusion using fresh frozen plasma, Haemaccel and normal saline. *J Med Assoc Thai* 1999; **82 (Suppl 1)**: S82–S86.

54. Wong W, Fok TF, Lee CH *et al.* Randomised controlled trial: comparison of colloid or crystalloid for partial exchange transfusion for treatment of neonatal polycythaemia. *Arch Dis Child Fetal Neonatal Edn* 1997; **77**: F115–F118.

Molly B. Sheridan Garry R. Cutting

11

Genetic and phenotypic variants of cystic fibrosis

Cystic fibrosis is the most common life-limiting genetic disorder in Caucasians. Sixteen years ago, the cystic fibrosis transmembrane conductance regulator (*CFTR*) was identified as the defective gene in cystic fibrosis patients with the classic form of the disease.[1] This discovery has revealed that the spectrum of disease associated with *CFTR* mutations is much broader than previously recognised. Knowledge of the molecular basis of a disease has important implications for the diagnosis, prognosis, and treatment of patients, especially those with an unusual phenotype. Furthermore, parsing of unusual phenotypes has permitted the identification of rare cystic fibrosis-like disorders caused by mutations in genes other than *CFTR*.

CLASSIC CYSTIC FIBROSIS

Cystic fibrosis is an autosomal recessive disorder which affects multiple organ systems including the respiratory tract, gastrointestinal tract, sweat gland, and male reproductive tract.[2] Most of our knowledge of the disease is derived from the study of patients with disease manifestations in each of the aforementioned organ systems defined as classic cystic fibrosis. Chronic obstructive pulmonary disease is the primary cause of mortality in cystic fibrosis. Cystic fibrosis lung disease is characterised by excessive sputum production, bronchiectasis, chronic cough, decreased mucociliary clearance and infection with unusual organisms including *Pseudomonas aeruginosa*, *Staphylococcus aureus*, *Haemophilus influenzae*,

Molly B. Sheridan BS
Graduate Student, McKusick–Nathans Institute of Genetic Medicine, Johns Hopkins University School of Medicine, BRB 559, 733 North Broadway, Baltimore, MD 21205, USA

Garry R. Cutting MD (for correspondence)
Professor of Pediatrics and Medicine, McKusick–Nathans Institute of Genetic Medicine, Johns Hopkins University School of Medicine, BRB 559, 733 North Broadway, Baltimore, MD 21205, USA
E-mail: gcutting@jhmi.edu

and *Burkholderia cepacia*. The progression of lung disease in cystic fibrosis patients is closely monitored through regular pulmonary function testing and sputum cultures. The nasal sinuses are also affected in classic cystic fibrosis with most patients developing chronic rhinosinusitis. Measurement of salt secretion across the respiratory epithelium lining the nasal turbinates has become a useful diagnostic test for cystic fibrosis. This test, termed the nasal potential difference measurement test, assesses *in vivo* CFTR function by measuring electrical potential across nasal respiratory epithelium.[3] Patients with classic cystic fibrosis have abnormal nasal potential difference measurements due to loss of chloride secretion through CFTR and increased activity of the epithelial sodium channel.

Patients with classic cystic fibrosis can manifest disease at a number of different locations in the gastrointestinal tract. Exocrine pancreatic dysfunction caused by obstruction of pancreatic ducts leads to fat and protein malabsorption. This complication usually manifests early in life as failure to thrive and deficiency of fat soluble vitamins. Clinical tests to assess pancreatic function are indirect, but include measurement of serum cationic trypsinogen and faecal fat analysis in stool. The symptoms of pancreatic insufficiency are minimised by pancreatic enzyme supplementation. Patients with classic cystic fibrosis are at risk for intestinal complications including meconium ileus (obstruction of the small intestine) at birth, distal intestinal obstruction syndrome, chronic constipation, rectal prolapse, and liver cirrhosis.

One of the defining characteristics of cystic fibrosis is an elevated concentration of chloride in the sweat. Patients with classic cystic fibrosis have a sweat chloride concentration above 60 mmol/l (normal < 40 mmol/l). The measurement of chloride in the sweat by quantitative pilocarpine iontophoresis is the standard diagnostic test for cystic fibrosis.[4] Patients with cystic fibrosis also have a decreased β-adrenergic stimulated sweat rate when compared to healthy controls. Measurement of cAMP-mediated sweat rate can be used along with the traditional sweat test as a quantitative measure of CFTR function *in vivo*.[5]

Most men with classic cystic fibrosis are infertile. This is due to obstructive azoospermia caused by congenital bilateral absence of the vas deferens. Congenital bilateral absence of the vas deferens can be diagnosed in prepubescent males by both palpation and transrectal ultrasonography. Semen analysis revealing low sperm count, low ejaculate volume, and abnormal semen chemistry can be indicative of congenital bilateral absence of the vas deferens in adults. Fertility is reduced in women with cystic fibrosis due to increased viscosity of cervical mucus and disrupted ovulary cycles.

Patients with the classic form of cystic fibrosis carry two deleterious mutations that significantly decrease the function of the cystic fibrosis transmembrane conductance regulator (CFTR). CFTR is a cAMP-activated chloride channel located in the apical membrane of epithelial tissues. Along with its role as a chloride channel, CFTR mediates the function of other ion channels, including the epithelial sodium channel.[6] Over 1200 disease-associated mutations have been identified in *CFTR*, with the most common mutation, a deletion of phenylalanine at position 508 of *CFTR* (ΔF508), accounting for about 70% of cystic fibrosis alleles.[1] This mutation causes CFTR misfolding and loss of functional CFTR at the apical membrane leading to classic cystic fibrosis when patients are homozygotes.[7] Despite the knowledge of the underlying genetic cause of cystic fibrosis, *CFTR* genotype does not account for all of the phenotypic variability seen in cystic fibrosis patients. Pancreatic disease and to a lesser extent sweat gland dysfunction are correlated with *CFTR* genotype. However, patients with the same *CFTR* genotype often have a highly variable lung phenotype. This variability may be attributed to other genetic (modifier genes or epigenetic factors) or environmental factors.[8]

Before the advent of genetic testing for cystic fibrosis, it was recognised that atypical forms of cystic fibrosis exist. These patients typically had later onset of pulmonary disease than classic cystic fibrosis patients, were pancreatic sufficient, and may have had normal or intermediate sweat chloride concentrations. The identification of *CFTR* mutations in patients with atypical forms of cystic fibrosis has further expanded the phenotypic spectrum of cystic fibrosis to include not only patients with disease in a subset of organ systems, but also those presenting with cystic fibrosis-like disease in only one organ system.

NON-CLASSIC CYSTIC FIBROSIS

Patients with characteristics of cystic fibrosis in two or three of the organ systems affected in classic cystic fibrosis have been classified as non-classic cystic fibrosis.[9,10] The non-classic cystic fibrosis phenotype is highly heterogeneous and patients can have disease in any combination of organ systems. Non-classic cystic fibrosis patients often present at a later age, have a milder course of disease, and overall better survival. Most patients retain some pancreatic function allowing them to escape the pancreatic insufficiency characteristic of classic cystic fibrosis. However, some non-classic cystic fibrosis patients manifest pancreatic disease in the form of pancreatitis. A subset of non-classic cystic fibrosis patients has been identified with normal sweat chloride concentration.

Most patients with non-classic cystic fibrosis have two mutations in *CFTR*. At least one mutation usually permits residual CFTR function that is sufficient to escape the classic cystic fibrosis phenotype. Some of these 'mild' mutations are included in the screens for common *CFTR* mutations, but most are rare and only identified after analysis of the exons and flanking intronic sequences of *CFTR*. The identification of one common *CFTR* mutation in a patient with non-classic cystic fibrosis indicates that a second, rare *CFTR* mutation likely occurs in the other *CFTR* gene.[11]

A number of studies report non-classic cystic fibrosis phenotypes that are unrelated to *CFTR* genotype. Mekus *et al.*[12] presented a patient who had laboratory and clinical evidence of cystic fibrosis in multiple organ systems in the absence of *CFTR* mutations. Linkage analysis argued against CFTR in the aetiology of disease in this patient. Another study analysed the entire coding region of *CFTR* in 31 non-classic cystic fibrosis patients and did not identify any *CFTR* mutations in 42% of patients.[13] In the most comprehensive study to date, Groman and colleagues[11,14] studied 158 non-classic cystic fibrosis patients and failed to identify any *CFTR* mutations in 40% of patients after sequencing of the coding region of *CFTR*. The study also identified two sets of siblings,

Table 1 Organ system involvement in *CFTR*-related phenotypes

Phenotype	CBAVD	Pancreas	Lung	Sinus	Sweat [Cl⁻] >60 mmol/l
Classic cystic fibrosis	+	+	+	+	+
Non-classic cystic fibrosis	±	±	±	±	±
CBAVD	+	–	±	±	±
Pancreatitis	–	+	–	–	–
Bronchiectasis	–	–	+	–	–
Allergic bronchopulmonary aspergillosis	–	–	+	–	–
Chronic rhinosinusitis	–	–	–	+	–
Isolated elevated sweat [Cl⁻]	–	–	–	–	+

CBAVD, Congenital bilateral absence of the vas deferens

both with non-classic cystic fibrosis, who inherited different *CFTR* genes. Patients without *CFTR* mutations in the former study could not be distinguished from non-classic cystic fibrosis patients with two *CFTR* mutations on the basis of clinical presentation or sweat chloride concentration. Taken together, these data indicate that factors other than CFTR dysfunction can cause non-classic cystic fibrosis. Indeed, mutations in each gene encoding the β-subunit of the epithelial sodium channel (*βENaC*) were found in two non-classic cystic fibrosis patients without mutations in the coding region of *CFTR*.[15] The latter study provided definitive evidence of genetic heterogeneity in non-classic cystic fibrosis.

MONOSYMPTOMATIC CYSTIC FIBROSIS PHENOTYPES

The phenotypic spectrum of cystic fibrosis also includes patients who present with clinical features of cystic fibrosis in only one organ system (Table 1). These phenotypes include congenital bilateral absence of the vas deferens, idiopathic chronic pancreatitis, brochiectasis, chronic rhinosinusitis, allergic broncho-pulmonary aspergillosis, and isolated elevated sweat chloride concentration.[16] Genetic factors play a role in the development of each disease. Because of the phenotypic overlap with cystic fibrosis, the *CFTR* gene was investigated in patients with each condition and some were found to carry one or two deleterious mutations in *CFTR*. However, in most cases, CFTR dysfunction contributes to, rather than causes, disease. Other genetic and/or environmental factors appear to play a substantial role in the development of these monosymptomatic phenotypes (Fig. 1).

CONGENITAL BILATERAL ABSENCE OF THE VAS DEFERENS

The concept of cystic fibrosis-like disease manifesting in only one organ system due to CFTR dysfunction is exemplified by males with congenital bilateral absence of the vas deferens.[17] In a study of 800 males with congenital bilateral absence of the vas deferens, two *CFTR* mutations were identified in 70.95% of patients, 15.9% had only one *CFTR* mutation, whereas 13.15% of patients had no identifiable *CFTR* mutations.[18] Each patient with two *CFTR* mutations carried at least one 'mild' *CFTR* mutation. The most common 'mild' mutation

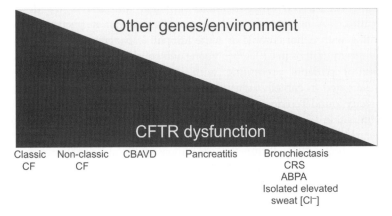

Classic CF	Non-classic CF	CBAVD	Pancreatitis	Bronchiectasis CRS ABPA Isolated elevated sweat [Cl⁻]	

Fig. 1 Spectrum of cystic fibrosis transmembrane regulator (CFTR) dysfunction in *CFTR*-related phenotypes. This graphic depicts the estimated contribution of *CFTR* genotype to the development of cystic fibrosis (CF) and other *CFTR* related phenotypes. CBAVD, congenital bilateral absence of the vas deferens; CRS, chronic rhinosinusitis; ABPA, allergic bronchopulmonary aspergillosis.

identified in congenital bilateral absence of the vas deferens males is the 5T allele of the polymorphic thymidine tract in the splice site acceptor of *CFTR* intron 8.[19] This allele is partially penetrant and associated with reduction of the number of *CFTR* transcripts containing exon 9 (those without exon 9 are not functional). Two studies have indicated that the length of a polymorphic TG tract found adjacent to the 5T variant can influence the penetrance of the 5T variant by modulating the amount of exon 9 skipping.[20,21] Thus, when screening for the 5T variant, it is imperative to also analyse TG tract length. While the 5T allele is common in congenital bilateral absence of the vas deferens, a fraction of men with congenital bilateral absence of the vas deferens carry at least one mutation which cannot be identified by standard screening methods. Mak *et al.*[22] emphasised the importance of analysis of the entire coding region of *CFTR* in patients with congenital bilateral absence of the vas deferens.

Men may present with congenital bilateral absence of the vas deferens and no other overt clinical signs of cystic fibrosis, while others may manifest subtle lung or sinus disease.[23] Thus, it is prudent to perform extensive clinical testing for signs of cystic fibrosis in males with congenital bilateral absence of the vas deferens. Furthermore, dysfunction of CFTR may be evident in asymptomatic patients by elevated or borderline sweat chloride concentration (between 40–60 mmol/l) or abnormal nasal potential difference.[24] The discovery of obstructive lung disease or CFTR dysfunction would fulfil the diagnostic criteria for cystic fibrosis and these men should be managed accordingly. Of the four organs affected in classic cystic fibrosis patients (lungs, pancreas, sweat gland, and vas deferens), the vas deferens appears to be the first to be affected when the level of CFTR function is decreased.

IDIOPATHIC PANCREATITIS

Idiopathic pancreatitis is defined as an acute or chronic inflammation of the pancreas without an apparent underlying cause of disease. Non-classic cystic fibrosis patients who are pancreatic sufficient are at risk for developing pancreatitis.[25] A number of studies have shown that a fraction of patients presenting with either chronic or acute idiopathic pancreatitis have one or two deleterious mutations in *CFTR*.[26,27] Noone and colleagues[28] demonstrated that the number of patients presenting with idiopathic chronic pancreatitis was underestimated in earlier studies that used standard *CFTR* screening methods. Their study found 9 compound heterozygotes and 8 patients who carried only one *CFTR* mutation after analysis of the coding region of *CFTR* in 41 patients with chronic pancreatitis. Furthermore, patients with one or two unusual *CFTR* mutations had CFTR dysfunction documented by abnormal sweat chloride concentration and/or nasal potential difference. These data confirm the usefulness of *CFTR* genotyping, sweat testing, and nasal potential difference measurements in patients who present with idiopathic pancreatitis. Patients with two *CFTR* mutations or evidence of CFTR dysfunction should be closely monitored for other cystic fibrosis manifestations. Indeed, a small percentage of non-classic cystic fibrosis patients present with pancreatitis before any other manifestation of disease.[25] However, mutations in *CFTR* do not account for all cases of idiopathic pancreatitis, suggesting a role for other genes or environmental factors.

IDIOPATHIC BRONCHIECTASIS

Idiopathic bronchiectasis is the irreversible dilation of the bronchi due to an unknown cause, often a result of chronic infection. Some studies of idiopathic bronchiectasis patients have identified more carriers of one *CFTR* mutation than expected,[29] while others have not.[30] However, the lack of association between *CFTR* and bronchiectasis in two studies may be the consequence of small sample size or incomplete analysis of the *CFTR* gene. Nevertheless, comprehensive studies on a larger cohort of bronchiectasis patients are needed to confirm the role of *CFTR* in bronchiectasis.

CHRONIC RHINOSINUSITIS

Most classic cystic fibrosis patients manifest disease in the nasal sinuses in the form of chronic rhinosinusitis, a persistent inflammation of the nasal and paranasal mucosa. In a study of 147 patients diagnosed with chronic rhinosinusitis in the absence of other overt symptoms of cystic fibrosis, 7% were found to carry one *CFTR* mutation in comparison to 2% of healthy controls (2/123).[31] One patient was identified with two *CFTR* mutations. Upon further clinical analysis of the latter patient, multiple features of cystic fibrosis were discovered and this patient was ultimately diagnosed with cystic fibrosis. Most of the chronic rhinosinusitis patients who were heterozygous for a *CFTR* mutation had other *CFTR* variants in their second *CFTR* allele, particularly the M470V polymorphism. A number of patients who carried one *CFTR* mutation had other symptoms of cystic fibrosis including borderline sweat chloride concentration or infection with *P. aeruginosa*. A similar study was performed in 58 children with chronic rhinosinusitis.[32] Mutations in *CFTR* were identified in 7 patients, a much larger number than expected based on the population frequency of *CFTR* mutations. Like the previous study, patients were identified with cystic fibrosis-like disease in other organ systems. In both studies, the frequency of CFTR mutations may be underestimated due to only screening for common mutations and not sequencing CFTR in all patients. On the other hand, a study of chronic rhinosinusitis patients in Finland failed to find a link between the two most common CFTR mutations in the general population in Finland and the development of chronic rhinosinusitis.[33] The concept that the presence of a single CFTR mutation predisposes to chronic rhinosinusitis has been validated in a study looking at the prevalence of chronic rhinosinusitis among CFTR mutation carriers. Wang et al.[34] found that there is an increased prevalence of chronic rhinosinusitis in cystic fibrosis carriers than in the general population. Taken together, these studies indicate that mutations in CFTR contribute to the aetiology of chronic rhinosinusitis in a fraction of patients, but other genetic or environmental factors are also implicated.

ALLERGIC BRONCHOPULMONARY ASPERGILLOSIS

Allergic bronchopulmonary aspergillosis is an inflammatory disorder of the airways caused by hypersensitivity to Aspergillosis fumigates, a common fungus. Allergic bronchopulmonary aspergillosis has been reported in up to 10% of classic cystic fibrosis patients.[2] Three studies have found that CFTR mutations are more common than expected in allergic bronchopulmonary aspergillosis patients.[35-37] Each of the patients enrolled in these studies met the diagnostic criteria for allergic bronchopulmonary aspergillosis in the absence of other symptoms of cystic fibrosis. As in the case of chronic rhinosinusitis, the number of CFTR mutation carriers may be underestimated because the entire coding region of CFTR was not analysed in the three studies. It appears likely that CFTR mutations account for only a small portion of allergic bronchopulmonary aspergillosis susceptibility and other factors play a significant role.

ELEVATED SWEAT CHLORIDE CONCENTRATION

While some patients with cystic fibrosis and two CFTR mutations can have a normal sweat chloride concentration (< 40 mmol/L), it has also been observed that mutations in CFTR can give rise to an abnormal sweat test in the absence of other features of cystic fibrosis. A mother and two daughters have been identified with an abnormal sweat test, but only one daughter had other clinical signs of cystic fibrosis.[38] Mutation analysis of CFTR identified S1455X in the mother and daughter with elevated sweat chloride concentration. Salvatore et al.[39] subsequently identified a set of sisters carrying S1455X and ΔF508. These patients appear clinically normal, yet each has a sweat chloride concentration in the cystic fibrosis range. It is possible that S1455X, in combination with a severe CFTR allele may also cause congenital bilateral absence of the vas deferens, but only one male has been identified with this genotype and his reproductive status is not known.[40] Thus, in females, it is possible for CFTR dysfunction to manifest as isolated elevated sweat chloride due to two mutations in CFTR. However, this only occurs in the context of a very specific CFTR mutation. Therefore, mutations in CFTR cannot account for disease in a large majority of patients who present with isolated elevated sweat chloride. It appears that other environmental or genetic factors are playing a substantial role.

Table 2 Causes of elevated sweat chloride concentration

- Anorexia nervosa
- Autonomic dysfunction
- Cystic fibrosis
- Environmental deprivation
- Familial cholestasis
- Fucosidosis
- Glucose-6-phosphate dehydrogenase deficiency
- Glycogen storage disease type I
- Klinefelter's syndrome
- Long-term prostaglandin E infusion
- Mauriac's syndrome
- Mucopolysaccharidosis type I
- Nephrogenic diabetes insipidus
- Nephrosis
- Protein-calorie malnutrition
- Pseudohypoaldosteronism
- Psychosocial failure to thrive
- Untreated adrenal insufficiency
- Untreated hypothyroidism

OTHER PHENOTYPES RELATED TO CFTR DYSFUNCTION

Neonatal screening has identified a cystic fibrosis-like phenotype in newborn carriers of one *CFTR* mutation. The initial neonatal screening test for cystic fibrosis is the measurement of immunoreactive trypsinogen in a blood spot. Neonates with classic cystic fibrosis have an elevated immunoreactive trypsinogen due to pancreatic dysfunction. A number of groups have noted that carriers of one *CFTR* mutation have higher neonatal immunoreactive trypsinogen values than non-carriers.[41,42] Newborns who carry only one *CFTR* mutation have immunoreactive trypsinogen values in the upper end of the normal range and normal sweat chloride concentrations. The role of *CFTR* has been studied in a number of additional phenotypes which overlap with the clinical spectrum of cystic fibrosis. A role for CFTR dysfunction has been suggested in asthma, the development of nasal polyps, and primary sclerosing cholangitis, a chronic progressive cholestatic liver disease.[43–45] Patients with these disorders may or may not have a slightly higher probability of carrying one *CFTR* mutation than the general population.

DIAGNOSIS OF CYSTIC FIBROSIS IN NON-CLASSIC PATIENTS

In 1998, the US Cystic Fibrosis Foundation Consensus Panel provided updated criteria for the diagnosis of cystic fibrosis.[46] The panel indicated that cystic fibrosis should be diagnosed on the basis of one or more clinical features of cystic fibrosis, a history of cystic fibrosis in a sibling, or a positive newborn screening test plus laboratory evidence of CFTR dysfunction by elevated sweat chloride concentration measured by pilocarpine iontophoresis or abnormal nasal epithelial ion transport or the identification of two *CFTR* mutations. Thus, the diagnosis of cystic fibrosis cannot be excluded in patients with cystic fibrosis-like features with evidence of CFTR dysfunction in the absence of two *CFTR* mutations.

A number of tests are useful in the evaluation of a patient presenting with features of non-classic cystic fibrosis. The measurement of sweat chloride by pilocarpine iontophoresis is the most common and most wide-spread test for demonstrating CFTR dysfunction. Age, diet, and measurement errors including low volume of sweat can have significant influence on sweat chloride concentration and can lead to false positive results. For these reasons, it is reasonable to perform testing on at least two separate occasions in patients with borderline abnormal results. It must also be noted that the sweat test is

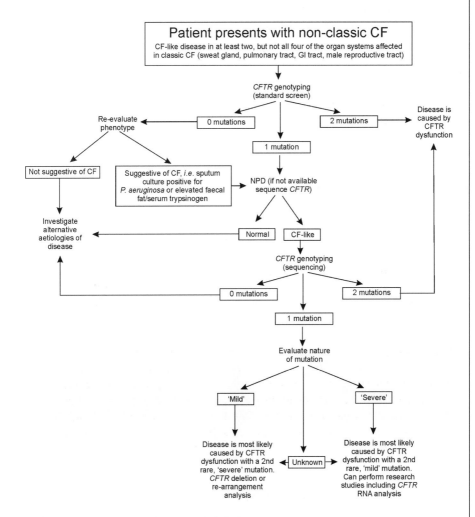

Fig. 2 Algorithm for the clinical and laboratory evaluation of patients with features of non-classic cystic fibrosis (CF). This diagram illustrates the recommended steps to follow for the evaluation of patients who present with cystic fibrosis-like symptoms in a subset of the four organ systems affected in classic cystic fibrosis. Sweat testing should be performed on two separate occasions and the presence of the vas deferens must be evaluated in male patients.

Table 3 Syndromes with clinical symptoms that overlap with non-classic cystic fibrosis in two or more organ systems

Disease	Sinopulmonary tract	Gastrointestinal tract	Male infertility	Sweat [Cl⁻]	Mode of inheritance
Non-classic cystic fibrosis	±	±	±	±	Most cases autosomal recessive with one *CFTR* mutation permitting partial function
Young syndrome	Chronic infections resulting in bronchiectasis	None	Yes, obstructive azoospermia caused by obstruction of the epididymis	Normal	Autosomal recessive?
Primary ciliary dyskinesia	Chronic infections resulting in bronchiectasis	None	Yes, caused by immotile spermatozoa	Normal	Autosomal recessive with extensive genetic heterogeneity. Can be caused by mutations in *DNAI1* or *DNAH5*
Immunodeficiency (*i.e.* bare lymphocyte syndrome, ICOS deficiency, immuno-deficiency with hyper IgM type 4)	Chronic bacterial infections	Chronic bacterial infections	None	Normal	Autosomal recessive
Schwachman–Diamond syndrome	Chronic bacterial infections (species of *Pseudomonas*, *Staphylococcus aureus*, *Haemophilus influenzae*)	Pancreatic insufficiency because of hyposecretion of pancreatic enzymes	None	Normal	Autosomal recessive, caused by mutations in *SBDS*
Pseudohypo-aldosteronism	Recurrent infections early in life (*Pseudomonas aeruginosa*, *Staphylococcus aureus*, *Haemophilus influenzae*)	None	None	Elevated (greater than 60 mmol/l)	Autosomal recessive, caused by mutations in α-, β-, or $\gamma ENaC$

not specific for cystic fibrosis (Table 2).[47] Conversely, there are some non-classic cystic fibrosis patients who have intermediate or normal sweat chloride concentration. Therefore, while an elevated sweat chloride concentration is highly predictive of cystic fibrosis, other clinical testing must be performed to confirm a cystic fibrosis diagnosis. It is also useful to evaluate the vas deferens in males presenting with non-classic cystic fibrosis. Because the vas deferens is especially sensitive to a low level of CFTR dysfunction, its presence or absence can be predictive of CFTR genotype. Nasal potential difference measurement is a measure of CFTR function in respiratory epithelium. Nasal potential difference can distinguish non-classic cystic fibrosis patients with disease due to two CFTR mutations and those without CFTR mutations. Patients with a normal nasal potential difference are unlikely to have disease caused by CFTR dysfunction and other aetiologies of disease should be investigated in these individuals. However, nasal potential difference testing is not widely available, whereas screening for common cystic fibrosis mutations is easy to perform. On this basis, we present an algorithm for the efficient evaluation of non-classic cystic fibrosis patients (Fig. 2).

The identification of CFTR mutations in patients with non-classic cystic fibrosis has important implications for diagnosis, prognosis, and treatment. Standard mutations screens incorporate about 20 of the most common cystic fibrosis mutations allowing identification of approximately 85% of the abnormal CFTR genes in Caucasians.[2] These panels include a combination of 'severe' and 'mild' mutations and are appropriate for the initial evaluation of a patient presenting with non-classic cystic fibrosis. A percentage of patients will be identified with only one common CFTR mutation after screening. In patients with non-classic cystic fibrosis, the presence of one common CFTR mutation predicts the presence of a second, rare mutation.[11] If available, nasal potential difference testing can be useful at this point and can distinguish patients with cystic fibrosis because of CFTR dysfunction from individuals who are carriers of only one CFTR mutation.[48] If no mutations are identified in CFTR after the initial screening, it is appropriate to re-evaluate the patient's phenotype to be certain that it is suggestive of cystic fibrosis.

If it is not feasible to perform a nasal potential difference or the nasal potential difference is abnormal, it is reasonable to consider sequencing CFTR. Most rare mutations can be identified through extensive sequencing of the coding regions of CFTR in an experienced diagnostic laboratory. However, there are limitations to the types of mutations which can be identified by standard sequencing methods. It is possible that patients may carry other rare mutations including gross deletions, gene re-arrangements or mutations in non-coding regions. In patients with only one identified CFTR mutation after sequencing who have a phenotype which is highly suggestive of cystic fibrosis or an abnormal nasal potential difference, additional steps can be taken to identify the second rare CFTR mutation. If the identified mutation is 'mild', the sample can be screened for genomic deletions or re-arrangements in the CFTR gene.[49] Mutations in CFTR non-coding regions can be identified through CFTR RNA analysis in a research setting. Patients who have no mutations identified after sequencing of CFTR should be re-evaluated and alternative aetiologies for disease should be investigated.

There are a number of different syndromes unrelated to CFTR dysfunction which have a clinical spectrum which overlaps with the non-classic cystic fibrosis phenotype (Table 3).[50-52] In most cases, patients with these disorders can be differentiated from cystic fibrosis patients based on clinical features. Patients with these syndromes will have a normal sweat chloride concentration in the presence of other clinical or laboratory findings which are not typical of cystic fibrosis. A notable exception is systemic pseudohypoaldosteronism Type I, an autosomal recessive disorder caused by mutations in the genes encoding the subunits of the epithelial sodium channel (α-, β-, or $\gamma ENaC$).[53] Patients with pseudo-hypoaldosteronism have elevated sweat chloride concentration and can have recurrent respiratory tract infections early in life which are characterised by bacteria commonly found in the lungs of cystic fibrosis patients (*i.e. P. aeruginosa*).[54] Usually, patients with pseudohypoaldosteronism can be distinguished from those with cystic fibrosis because they typically present in the first weeks of life with severe renal salt wasting characterised by elevated serum aldosterone and renin. However, mutations in the β-subunit of *ENaC* have been identified in two non-classic cystic fibrosis patients with elevated sweat chloride concentration and cystic fibrosis-like pulmonary disease in the absence of renal salt wasting.[15] These data suggest that *βENaC* can play a role in the development of cystic fibrosis-like disease and should be evaluated in patients with elevated sweat chloride and cystic fibrosis-like pulmonary disease who do not have mutations in *CFTR* after sequencing of the coding region. Groman *et al.*[11] identified one patient who presented with a non-classic cystic fibrosis phenotype in the absence of *CFTR* mutations who had mutations in each Schwachman-Bodian-Diamond Syndrome gene. This patient was ultimately diagnosed with an atypical form of Schwachman Diamond Syndrome which presented as steatorrhea, low serum trypsinogen, chronic sinusitis, frequent pulmonary tract infections, and transient neutropenia. This patient had a borderline abnormal sweat chloride concentration, possibly due to insufficient quantity of sweat, illustrating the importance of sweat volume for accurate sweat testing.

Key points for clinical practice

- Classic cystic fibrosis is an autosomal recessive disorder which affects the sweat gland, pulmonary tract, gastrointestinal tract, and male reproductive tract. Classic cystic fibrosis patients have mutations in the gene encoding the cystic fibrosis transmembrane conductance regulator (CFTR), a cAMP-activated chloride channel found in the apical membrane of epithelial tissues.

- Non-classic cystic fibrosis patients manifest disease in only a subset of the organ systems affected in classic cystic fibrosis. Most patients have two deleterious mutations in *CFTR*, including one which permits some CFTR function.

- Rare patients presenting with a non-classic cystic fibrosis phenotype do not have *CFTR* mutations.

- The accurate diagnosis of non-classic cystic fibrosis has important implications for prognosis, family counselling, and treatment. A combination of clinical and genetic testing can aid in the diagnosis in atypical patients.

Key points for clinical practice*(continued)*

- Elevation of sweat chloride concentration can be indicative of CFTR dysfunction. However, there are a subset of non-classic cystic fibrosis patients who have normal sweat chloride concentrations.

- Nasal potential difference measurements are useful in distinguishing patients with non-classic cystic fibrosis caused by CFTR dysfunction from those with disease caused by mutations in genes other than *CFTR*.

- Standard *CFTR* mutation screens will identify two mutations in only a subset of patients with non-classic cystic fibrosis. Rare mutations can be identified through sequencing of the coding regions of *CFTR* in patients with evidence of CFTR dysfunction.

- Males with infertility due to congenital absence of the vas deferens often have one or two deleterious *CFTR* mutations. Comprehensive clinical and laboratory examination of these patients can reveal other symptoms of cystic fibrosis.

- Patients with idiopathic pancreatitis may have one or two deleterious *CFTR* mutations in the absence of other cystic fibrosis clinical symptoms.

- CFTR dysfunction appears to plays a role in the development of idiopathic bronchiectasis, chronic rhinosinusitis, allergic broncho-pulmonary aspergillosis, and elevated sweat chloride concentration. However, it seems that CFTR dysfunction contributes to, rather than causes disease in most patients with these phenotypes.

References

1. Riordan JR, Rommens JM, Kerem B et al. Identification of the cystic fibrosis gene: cloning and characterization of complementary DNA. *Science* 1989; **245**: 1066–1073.
2. Welsh MJ, Ramsey BW, Accurso FJ, Cutting GR. Cystic fibrosis. In: Scriver CR, Beaudet AL, Valle D, Sly WS. (eds) *The Metabolic and Molecular Bases of Inherited Disease*. New York: McGraw-Hill, 2001; 5121–5188.
3. Knowles MR, Paradiso AM, Boucher RC. *In vivo* nasal potential difference: techniques and protocols for assessing efficacy of gene transfer in cystic fibrosis. *Hum Gene Therapy* 1995; **6**: 445–455.
4. Gibson LE, Cooke RE. A test for concentration of electrolytes in sweat in cystic fibrosis of the pancreas utilizing pilocarpine by iontophoresis. *Pediatrics* 1959; **23**: 545–549.
5. Callen A, Diener-West M, Zeitlin PL, Rubenstein RC. A simplified cyclic adenosine monophosphate-mediated sweat rate test for quantitative measure of cystic fibrosis transmembrane regulator (CFTR) function. *J Pediatr* 2000; **137**: 849–855.
6. Stutts MJ, Canessa CM, Olsen JC et al. CFTR as a cAMP-dependent regulator of sodium channels. *Science* 1995; **269**: 847–850.
7. Cheng SH, Gregory RJ, Marshall J *et al.* Defective intracellular transport and processing of CFTR is the molecular basis of most cystic fibrosis. *Cell* 1990; **63**: 827–834.
8. Cutting GR. Modifier genetics: cystic fibrosis. *Annu Rev Genomics Hum Genet* 2005; **6**: 237–260.
9. Cutting GR. *Cystic Fibrosis. Emery and Rimon's Principles and Practice of Medical Genetics*, 4th edn. London: Churchill-Livingstone, 2002.

10. Knowles MR, Durie PR. What is cystic fibrosis? *N Engl J Med* 2002; **347**: 439–442.
11. Groman JD, Karczeski B, Sheridan M, Robinson TE, Fallin MD, Cutting GR. Phenotypic and genetic characterization of patients with features of 'nonclassic' forms of cystic fibrosis. *J Pediatr* 2005; **146**: 675–680.
12. Mekus F, Ballmann M, Bronsveld I, Dörk T, Bijman J, Tummler B. Cystic-fibrosis-like disease unrelated to the cystic fibrosis transmembrane conductance regulator. *Hum Genet* 1998; **102**: 582–586.
13. Hughes D, Dork T, Stuhrmann M, Graham C. Mutation and haplotype analysis of the CFTR gene in atypically mild cystic fibrosis patients from Northern Ireland. *J Med Genet* 2001; **38**: 136–139.
14. Groman JD, Meyer ME, Wilmott RW, Zeitlin PL, Cutting GR. Variant cystic fibrosis phenotypes in the absence of CFTR mutations. *N Engl J Med* 2002; **347**: 401–407.
15. Sheridan MB, Fong P, Groman JD *et al*. Mutations in the beta subunit of the epithelial Na⁺ channel in patients with a cystic fibrosis-like syndrome. *Hum Mol Genet* 2005; **14**: 3493–3498.
16. Noone PG, Knowles MR. 'CFTR-opathies': disease phenotypes associated with cystic fibrosis transmembrane regulator gene mutations. *Respir Res* 2001; **2**: 328–332.
17. Cuppens H, Cassiman JJ. CFTR mutations and polymorphisms in male infertility. *Int J Androl* 2004; **27**: 251–256.
18. Claustres M, Guittard C, Bozon D *et al*. Spectrum of CFTR mutations in cystic fibrosis and in congenital absence of the vas deferens in France. *Hum Mutat* 2000; **16**: 143–156.
19. Chillon M, Casals T, Mercier B *et al*. Mutations in the cystic fibrosis gene in patients with congenital absence of the vas deferens. *N Engl J Med* 1995; **332**: 1475–1480.
20. Cuppens H, Lin W, Jaspers M *et al*. Polyvariant mutant cystic fibrosis transmembrane conductance regulator genes: The polymorphic (TG)m locus explains the partial penetrance of the 5T polymorphism as a disease mutation. *J Clin Invest* 1998; **101**: 487–496.
21. Groman JD, Hefferon TW, Casals T *et al*. Variation in a repeat sequence determines whether a common variant of the cystic fibrosis transmembrane conductance regulator gene is pathogenic or benign. *Am J Hum Genet* 2004; **74**: 176–179.
22. Mak V, Zielenski J, Tsui LC *et al*. Proportion of cystic fibrosis gene mutations not detected by routine testing in men with obstructive azoospermia. *JAMA* 1999; **281**: 2217–2224.
23. De Rose AF, Giglio M, Gallo F, Romano L, Carmignani G. Congenital bilateral absence of the vasa deferentia and related respiratory disease. *Arch Ital Urol Androl* 2003; **75**: 214–216.
24. Pradal U, Castellani C, Delmarco A, Mastella G. Nasal potential difference in congenital bilateral absence of the vas deferens. *Am J Respir Crit Care Med* 1998; **158**: 896–901.
25. Durno C, Corey M, Zielenski J, Tullis E, Tsui LC, Durie P. Genotype and phenotype correlations in patients with cystic fibrosis and pancreatitis. *Gastroenterology* 2002; **123**: 1857–1864.
26. Cohn JA, Mitchell RM, Jowell PS. The role of cystic fibrosis gene mutations in determining susceptibility to chronic pancreatitis. *Gastroenterol Clin North Am* 2004; **33**: 817–837, vii.
27. Bishop MD, Freedman SD, Zielenski J *et al*. The cystic fibrosis transmembrane conductance regulator gene and ion channel function in patients with idiopathic pancreatitis. *Hum Genet* 2005; **118**: 372–381.
28. Noone PG, Zhou Z, Silverman LM, Jowell PS, Knowles MR, Cohn JA. Cystic fibrosis gene mutations and pancreatitis risk: relation to epithelial ion transport and trypsin inhibitor gene mutations. *Gastroenterology* 2001; **121**: 1310–1319.
29. Pignatti PF, Bombieri C, Marigo C, Benetazzo M, Luisetti M. Increased incidence of cystic fibrosis gene mutations in adults with disseminated bronchiectasis. *Hum Mol Genet* 1995; **4**: 635–639.
30. Divac A, Nikolic A, Mitic-Milikic M *et al*. CFTR mutations and polymorphisms in adults with disseminated bronchiectasis: a controversial issue. *Thorax* 2005; **60**: 85.
31. Wang X, Moylan B, Leopold DA *et al*. Mutation in the gene responsible for cystic fibrosis and predisposition to chronic rhinosinusitis in the general population. *JAMA* 2000; **284**: 1814–1819.
32. Raman V, Clary R, Siegrist KL, Zehnbauer B, Chatila TA. Increased prevalence of mutations in the cystic fibrosis transmembrane conductance regulator in children with chronic rhinosinusitis. *Pediatrics* 2002; **109**: E13.
33. Hytonen M, Patjas M, Vento SI *et al*. Cystic fibrosis gene mutations deltaF508 and 394delTT in patients with chronic sinusitis in Finland. *Acta Otolaryngol* 2001; **121**: 945–947.

34. Wang XJ, Kim J, McWilliams R, Cutting GR. Increased prevalence of chronic rhinosinusitis in carriers of a cystic fibrosis mutation. *Arch Otolaryngol Head Neck Surg* 2005; **131**: 237–240.

35. Miller PW, Hamosh A, Macek Jr M *et al*. Cystic fibrosis transmembrane conductance regulator (CFTR) gene mutations in allergic bronchopulmonary aspergillosis. *Am J Hum Genet* 1996; **59**: 45–51.

36. Marchand E, Verellen-Dumoulin C, Mairesse M *et al*. Frequency of cystic fibrosis transmembrane conductance regulator gene mutations and 5T allele in patients with allergic bronchopulmonary aspergillosis. *Chest* 2001; **119**: 762–767.

37. Eaton TE, Weiner Miller P, Garrett JE, Cutting GR. Cystic fibrosis transmembrane conductance regulator gene mutations: do they play a role in the aetiology of allergic bronchopulmonary aspergillosis? *Clin Exp Allergy* 2002; **32**: 756–761.

38. Mickle J, Macek Jr M, Fulmer-Smentek SB *et al*. A mutation in the cystic fibrosis transmembrane conductance regulator gene associated with elevated sweat chloride concentrations in the absence of cystic fibrosis. *Hum Mol Genet* 1998; **7**: 729–735.

39. Salvatore D, Tomaiuolo R, Vanacore B, Elce A, Castaldo G, Salvatore F. Isolated elevated sweat chloride concentrations in the presence of the rare mutation S1455X: an extremely mild form of CFTR dysfunction. *Am J Med Genet* 2005; **133A**: 207–208.

40. Epaud R, Girodon E, Corvol H *et al*. Mild cystic fibrosis revealed by persistent hyponatremia during the French 2003 heat wave, associated with the S1455X C-terminus CFTR mutation. *Clin Genet* 2005; **68**: 552–553.

41. Laroche D, Travert G. Abnormal frequency of F508 mutation in neonatal transitory hypertyrosinaemia. *Lancet* 1991; **337**: 55.

42. Castellani C, Picci L, Scarpa M *et al*. Cystic fibrosis carriers have higher neonatal immuno-reactive trypsinogen values than non-carriers. *Am J Med Genet* 2005; **135A**: 142–144.

43. Lazaro C, de Cid R, Sunyer J *et al*. Missense mutations in the cystic fibrosis gene in adult patients with asthma. *Hum Mutat* 1999; **14**: 510–519.

44. Kostuch M, Klatka J, Semczuk A, Wojcierowski J, Kulczycki L, Oleszczuk J. Analysis of most common CFTR mutations in patients affected by nasal polyps. *Eur Arch Otorhinolaryngol* 2005; **262**: 982–986.

45. Sheth S, Shea JC, Bishop MD *et al*. Increased prevalence of CFTR mutations and variants and decreased chloride secretion in primary sclerosing cholangitis. *Hum Genet* 2003; **113**: 286–292.

46. Rosenstein BJ, Cutting GR. The diagnosis of cystic fibrosis: a consensus statement. *J Pediatr* 1998; **132**: 589–595.

47. LeGrys VA, Burritt MF, Gibson LE, Hammond KB, Kraft K, Rosenstein BJ. *Sweat Testing: Sample Collection and Quantitative Analysis; Approved Guideline*. Villanova, PA: NCCLS, 1994.

48. Wilschanski M, Famini H, Strauss-Liviatan N *et al*. Nasal potential difference measurements in patients with atypical cystic fibrosis. *Eur Respir J* 2001; **17**: 1208–1215.

49. Audrezet MP, Chen JM, Raguenes O *et al*. Genomic rearrangements in the CFTR gene: extensive allelic heterogeneity and diverse mutational mechanisms. *Hum Mutat* 2004; **23**: 343–357.

50. Schanker HM, Rajfer J, Saxon A. Recurrent respiratory disease, azoospermia, and nasal polyposis. A syndrome that mimics cystic fibrosis and immotile cilia syndrome. *Arch Intern Med* 1985; **145**: 2201–2203.

51. Bush A, Cole P, Hariri M *et al*. Primary ciliary dyskinesia: diagnosis and standards of care. *Eur Respir J* 1998; **12**: 982–988.

52. Boocock GR, Morrison JA, Popovic M *et al*. Mutations in SBDS are associated with Shwachman-Diamond syndrome. *Nat Genet* 2003; **33**: 97–101.

53. Chang SS, Grunder S, Hanukoglu A *et al*. Mutations in subunits of the epithelial sodium channel cause salt wasting with hyperkalaemic acidosis, pseudohypoaldosteronism type 1. *Nat Genet* 1996; **12**: 248–253.

54. Marthinsen L, Kornfalt R, Aili M, Andersson D, Westgren U, Schaedel C. Recurrent *Pseudomonas* bronchopneumonia and other symptoms as in cystic fibrosis in a child with type I pseudohypoaldosteronism. *Acta Paediatr* 1998; **87**: 472–474.

Ronit M. Pressler

12

Behaviour problems in children with epilepsy

Behaviour, in the broadest sense, encompasses all activities concerning autonomic responses and integrated reactions to dynamic situations, the experiencing and expressing of emotions and the forming and maintaining of interpersonal relationships. Epilepsy can be defined as two or more unprovoked seizures of any type. Therefore, febrile seizures and seizures in the course of acute trauma or infection are not classified as epilepsy.

Population-based studies have shown that febrile seizures in early childhood do not have an adverse effect on behaviour.[1] However, children with epilepsy are at a higher risk of developing behavioural problems and psychiatric disorders than their healthy peers. In the Isle of White study, psychiatric disorders, including significant behavioural problems occurred in 7% (*n* = 2189) of school children in the general population, in 16% of children with chronic medical disorders, 29% of children suffering from idiopathic epilepsy, and in 58% of epilepsy cases associated with structural cerebral abnormalities.[2] Psychiatric disorders are co-morbid with epilepsy due to selection bias, genetic factors or environmental factors and may precede, co-occur or follow the onset of epilepsy.[3,4]

Austin *et al.*[5] compared quality of life in children with epilepsy and those with asthma, another chronic disease with unpredictable episodes that requires medication and regular visits to a physician. Children with epilepsy showed a more compromised quality of life in psychological, social and educational domains, even though they developed their condition at a later age and were having fewer episodes. In contrast, children with asthma had a more compromised quality of life in the physical domain. This suggests that, in addition to dealing with a chronic disorder, other aspects of epilepsy are related to a poor quality of life.

Ronit M. Pressler MD MRCPCH
SpR Clinical Neurophysiology, Department of Clinical Neurophysiology, The National Hospital for
Neurology, Queen Square, London WC1N 3BG, UK
E-mail: ronit.pressler@uclh.org

Though the increased prevalence of behavioural problems has often been documented in children with chronic seizures, several studies have also shown an increased prevalence of behavioural problems in children with new-onset seizures or children whose seizures respond well to anti-epileptic drug treatment and are educated in mainstream schools. Of children with new onset epilepsy, 30–50% were at risk or having clinical behavioural problems,[6,7] in contrast to less than 20% of children with new-onset diabetes.[6] This may be due to previously unrecognised seizures or due to neurological dysfunction responsible for both seizures and behavioural problems. Children with epilepsy attending mainstream schools have been found to have more learning and behavioural problems in school compared to healthy matched controls and achieve less than expected for their age and IQ.[8,9] This is in contrast to a population-based study in Australia which suggested that behavioural problems are mainly related to intellectual disability.[10]

Increased behavioural problems in children with epilepsy are a consequence of a range of multifaceted and overlapping influences including underlying brain lesion, age of onset of seizures, anti-epileptic drugs, psychosocial issues, seizure type and frequency, and interictal EEG abnormalities (Fig. 1).

SPECIFIC BEHAVIOURAL PROBLEMS

Epilepsy in childhood has been associated with specific behavioural problems and psychiatric co-morbidity, with mood disorders and disruptive behaviours being found most commonly. Boys with epilepsy, particularly those with partial seizures, are more likely to have inattentive and conduct problems.[11] Adolescent girls, particularly those with severe epilepsy during the transition to adolescence, are at a high risk of internalising and externalising behavioural problems.[12] As found in adults with epilepsy, there appears to be an association between depression and epilepsy in children and adolescents.[3] Around a quarter of school children wit epilepsy have been found to have symptoms of depression.[13] Neurosis is also more common in children and adolescent with epilepsy.

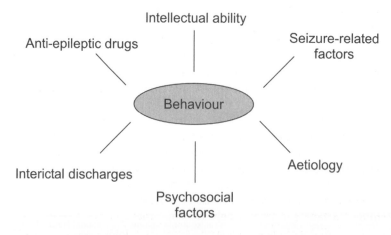

Fig. 1 Factors influencing behaviour in children with epilepsy.

Of the disruptive disorders, the association between attention-deficit/hyperactivity disorder (ADHD) and epilepsy has the best support from research data. Inattentive behaviour and co-morbid ADHD were found in 10–60% of children depending of the population studied.[14] More children with generalised tonic–clonic seizures had ADHD compared to children with partial seizures or absences.[14]

There seems to be an association between autism and epilepsy, with seizures occurring in up to one-third of children with autism. The incidence is higher in the presence of other neurological disability such as cerebral palsy. Tuchman and Rapin[15] have suggested that epilepsy and interictal discharges may be implicated in the pathophysiology of a minority of children with autism. However, symptoms of psychiatric disorders in children with epilepsy are poorly recognised and very few children receive a diagnosis or appropriate treatment.

FACTORS INFLUENCING BEHAVIOUR

AETIOLOGY

Several large studies have shown that children with symptomatic epilepsy are more likely to develop intellectual impairment, psychiatric disturbances and behavioural problems compared to patients with idiopathic epilepsy.[2] Brain dysfunction may be independent of the epilepsy (e.g. in children with cortical dysplasia) or may be caused by the epilepsy (e.g. in children with epileptic encephalopathy). Besag[16] has recently reviewed behavioural aspects of paediatric epilepsy syndromes.

There is little doubt that localisation of brain lesions can cause specific behavioural dysfunction. Frontal lobe dysfunction may result in grossly disinhibited behaviour, which may present with features resembling attention-deficit disorder. Dominant temporal damage may result in poor language function with accompanying frustration and behavioural disturbances. Non-dominant dysfunction may cause significant visuospatial problems. If their verbal abilities are intact, their problems are usually much more difficult to estimate for others.[17] Consequently, parents and teachers will set expectations too high and the children will fail repeatedly which has great implications for their self-esteem. Stores and colleagues[11] demonstrated significantly more behavioural disturbances in boys with left temporal discharges than in boys with epilepsy but without inter-ictal discharges.

Several symptomatic epilepsy syndromes are also associated with behaviour disturbances.

In **infantile spasms**, there is initially cognitive arrest or regression which can be autistic. Neuropsychological outcome is variable but the proportion of cases with behavioural problems or psychiatric disorders such as autism and ADHD is high. In tuberous sclerosis, autism is related to temporal lobe tubers.[18]

In children with **severe myoclonic epilepsy**, behavioural problems are commonly found, but there are no systematic reviews.

In **Lennox-Gastaut syndrome**, behavioural problems are frequent with hypokinesia and distractibility. Psychosis, aggressive behaviour and autistic feature are common.

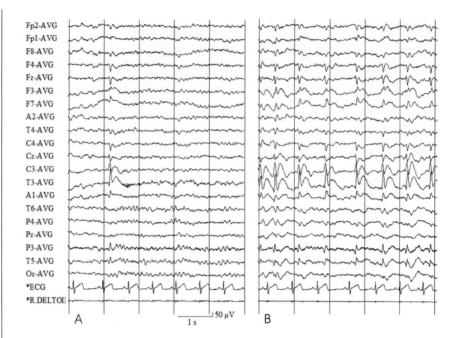

Fig. 2 Boy aged 5 years with nocturnal oro-facial seizures and behavioural problems. (A) EEG during wakefulness shows occasional discharges in the centro-temporal region. (B) EEG during drowsiness where sleep discharges become nearly continuous.

Epilepsy with continuous spike and wave during slow-wave sleep is characterised by intellectual disturbance and behavioural problems in a previously normal child, but may also be seen in children with early thalamic injury.[19] The EEG shows electrical status epilepticus in slow-wave sleep with at least 85% of non-REM sleep occupied by spike and wave discharges (Fig. 2).

Landau-Kleffner syndrome presents with language regression (verbal auditory agnosia) and prolonged epileptiform discharges during non-REM sleep. Seizure may be infrequent; indeed, up to 30% of children with continuous spike and wave during slow wave sleep and Landau-Kleffner syndrome do not have overt seizures. Behavioural disturbances are the presenting symptoms in epilepsy with continuous spike and wave during slow wave sleep but are also very common Landau-Kleffner syndrome and include hyperkinesias, depression, aggressiveness and psychotic conditions. These difficulties may be secondary to the language difficulties; however, in a proportion of children, these problems precede the onset of agnosia. Continuous nocturnal EEG abnormalities are likely to contribute to behavioural and cognitive disturbances. Early intervention with anti-epileptic drugs such as steroids is associated with better outcome.[20]

Children with **idiopathic epilepsy** are also at risk of behavioural disturbances.[2] Benign partial epilepsy with centro-temporal spikes (Rolandic epilepsy) is one of the most common idiopathic epilepsy syndromes in childhood. It has been traditionally considered benign without mental retardation and neurological deficits. However, several studies have reported impaired cognition and behaviour.[21,22] Weglage *et al.*[21] assessed the behavioural status of 40 children with centro-temporal spikes with and without obvious seizures and compared them with 20 matched controls. The global behavioural scores of children with discharges (with or without seizures) were significantly worse than controls suggesting that EEG abnormalities play a more important role in the aetiology of behavioural dysfunction than the seizures. In a longitudinal study in children with benign partial epilepsy with centro-temporal spikes, atypical features were found in 10 of 35 children including deterioration of academic abilities and sociofamilial maladjustment.[23] This complicated evolution was associated with the following EEG criteria: intermittent slow-wave focus, asynchronous foci, long spike and wave clusters, generalised 3/s spike and wave discharges and prolonged discharges during sleep. Another explanation for neuropsychological deficits is a hereditary cerebral maturation disorder.[24]

Juvenile myoclonic epilepsy is one of the most important idiopathic generalised epilepsies in childhood and adolescence. In the original paper by Janz[25] in the late 1950s, patients were described as unstable, suggestive, unreliable and immature, often resulting in inadequate social adjustment. An increased rate of psychiatric disorders in juvenile myoclonic epilepsy compared to people with diabetes has been confirmed, even though there are no studies on behavioural and personality disturbances using standardised scales.[26]

SEIZURE-RELATED FACTORS

Seizure control is the most significant predictor of behavioural problems.[27] An earlier age of onset of seizures and a higher seizure frequency have also been associated with both lower cognitive abilities and increased behavioural problems.[6]

Children with temporal lobe epilepsy are more likely to develop behavioural problems and emotional problems (including neurosis, psychosis and personality disorders) than children with generalised seizures.[28] Pre-ictal changes (prodrome) can manifest as mood or behavioural disturbances lasting minutes to hours and in some children even days. An aura is often considered as a warning, but is, in fact, a simple partial seizure which may or may not progress to a complex partial seizure or a secondary generalised seizure. The child is fully conscious during the aura and symptoms often cause anxiety and the feeling of being out of control. Similarly, complex partial seizures arising from the amygdale can manifest with anxiety. Postictal changes are more common after complex partial seizure or generalised tonic–clonic seizure and include confusion, irritability or psychotic symptoms.

The threat of unpredictable seizures and the experience of being out of control during the seizure are features that make epilepsy unique among the chronic illnesses in childhood. The fear associated with this has major implications on family relationships and social integration as well as individual coping capacity.

ANTI-EPILEPTIC DRUGS

Anti-epileptic drugs interact with behaviour mainly in three ways:

1. Anti-epileptic drugs improve behaviour by treating seizures and suppressing interictal discharges in most children with epilepsy.

2. Some anti-epileptic drugs (*e.g.* sodium valproate, carbamazepine, lamotrigine and gabapentin) improve mood and play a role in the treatment of depression. Sodium valproate and lamotrigine are also used in bipolar disorders.[4]

3. Some anti-epileptic drugs have adverse cognitive and behavioural effects, particularly if titrated rapidly, high doses are given or the inadequate anti-epileptic drugs is used for a specific syndrome.

Unfortunately, there is a misconception between parents and doctors about the relevance of these factors. Initially, the most important aim in the management of epilepsy must be treating the seizures; in 60–70% of children, good seizure control can be achieved with one or two anti-epileptic drugs with consequently improved psychosocial functioning. Poor seizure control is closely related to behavioural problems.[27] Some anti-epileptic drugs can cause behavioural disturbances if used inadequately by increasing seizures; for example, carbamazepine and phenytoin in some idiopathic generalised epilepsies. Carbamazepine can increase nocturnal discharges in some children with benign partial epilepsy with centro-temporal spikes and may be associated with a deterioration of language abilities and behaviour.

Nevertheless, many parents and doctors are concerned about behavioural effects and this is reflected in a large number of studies, most in adults.[29] However, there is still much uncertainty because of methodical shortcomings in many studies. These include: small sample size, short observation period, open label studies, no or inappropriate controls, no or inadequate randomisation, inappropriate statistical methods and emphasising statistical significance over clinical relevance. The situation is even more uncertain in children with epilepsy.[29] There is convincing evidence that phenobarbital and clonazepam have a negative effect on behaviour in children with epilepsy.[30] The effects of other established anti-epileptic drugs in children are largely unclear due to the above-mentioned methodological problems. Some

Table 1 The effects of anti-epileptic drugs on behaviour[29,32]

Drug	Behavioural disturbances
Carbamazepine	No definite effect
Clonazepam	Restlessness, hyperactivity, behavioural disturbances
Gabapentin	Aggressive behaviour, hyperactivity
Ethosuximide	Psychosis
Lamotrigine	No definite effect. Restlessness and aggression in some children with learning difficulties have been described
Oxcarbazepine	Similar to carbamazepine
Phenobarbital	Hyperactivity, attention difficulty, conduct disturbances
Phenytoin	Little or no behavioural side effects. Some studies indicate attention difficulty and personality changes
Sodium valproate	No definite effect
Tiagabine	No definite effect
Topiramate	Psychosis, attention difficulty
Vigabatrine	Psychosis, depression, aggression, irritability

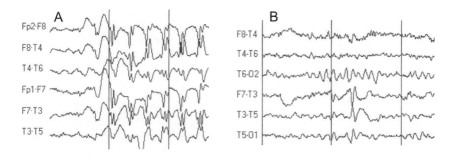

Fig. 3 Interictal discharges. (A) Generalised spike-and-wave in a teenager with juvenile absence epilepsy. (B) Focal sharp wave over left temporal region in a child with complex partial seizures.

behavioural disturbances are likely to occur with phenytoin, but are less evident with sodium valproate and carbamazepine. Further, there are very few studies of the more recently introduced anti-epileptic drugs in children using formal testing, although psychotic symptoms have been observed in children on topiramate and vigabatrine. Aggressive behaviour has been associated with lamotrigine, particularly in some children with learning difficulties. In an international, multicentre study, 2.5% of children were found to have behavioural side effects. The authors contributed this behaviour to patients becoming more alert, active, and demanding.[31] They argued that this may be a necessary stage in the rehabilitation of such patients following an improvement in seizure control. Psychotic symptoms have been described with ethosuximide, topiramate, and vigabatrine. Table 1 summarises the most important behavioural effects of old and new anti-epileptic drugs.

Side effects depend on speed of initial dose escalation dose of drug and, particularly in the case of phenytoin, on the duration of treatment. Polytherapy is more likely to cause behavioural problems than monotherapy.

INTERICTAL DISCHARGES

Subclinical or interictal discharges are epileptiform EEG discharges (Fig. 3) not accompanied by clinical events using available methods of clinical observation.[33] These discharges occur in up to 80% of patients with on-going epilepsy although they are not seen in every EEG recording. Interictal discharges have been associated with behavioural and cognitive dysfunction in both symptomatic and idiopathic epilepsy syndromes.[11,17] This association may be due to prolonged discharges during day-time causing non-convulsive status epilepticus, prolonged nocturnal discharges (electrical status epilepticus during slow-wave sleep) or a transitory impairment of cognitive function at the time of the discharge (transitory cognitive impairment or TCI).

Continuous epileptiform EEG activity without motor components lasting for hours, days, or even weeks is often referred to as non-convulsive status epilepticus. It may have a rather dramatic presentation as 'pseudo-dementia' but often the changes are more subtle. Unfortunately, there has been little systematic research of the effects of such prolonged discharges on mental function.

Electrical status epilepticus during slow-wave sleep is an EEG phenomenon, describing the occurrence of epileptiform discharges during no less than 85% of non-rapid eye movement (non-REM) sleep of continuous, bilateral diffuse slow spike and wave activity, which abates during REM periods. It occurs in the following four epileptic syndromes: (i) epilepsy with continuous spike and wave during slow-wave sleep; (ii) Landau-Kleffner syndrome; (iii) unilateral polymicrogyria; and (iv) some cases of benign partial epilepsy with centro-temporal spikes. Electrical status epilepticus has been associated with behavioural and cognitive dysfunction seen in these syndromes.[34] It has been suggested that benign partial epilepsy with centro-temporal spikes, Landau-Kleffner syndrome and epilepsy with continuous spike and wave during slow-wave sleep represent a spectrum with benign partial epilepsy with centro-temporal spikes forming the benign common and Landau-Kleffner syndrome and continuous spike and wave during slow-wave sleep the severe uncommon end.

Even brief discharges can cause brief disruptions of cognitive function. As early as 1939, Schwab[35] developed a method to measure visual reaction times during EEG recording. He found delayed or missing reactions during EEG discharges compared to presentations occurring without discharges. About 50 studies subsequently confirmed a direct temporal association between EEG discharges and brief impairment of cognitive function only detectable with appropriate psychological testing.[33,36] This was termed transitory cognitive impairment. Generalised bursts lasting at least 3 s are most likely to produce demonstrable cognitive impairment, but transitory cognitive impairments are also found during briefer and focal discharges.[33] The laterality of discharges has implications on the type of impairment: right-sided discharges are more likely to produce impairment of non-verbal tasks whereas left-sided discharges cause impairment of verbal performance. This means that transitory cognitive impairment is not a global impairment of attention but a specific impairment of cognitive function of the brain region involved in interictal discharges. Transitory cognitive impairment may affect day-to-day psychosocial function.[36] In children with benign partial epilepsy with centro-temporal spikes, epileptiform discharges causing transitory cognitive impairment are associated with an increased risk of behavioural problems.[37]

The concept of transitory cognitive impairment is still controversial. It has been argued that the EEG abnormalities are a co-existing but independent phenomena simply indicating the relative severity and distribution of cerebral pathology or pathophysiology among groups rather than reflecting a specific cause. The only way to differentiate between the two views is by finding an improvement of cognition and behaviour when EEG discharges are suppressed. Single observations and uncontrolled reports have claimed an improvement of cognitive functioning by suppressing discharges with anti-epileptic drugs in patients with epilepsy.[33] In a preliminary study, sodium valproate or clobazam add-on was used to suppress discharges in 10 children with uncontrolled epilepsy. A reduction of discharge rate was associated with improvement in global rating of psychosocial function in 8 out of 10 children.[38] However, all but one patient showed an unexpected reduction in seizure frequency on active treatment. This confounding factor made it difficult to interpret the results. In a recent double-blind, placebo-controlled, cross-over study, 61 children with well-controlled or mild epilepsy were randomly assigned to add-on therapy with lamotrigine.[39] Global rating of behaviour improved only in patients who showed a reduction in either frequency or duration of discharges ($P < 0.05$) during active treatment, but not in patients without a change in discharge rate. This suggests that suppressing interictal discharges can improve behaviour in some children with behavioural problems and epilepsy. These findings have to be used with caution and 'treating the EEG' remains controversial. However, the point at issue is not whether to treat the EEG, but whether seizures, so subtle as to be recognisable only by EEG and behavioural monitoring, produce disability sufficient to justify treatment. Further studies, with larger numbers of patients and long-term follow-up are needed to assess the benefit of treating the EEG in patients with interictal discharges.

INTELLECTUAL ABILITIES

It is obvious that cognitive dysfunction and behavioural problems are closely related. In a recent cross-sectional survey of behavioural problems in children with epilepsy, patients with abnormal behavioural scores were more likely to have learning difficulties.[40] Often, the same underlying brain dysfunction will cause both cognitive and behavioural problems. However, it is important to realise that learning difficulties themselves can lead to significant behavioural difficulties. This may be due to teasing, frustration, damaged self-esteem, stigmatisation or dysfunctional child–parent relationships. Particularly in children with mild or specific learning difficulties, the relevance is often underestimated. In return, behavioural problems in school and at home will have implications on learning leading to a viscous circle.

PSYCHOSOCIAL FACTORS

Adverse social attitudes play a major part, particularly the belief that a child with epilepsy is fundamentally incapable of the same levels of attainment as other children. As a consequence, parents' and teachers' expectations are set too low and this can negatively affect the child's effort, the child's attitude about his or her abilities, or the child's academic performance. Equally to be avoided is setting targets too high – unrealistic expectations. Some parents blame decreased achievement on seizures or medication and expect that changes in medical management will result in better performance. If the child's ability is within the lower range, these expectations may not be realistic and cause undue stress on the child resulting in low self-esteem. Such psychological factors have been relatively neglected in research on cognitive function in children with epilepsy, in favour of studies into biological influences.[41] Furthermore, the restrictions imposed by parents and doctors to avoid seizure-related injuries can impair quality of life and development, even though restrictions were often not adequately adapted to seizure-related risks and were, therefore, unnecessary.[42]

The threat of unpredictable seizures and the feeling of being out of control during the seizure are experienced by both child and parent. Even when seizures are well controlled, parental fear and expectations and the anxiety

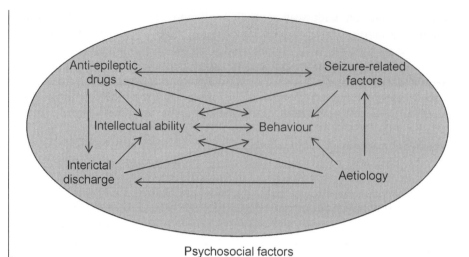

Fig. 4 Complex framework of factors affecting behaviour in children.

regarding the possibility of recurrence of seizures contribute to the long-term process of adjustment to the disease and to the child–parent relationship. Parent–child relationship and communication have been implicated as important predictors of outcomes such as self-esteem, dependency and academic achievement. It has been suggested that mothers' restrictions, overprotection or intrusive behaviour as well as her emotional support contribute to the children's lack of competence.[43]

As in the normal population the integrity of the family is one of the most important predictors of behavioural problems and has implications on coping mechanisms within the family. Social competence was associated most strongly with good seizure control, followed by shorter duration of epilepsy and higher family income.[27]

CONCLUSIONS

It is generally acknowledged that behavioural disturbances are common in children with epilepsy. These problems provide a major management challenge and can affect social outcome. However, limitations of studies on behaviour in children with epilepsy are small sample size, cross-sectional design, lack of control group and highly selected populations. It has been argued that if behavioural problems are present at the onset of seizures, then central nervous system dysfunction would be the most likely aetiology for both seizures and emotional problems. If behavioural problems develop later, then anti-epileptic drug side effects, the effects of recurrent seizures or problems with adaptation would be more likely causes.[7] However, this concept does not take into account that the child may have had unrecognised seizures before the diagnosis of epilepsy or indeed interictal discharges either during day-time causing transitory cognitive impairment or during sleep causing electrical status epilepticus during slow wave sleep.

All factors interact in complex ways and it is usually impossible to determine a specific factor responsible for psychosocial dysfunction. Aetiology, co-morbidity, epilepsy-related factors and anti-epileptic drugs build a framework (Fig. 4), which has to be considered in each child. Understanding the inter-relationships between these factors is essential in the management of these children.

Key points for clinical practice

- Children and adolescents with epilepsy have an increased risk of developing behavioural problems compared to healthy children and children with other chronic disease.

- Epilepsy in childhood has been associated with specific behavioural problems and psychiatric co-morbidity, with mood disorders and disruptive behaviours being found most commonly.

- The reasons for behaviour problems in epilepsy are multifactorial and interacting and include aetiology, age of onset of seizures, anti-epileptic drugs, psychosocial issues, seizure type and frequency, and interictal EEG abnormalities.

- Anti-epileptic drugs may improve behaviour by controlling seizures or an independent psychotropic effect. Some anti-epileptic drugs have adverse cognitive and behavioural effects, particularly if titrated rapidly, given in high doses or inadequate anti-epileptic drugs are used.

- Interictal discharges can cause transitory cognitive impairment which has been associated with behavioural problems. Treatment of interictal discharges may improve behaviour in some children with epilepsy.

- The threat of unpredictable seizures and the feeling of being out of control during seizures have major implications on self-esteem, child–parent relationships and social integration.

- Symptoms of psychiatric disorders in children with epilepsy are poorly recognised and very few children receive a diagnosis or appropriate treatment.

- Understanding the inter-relationships between these factors is essential in the management of these children.

References

1. Chang YC, Guo NW, Huang CC, Wang ST, Tsai JJ. Neurocognitive attention and behavior outcome of school-age children with a history of febrile convulsions: a population study. *Epilepsia* 2000; **41**: 412–420.
2. Rutter M, Graham P, Yule W. A neuropsychiatric study in childhood. *Clin Dev Med* 1970; **35/36**: 1–265.
3. Gaitatzis A, Trimble MR, Sander JW. The psychiatric comorbidity of epilepsy. *Acta Neurol Scand* 2004; **110**: 207–220
4. Pellock JM. Defining the problem: psychiatric and behavioral comorbidity in children and adolescents with epilepsy. *Epilepsy Behav* 2004; **5 (Suppl 3)**: S3–S9.
5. Austin JK, Smith MS, Risinger MW, McNelis AM. Childhood epilepsy and asthma: comparison of quality of life. *Epilepsia* 1994; **35**: 608–615.

6. Hoare P. Does illness foster dependency? A study of epileptic and diabetic children. *Dev Med Child Neurol* 1984; **26**: 20–24.
7. Dunn DW, Austin JK, Huster GA. Behaviour problems in children with new-onset epilepsy. *Seizure* 1997; **6**: 283–287.
8. Seidenberg M, Beck N, Geisser M *et al*. Academic achievement of children with epilepsy. *Epilepsia* 1986; **27**: 753–759.
9. Aman MG, Werry JS, Turbott SH. Behavior of children with seizures. Comparison with norms and effect of seizure type. *J Nerv Ment Dis* 1992; **180**: 124–129.
10. Lewis JN, Tonge BJ, Mowat DR, Einfeld SL, Siddons HM, Rees VW. Epilepsy and associated psychopathology in young people with intellectual disability. *J Paediatr Child Health* 2000; **36**: 172–175.
11. Stores G. School-children with epilepsy at risk for learning and behaviour problems. *Dev Med Child Neurol* 1978; **20**: 502–508.
12. Austin JK, Dunn DW, Huster GA. Childhood epilepsy and asthma: changes in behavioural problems related to gender and change in condition severity. *Epilepsia* 2000; **41**: 615–623.
13. Ettinger AB, Weisbrot DM, Saracco J, Dhoon A, Kanner A, Devinsky O. Positive and negative psychotropic effects of lamotrigine in patients with epilepsy and mental retardation. *Epilepsia* 1998; **39**: 874–877.
14. Dunn DW, Austin JK, Harezlak J, Ambrosius WT. ADHD and epilepsy in childhood. *Dev Med Child Neurol* 2003; **45**: 50–54.
15. Tuchman RF, Rapin I. Regression in pervasive developmental disorders: seizures and epileptiform electroencephalogram correlates. *Pediatrics* 1997; **99**: 560–566.
16. Besag F. Behavioural aspects of paediatric epilepsy syndromes. *Epilepsy Behav* 2004; **5**: 3–13.
17. Besag FM. Childhood epilepsy in relation to mental handicap and behavioural disorders. *J Child Psychol Psychiatry* 2002; **43**: 103–131.
18. Bolton PF, Park RJ, Higgins JN, Griffiths PD, Pickles A. Neuro-epileptic determinants of autism spectrum disorders in tuberous sclerosis complex. *Brain* 2002; **125**: 1247–1255.
19. Guzzetta F, Battaglia D, Veredice C *et al*. Early thalamic injury associated with epilepsy and continuous spike-wave during slow sleep. *Epilepsia* 2005; **46**: 889-900.
20. Robinson RO, Baird G, Robinson G, Simonoff E. Landau-Kleffner syndrome: course and correlates with outcome. *Dev Med Child Neurol* 2001; **43**: 243–247.
21. Weglage J, Demsky A, Pietsch M, Kurlemann G. Neuropsychological, intellectual, and behavioral findings in patients with centrotemporal spikes with and without seizures. *Dev Med Child Neurol* 1997; **39**: 646–651.
22. Croona C, Kihlgren M, Lundberg S, Eeg-Olofsson O, Eeg-Olofsson KE. Neuropsychological findings in children with benign childhood epilepsy with centrotemporal spikes. *Dev Med Child Neurol* 1999; **41**: 813–818.
23. Massa R, Saint-Martin A, Carcangiu R *et al*. EEG criteria predictive of complicated evolution in idiopathic Rolandic epilepsy. *Neurology* 2001; **57**: 1071–1079.
24. Doose H, Neubauer BA, Petersen B. The concept of hereditary impairment of brain maturation. *Epileptic Disord* 2000; **2 (Suppl 1)**: S45–S49.
25. Janz D, Christian W. Impulsive-petit mal. *Dtsch Z Nervenheilk* 1957; **176**: 346.
26. Perini GI, Tosin C, Carraro C *et al*. Interictal mood and personality disorders in temporal lobe epilepsy and juvenile myoclonic epilepsy. *J Neurol Neurosurg Psychiatry* 1996; **61**: 601–605.
27. Herman BP, Whitman S, Hughes JR, Melyn MM, Dell J. Multietiological determinants of psychopathology and social competence in children with epilepsy. *Epilepsy Res* 1988; **2**: 51–60.
28. Shukla GD, Srivastava ON, Katiyar BC, Joshi V, Mohan PK. Psychiatric manifestations in temporal lobe epilepsy: a controlled study. *Br J Psychiatry* 1979; **135**: 411–417.
29. Loring DW, Meador KJ. Cognitive side effects of antiepileptic drugs in children. *Neurology* 2004; **62**: 872–877.
30. Vining EP, Mellitis ED, Dorsen MM *et al*. Psychologic and behavioral effects of antiepileptic drugs in children: a double-blind comparison between phenobarbital and valproic acid. *Pediatrics* 1987; **80**: 165–174.
31. Besag FM, Wallace SJ, Dulac O, Alving J, Spencer SC, Hosking G. Lamotrigine for the treatment of epilepsy in childhood. *J Pediatr* 1995; **127**: 991–997.

32. Besag FM. Behavioural effects of the newer antiepileptic drugs: an update. *Expert Opin Drug Safety* 2004; **3**: 1–8.
33. Aarts JH, Binnie CD, Smit AM, Wilkins AJ. Selective cognitive impairment during focal and generalized epileptiform EEG activity. *Brain* 1984; **107**: 293–308.
34. Deonna T, Zesinger P, Davidoff V, Meader M, Roulet E. benign partial epilepsy of childhood: a longitudinal neuropsychological and EEG study of cognitive function. *Dev Med Child Neurol* 2000; **42**: 595–603.
35. Schwab RS. A method of measuring consciousness in petit mal epilepsy. *J Nerv Ment Dis* 1939; **89**: 690–691.
36. Binnie CD. Cognitive impairment during epileptiform discharges: is it ever justifiable to treat the EEG? *Lancet Neurol* 2003; **2**: 725–730.
37. Binnie CD, de Silva M, Hurst A. Rolandic spikes and cognitive function. *Epilepsy Res Suppl* 1992; **6**: 71–73.
38. Marston D, Besag F, Binnie CD, Fowler M. Effects of transitory cognitive impairment on psychosocial functioning of children with epilepsy: a therapeutic trial. *Dev Med Child Neurol* 1993; **35**: 574–581.
39. Pressler RM, Robinson RO, Wilson GA, Binnie CD. Treatment of interictal epileptiform discharges can improve behavior in children with behavioral problems and epilepsy. *J Pediatr* 2005; **146**: 112–117.
40. Keene DL, Manion I, Whiting S *et al*. A survey of behavior problems in children with epilepsy. *Epilepsy Behav* 2005; **6**: 581–586.
41. Whitman S, Hermann BP, Black RB, Chhabria S. Psychopathology and seizure type in children with epilepsy. *Psychol Med* 1982; **12**: 843–853.
42. Carpay HA, Vermeulen J, Stroink H *et al*. Disability due to restrictions in childhood epilepsy. *Dev Med Child Neurol* 1997; **39**: 521–526.
43. Lothman DJ, Pianta RC. Role of child-mother interaction in predicting competence of children with epilepsy. *Epilepsia* 1993; **34**: 658–669.

Marsha D. Rappley

13

Attention deficit hyperactivity disorder

Attention deficit hyperactivity disorder (ADHD) is one of the most common reasons for a school-aged child to visit a physician's office. Medications used to treat ADHD are among the most common of all medications prescribed for children. Both European and American organisations offer consistent, evidence-based guidelines that together offer a standard of care. New research reveals the genetic basis of ADHD and the influence of environment. Stimulant medications remain the first-line treatment and newer medications provide extended options for children, families and physicians. The role of behavioural therapy is better defined as an adjunct to medication. Research also indicates that ADHD persists into adulthood and broadens our concept of ADHD as a life-long condition.[1,2]

UNDERSTANDING ATTENTION DEFICIT HYPERACTIVITY DISORDER

ADHD is a chronic health condition, with symptoms experienced over a life-time, characterised by impairment of attention, hyperactivity, and impulsivity. ADHD is a neurobehavioural condition, with pathophysiology involving frontal lobe areas of the brain responsible for executive function and the central neurotransmitter systems of dopamine and norepinephrine. In addition, ADHD is a developmental condition – symptoms change as children grow through childhood, adolescence and become adults. Brain structure, function and response to stimulants differ for children and adults with ADHD, but these studies do not yet have implications for diagnosis and treatment.[3] For example, imaging studies indicate up to 5% less overall brain volume for children with ADHD; differences are apparent when the cerebellum is examined, as well. However, it is not known if these differences are clinically significant.

Genetics accounts for 60–80% of variance in susceptibility to ADHD, with strong interplay of genes and environment.[4] Children of parents with ADHD

Marsha D. Rappley MD
Acting Dean, College of Human Medicine, A110 E. Fee, Michigan State University, East Lansing, MI
48824, USA. E-mail: rappley@msu.edu

and siblings of children with ADHD are at a 3–5-fold higher risk for ADHD. Studies of dopamine and norepinephrine receptors and transporter genes indicate familial transmission of both the behavioural phenotype and genetic markers.[5] Environmental causes of symptoms include very low birth weight, exposure to tobacco and other substances *in utero*, head trauma, and lead toxicity.[6] However, most children with ADHD do not have a history of neonatal or central nervous system injury.

The prevalence of ADHD is 3–7% according to the *Diagnostic and Statistical Manual of Mental Disorders*, 4th edn, text revision (*DSM IV-TR*).[7] When isolated symptoms were examined, 9% of children in Ontario were reported to have such problems.[8] A higher prevalence is noted among children with specific problems, such as juvenile offenders or children from psychiatry referral clinics. In all studies, boys are more often affected than girls; the ratio varies from 9:1 to 2.5:1, with more girls identified in community samples.[9]

MAKING A DIAGNOSIS

Evidence-based recommendations are available to guide diagnosis and treatment of ADHD (Table 1). These promote consistent and informed decision-making with

Table 1 Major recommendations of guidelines for attention deficit hyperactivity disorder[1,10–15]

DIAGNOSIS
- Comprehensive history, including developmental, social and family history
- Standardised checklists assist in assessing behaviours
- Consideration of co-existing mental health disorders through history
- Physical examination not diagnostic but considers genetic and other conditions

TREATMENT
- Management of ADHD as chronic health condition
- Mutual treatment goals established with child, family, school
- Stimulant medication for symptom management, monotherapy (Atomoxetine possible alternative*)
- Behavioural therapy for parent–child conflict and persistent oppositional behaviour

DESIRED OUTCOMES OF TREATMENT
- Improvement in relationships with family, teachers and peers
- Decreased incidents of disruptive behaviour
- Increased quality, quantity, efficiency and completion of academic work
- Increased independence in caring for self and carrying out age-appropriate activity
- Improved self esteem
- Enhanced safety: crossing streets, staying with adult in public places, risk-taking behaviour

Compiled from the American Academy of Pediatrics, American Academy of Child and Adolescent Psychiatry, European Society for Child and Adolescent Psychiatry, and the Scottish Intercollegiate Guidelines Network.

*Recommended as alternative by American Academy of Child and Adolescent Psychiatry.

emphasis on a comprehensive history from multiple domains of the child's life, the utility of standardised collection instruments, the consideration of co-existing mental health conditions, and first-line treatment with stimulant medications and behaviour management as needed.[10-15]

Criteria of the *DSM IV TR* are grouped into two categories, inattention and hyperactivity/impulsivity (Table 2). A child must have six behaviours in each group that exceed expectations for children of the same age. Symptoms must be present before 7 years of age, evidence of significant impairment must exist in two or more settings, and the symptoms cannot be better explained by another disorder.

The diagnosis of ADHD is classified into subtypes. The **ADHD, combined inattentive/hyperactive-impulsive subtype** is the most common, accounting for about 80% of cases. Children typically present in early school years due to disruptive behaviour and difficulty with academic progress. **ADHD, predominantly inattentive subtype** is characterised by problems with inattention and distractibility, accounting for about 10–15% of cases. While girls are often diagnosed in this category, the ratio still favours boys. This diagnosis can be overlooked, as children are not typically disruptive and problems may not become apparent until the child fails to make academic progress in later school years. The least common subtype is **ADHD, predominantly hyperactive-impulsive**, in which inattention does not meet diagnostic criteria. This may account for 5% of cases. Exclusively hyperactive and impulsive behaviours warrant careful investigation for conditions other than ADHD, as this is an unusual presentation.

THE IMPORTANCE OF THE HISTORY

The single most important aspect of the diagnostic process in evaluation of a child for ADHD is the comprehensive history. This may be acquired over multiple visits, and indeed for younger children, over many months. A chronology of these behaviours is obtained, similar to descriptions of other symptoms in a medical history: duration, onset, triggering and ameliorating factors, intensity, and impairment of daily function. Careful attention is paid to the sleep history. An inadequate amount of sleep can result in irritability, poor attention and day-time sleepiness. Children with disorders of sleep, including snoring, sleep apnoea and periodic limb movements typically have such symptoms. A smaller subset of children with ADHD will also have disorders of sleep that should be identified.[16] Absence seizures may be suspected in a history of intermittent episodes of inattentiveness, while the inattention of ADHD is a pervasive finding. The combination of sleep disorders, seizures and behavioural disorders is found in many genetic disorders and mental retardation of unknown aetiology.

The developmental history is obtained from birth to reveal problems with language, motor or social development. The family history may suggest heritable genetic disorders associated with behavioural problems. Specific inquiry is made of mental health disorders because these place the child at risk in two ways: an increased chance of inheriting the disorder, and difficulty in the home environment and relationships that result from the parent's condition.

Table 2 Attention deficit hyperactivity disorder: diagnostic criteria[15]

A. Either (1) or (2)

(1) Inattention: six or more of the following, persisting for at least 6 months, maladaptive and inconsistent with developmental level: often fails to give close attention to details, makes careless mistakes

- often has difficulty sustaining attention
- often does not seem to listen
- often does not seem to follow through
- often has difficulty organising
- often avoids tasks that require sustained attention
- often loses necessary things
- often easily distracted
- often forgetful

(2) Hyperactivity/impulsivity: six or more of the following, persisting for at least 6 months, maladaptive and inconsistent with developmental level:

Hyperactivity
- often fidgets
- often leaves seat
- often runs about or climbs excessively
- often has difficulty in quiet leisure activities
- often 'on the go' or 'driven by a motor'
- often talks excessively

Impulsivity
- often blurts out answers
- often has difficulty awaiting turn
- often interrupts or intrudes

B. Some symptoms that caused impairment were present before age 7 years

C. Some impairment is present in two or more settings (*e.g.* home, school, work)

D. Evidence of clinically significant impairment in social, academic or occupational functioning

E. Symptoms do not occur exclusively during the course of a pervasive developmental disorder, schizophrenia or other psychotic disorder and are not better accounted for by another mental disorder (*e.g.* mood disorder, anxiety disorder)

ICD-9 Code based on type:
   314.01 Attention Deficit/Hyperactivity Disorder, Combined Type: per both criteria A1 and A2
   314.00 Attention Deficit Hyperactivity Disorder, Predominantly Inattentive Type: criterion A1 is met but not criterion A2
   314.01 Attention Deficit/Hyperactivity Disorder, Predominantly Hyperactive-Impulsive Type: criterion A2 is met but not criterion A1

'Partial remission' may be specified for those who have symptoms but no longer meet full criteria

Adapted from American Psychiatric Association. *Diagnostic and Statistical Manual of Mental Disorders*, 4th edn, text revision edn.[7]

Standardised checklists supplement the history. They allow comparison of the symptoms to children of similar age. The American Academy of Pediatrics provides the *ADHD Toolkit* using the Vanderbilt Scales for reporting of symptoms from parents and teachers.[17] Another widely used checklist is the Conner's Parent and Teacher Rating Scale.[18] These checklists do not require special scoring devices or sophisticated training to interpret results. Concentration, attention, and control of impulse and activity emerge for all children in a developmental process. Despite the subjective nature of the observations of the person completing the checklist, these are the best available tool to compare children of the same age in specific areas, such as attention and activity level. Standardised checklists also help identify impairment, either directly or by guiding the history.

Other diagnoses have symptoms similar to those of ADHD, which complicates the initial diagnosis and on-going assessment (Table 3).[10] According to the *DSM IV TR*, the behaviours of concern should not be better explained by another diagnosis, such as autism or mental retardation. However, such children may have symptoms that meet criteria for ADHD beyond the primary diagnosis and impair functioning to the degree that the child cannot benefit from a therapeutic school or home environment. It may be appropriate to diagnosis the child with two disorders. However, the clinician must be clear with parents that these conditions have different implications for prognosis and treatment.

Often a question arises as to whether a child really has ADHD or is simply living in a difficult social circumstance that results in problematic behaviours. Symptoms of ADHD may be mimicked or aggravated by reactions to social circumstances. Research with families indicates that ADHD is both exacerbated by, and contributes to, anxiety and stress experienced by the family.[19] Any adverse social circumstance such as disruption in the family or financial duress will aggravate symptoms for the child struggling to maintain attention, modulate activity and control impulsive actions. Behaviours of aggression, running away or distraction may be signals of other disturbances in the child's life. It is also possible that parents or teachers have unreasonable and unrealistic expectations of a child.

THE ROLE OF TESTING

Achievement and intelligence testing do not diagnosis ADHD but may assist in the identification of symptoms, the diagnosis of specific learning disorders, and planning for school services. Other tests are not routinely recommended for evaluation of ADHD. Computerised or manual performance tests of attention and impulsivity may offer supportive information, but they are not diagnostic of ADHD. Electroencephalogram, thyroid function, genetic testing, and a complete blood count are obtained when disorders such as seizures, thyroid dysfunction, dysmorphology or lead exposure are specifically suggested by the clinical presentation. These tests are not diagnostic of ADHD.[10] There are no specific physical findings which are characteristic of ADHD. However, the physical examination is important to reveal other conditions that might be associated with ADHD symptoms, such as Fragile X syndrome.

Table 3 Examples of mental health conditions that mimic or co-exist with attention deficit hyperactivity disorder[1]

Learning disorders	
Symptoms that may overlap with ADHD	Underachievement in school. Disruptive behaviour during academic activity. Refusal to engage with academic tasks and materials
Features not characteristic of ADHD	Predominantly occurs in academic work rather than in multiple settings and activities
Diagnostic dilemma	Difficult to determine which to evaluate first, a learning disorder or ADHD – follow preponderance of symptoms
Oppositional defiant disorder	
Symptoms that may overlap with ADHD	Disruptive behaviour, especially in regard to rules. Not following directions
Features not characteristic of ADHD	Defiance is the predominant quality, rather than unsuccessful attempts to co-operate
Diagnostic dilemma	Defiant behaviour is often associated with high activity level. Difficult to determine child's effort to comply in negative parent/child or teacher/child relationship
Conduct disorder	
Symptoms that may overlap with ADHD	Disruptive behaviour. Encounters with law enforcement and legal systems
Features not characteristic of ADHD	Lack of remorse. Intent to harm or do wrong. Aggression and hostility. Antisocial behaviour
Diagnostic dilemma	Fighting, running away may be reasonable reactions to adverse social circumstances
Anxiety, obsessive compulsive disorder, post-traumatic stress disorder	
Symptoms that may overlap with ADHD	Poor attention. Fidgety. Difficulty with transitions. Physical reactivity to stimuli
Features not characteristic of ADHD	Excessive worries. Fearfulness. Obsessions or compulsions. Nightmares. Re-experiencing trauma
Diagnostic dilemma	Anxiety may be source of high activity and inattention
Depression	
Symptoms that may overlap with ADHD	Irritability. Reactive impulsivity. Demoralisation
Features not characteristic of ADHD	Pervasive and persistent feelings of irritability or sadness
Diagnostic dilemma	May be difficult to distinguish from reaction to repeated failure associated with ADHD
Bipolar disorder	
Symptoms that may overlap with ADHD	Poor attention. Hyperactivity. Impulsivity. Irritability
Features not characteristic of ADHD	Expansive affect. Grandiosity. Manic quality
Diagnostic dilemma	Difficult to distinguish severe ADHD from early-onset bipolar disorder
Tic disorder	
Symptoms that may overlap with ADHD	Poor attention. Impulsive verbal or motor actions. Disruptive activity
Features not characteristic of ADHD	Repetitive vocal or motor movements
Diagnostic dilemma	Tics may not be apparent to patient, family or casual observer
Adjustment disorder	
Symptoms that may overlap with ADHD	Poor attention. Hyperactivity. Disruptive behaviour. Impulsivity. Poor academic performance
Features not characteristic	Recent onset. Precipitating event
Diagnostic dilemma	Chronic stressors, such as sibling with mental illness, or attachment and loss issues may also produce symptoms of anxiety and depression

DEVELOPMENTAL ASPECTS OF SYMPTOMS

The physician can expect that a child's ADHD symptoms will be expressed differently over time, and vary with developmental age, circumstances of life, and other co-existing medical and mental health problems.[20] Problems of younger children are remarkable most often for hyperactivity and impulsivity. The school-aged child may be disruptive, but the greater impairment for many is lack of academic progress due to inattention and distractibility. Hyperactivity might lessen in severity over teenage years while problems with inattention and impulsivity persist into adulthood for at least half of those affected.

Each age has particular challenges in dealing with ADHD. The younger child may have a relationship with a parent that is characterised by scolding and limit-setting, without opportunity for positive interaction. The school-aged child may experience isolation from peers due to impulsive behaviours and demoralisation after repeated failure. The high-school student may desire a college preparatory course but have difficulty keeping good grades. Issues around control and separation from parents can be especially difficult for these families. Transitioning into adult life is a challenge as young people seek employment, further education and begin families of their own.

ORGANISING A TREATMENT PLAN

ADHD has consequences throughout a child's life and affects all major institutions of society: individuals, families, the work place, the school, medical systems, social service institutions, and the juvenile justice system. Management focuses on patient education, improvement of symptoms that will vary with development and context, anticipatory guidance, short- and long-term planning for education, interpersonal relationships, transition to adult life, and career development.

MEDICATION

Stimulants
Stimulant medications are most strongly supported by evidence of effective management of inattention, impulsivity and hyperactivity (Table 4). Stimulants increase dopamine and norepinephrine neurotransmitters which modulate activity and attention in the nigrostriatal and frontal lobe areas of the brain. The Centre for Evidenced-based Medicine, Oxford, classifies evidence from randomised controlled trials of methylphenidate at the highest level, 1a.[21] Stimulants are consistently demonstrated to have efficacy and safety when compared to placebo in improving symptoms of ADHD.

Two recent studies contribute greatly to our understanding of stimulant treatment of ADHD. The Multimodal Treatment Study of ADHD (MTA), involved 597 children, at 6 centres, followed for 24 months, including a 14-month treatment phase.[22] A second study by Abikoff et al.[23] involved 103 children, at 2 centres, randomised to 24 months of treatment. Both studies included children aged 7–9 years, and randomised pharmacological and psychological interventions. Both assessed behavioural outcomes in the home and school setting. These trials demonstrated that 68–80% of children treated

Table 4 Recommended medications for attention deficit hyperactivity disorder[1]

Medication	Dosing
Methylphenidate*	
Generic, Ritalin®, Methylin®	Start: 5–10 mg bid to tid Usual: 10–20 mg bid to tid
Concerta®	Start: 18–27 mg qd Usual: 27–54 mg qd
Metadate ER®, Metadate CD® Methylin ER®	Start: 10 mg qd Usual: 10–20 mg qd
Ritalin LA®	Start: 20 mg qd Usual: 20–40 mg qd
Focalin® (dextro isomer of methylphenidate, lower mg dose)	Start: 2.5– 5 mg bid to tid Usual: 2.5 mg to 10 mg tid
MethyPatch® (not yet available)	Sustained action transdermal patch
	With use of a long-acting product, a short-acting may be added 5–6 p.m. for home work or special activities; appetite and sleep onset then monitored carefully

Side effects
Appetite suppression, stomach aches, headaches, irritability, weight loss, growth rate deceleration, exacerbation of psychosis, exacerbation of tics,* mild increase in blood pressure and pulse
Contra-indications
Marked anxiety, tension, agitation, glaucoma, monoamine oxidase inhibitors. Seizures*. Tics*

Dextroamphetamine and mixed amphetamine salts*	
Generic, Dexedrine®	Start: 5 mg bid to tid Usual: 5–20 mg tid
Dexedrine Spanusles®	Start: 5–10 mg qd to bid Usual: 5–15 mg bid
Adderall®	Start: 5–10 mg qd to bid Usual: 5–30 mg bid
Adderall XR®	Start: 5–10 mg qd Usual: 10–30 mg qd
	With use of a long-acting product, a short-acting may be added 5–6 p.m. for home work or special activities; appetite and sleep onset then monitored carefully

Side effects
Appetite suppression, weight loss, stomach aches, headaches, irritability, possible growth inhibition, exacerbation of psychosis, exacerbation of tics,* mild increase in blood pressure and pulse. Warning for XR: increased risk of sudden death in children with underlying heart defects
Contra-indications
Cardiovascular disease, hypertension, hyperthyroidism, glaucoma, drug dependence, monoamine oxidase inhibitors

Atomoxetine	
Strattera®	Start: 10–25 mg qd Usual: 18–60 mg qd Younger children may need bid

Side effects
Decreased appetite, nausea, vomiting, fatigue, weight loss, jaundice, growth deceleration, mild increase in blood pressure and pulse
Contra-indications
Jaundice, other laboratory evidence of liver injury, monoamine oxidase inhibitors, narrow angle glaucoma

Table 4 *(cont'd)* Recommended medications for attention deficit hyperactivity disorder[1]

Medication	Dosing
Bupropion Only SR or XL recommended	
Wellbutrin SR®	Start: 100–150 mg qd Usual: 150 mg qd or bid
Wellbutrin XL®	Start: 150 mg qd Usual: 150–300 mg qd

Side effects
Not approved for paediatric use
Higher incidence of side effects with immediate release preparation
Weight loss, insomnia, agitation, anxiety, dry mouth, seizures, others
Contra-indications
Seizures, bulimia, anorexia nervosa, abrupt d/c alcohol or benzodiazepines, monoamine oxidase inhibitors, other bupropion products (Zyban®)

*Manufacturer states seizures and tic disorder are contra-indications; research supports use in children with seizures stabilised on anticonvulsants, and in tic or Tourette's syndrome.

with stimulants had improvement in behaviour such that the children no longer met criteria for a diagnosis of ADHD at the end of the treatment phase. The benefit of treatment with stimulants was reduced in the MTA trial after children completed the 14-month active study phase. However, benefit was sustained in the Abikoff *et al.* study throughout 24 months of treatment.

Existing research evidence supports either methylphenidate or dextroamphetamine as a first choice; 70–80% of children will respond with improved attention to one or the other.[11] Randomised trials directly comparing methylphenidate and dextroamphetamine have demonstrated similar benefit from both medications, but mild side effects were more often seen with dextroamphetamine. Preparations of both are available as short-, intermediate- and long-acting, with duration of 3–10 h and comparable efficacy. Short-acting medications allow targeting of specific activities and times of day. Long-acting medications obviate the need for doses during the school day. This is more than convenience, as issues surrounding a school dose include compliance, consistent administration and loss of privacy. Short- and long-acting preparations have similar safety profiles and are metabolised and excreted by the end of the day for most children. The pharmacodynamic properties of all preparations of methylphenidate and dextroamphetamine provide the flexibility of allowing weekends, holidays and summers off medication, or intermittent use for specific occasions during these times. Laboratory studies are not routinely performed prior to or during the course of treatment with stimulants.

In February 2005, Health Canada withdrew Adderall XR® from the Canadian market to analyse reports of sudden death in young people taking this medication (the immediate release Adderall® was never available in Canada). The US Food and Drug Administration (FDA) reviewed these data in 2004 and decided that the occurrence of sudden death among those taking Adderall® or Adderall XR® was not above that of the general population, and these remain available in the US. In 2004, The FDA changed the label of

Adderall XR® to include a warning that children with underlying cardiac structural defects may be at higher risk with this medication. The stimulant magnesium pemoline remains available; however, the occurrence of idiopathic and fatal hepatotoxicity has limited its use.

Dosing of methylphenidate and dextroamphetamine is not weight-based. Guidelines consistently recommend starting with lower doses and titrating to an effective dose that does not cause side effects (Table 4). The usual dosing intervals are 2–4 times a day for short-acting, once a day for long-acting, and sometimes a morning dose of a long-acting with an early evening dose of short-acting of the same generic medication. There is no evidence to support using both methylphenidate and dextroamphetamine simultaneously. Dextroamphetamine products are more potent; 10 mg of methylphenidate is approximately equivalent to 7.5 mg dextroamphetamine.

The use of medication on the weekend and summers depends on the target behaviours decided upon by the physician, parent and child.(Table 1) If a child's symptoms interfere with peer and family relationships, it is reasonable to continue medication 7 days a week. If symptoms only occasionally interfere with family activities, such as church or large gatherings, a short-acting preparation can be used for those activities. An important role for the physician is to help families remain clear about why medication is used, what benefit is expected regarding specific target behaviours, and what side effects to observe. With this knowledge, families learn how to use medication in a safe and predictable manner to achieve maximum effectiveness for the child. This is especially important in the high-school student who will manage his or her own medications within a few years.

Side effects of stimulants are generally mild and managed by attention to dose and timing. The most common are appetite suppression, stomach ache and headache, leading to discontinuation of medication in about 1–4% of children.[11] Delayed sleep onset, previously thought to be associated with treatment, may be associated with the underlying disorder. Less common side effects are exacerbation of tics and weight loss. Despite early beliefs that stimulants should not be used in the presence of a tic disorder, the two conditions often co-exist and studies indicate that stimulants do not necessarily aggravate the tic disorder.[24] Research also indicates that stimulants can be used for children who have both ADHD and epilepsy when they are stabilised on anti-convulsants.[25]

Weight loss is often prevented by close follow-up and by alerting the family to the importance of taking medication with meals and making food available to the child when the medication wears off. This problem is more difficult to manage in the younger child. Decrease in height velocity of 1 cm/year associated with stimulant use is now described in follow-up studies of the MTA trial.[26] While this may still be within the range of normal growth for most children, this effect nonetheless warrants discussion and consent by parents and child. It is not yet clear if this decrement in growth velocity can be ameliorated during intervals off medication, such as summer.

Longer acting medications

In addition to stimulants, two other longer acting medications are effective with the core symptoms of ADHD. Atomoxetine is not classified as a stimulant medication; it is a selective norepinephrine re-uptake inhibitor. Randomised trials including more than 1000 children and adults indicate that 58–64% of children achieved 25–30% or greater improvement in symptoms.[27] A study conducted in several countries showed treatment benefit sustained over 9 months.[28] Reports of liver toxicity prompted a warning label for atomoxetine, stating that it should not be used in the presence of jaundice or other laboratory evidence of liver injury. This rare adverse effect appears to be reversible with discontinuation of atomoxetine. Other side effects such as appetite suppression and weight loss are reported at a frequency similar to methylphenidate. Seizures and prolonged QTc intervals are reported with overdose of atomoxetime, but not with therapeutic doses. Cases of tics developing during treatment with atomoxetine were recently reported, but were not found in randomised trials. Bupropion, an aminoketone antidepressant, is also effective for inattention and impulsivity, but is not approved by the US FDA for use in children. Contra-indications include seizures and eating disorders. Two randomised trials comparing bupropion with methylphenidate reported a smaller treatment effect and more side effects with bupropion, among a total of 124 children and adolescents (Table 4).[29] Atomoxetine and bupropion might be effective for children who require control of symptoms 24 hours a day and for those who do not respond to methylphenidate or dextroamphetamine. Atomoxetine and bupropion require about 3–4 weeks to achieve a therapeutic level, and cannot be used intermittently. Laboratory assessments of complete blood count, renal and liver function are appropriate during treatment with these medications. It is important to caution families who are accustomed to the flexible use of stimulants, that atomoxetine and bupropion must be consistently taken every day, doses cannot be adjusted according to a day's activities, and advice should be sought from the physician before discontinuing the medication.

Other medications

Two other classes of medications used as alternatives in the treatment of ADHD are the tricyclic antidepressants, imipramine and desipramine, and the α-agonist clonidine. Both have side effects related to cardiac and cardiovascular function. Other antidepressants, such as the serotonin re-uptake inhibitors, may be helpful for other diagnoses, such as depression, obsessive compulsive disorder or anxiety, but these are not effective with the symptoms of ADHD.

A single medication is usually adequate for ADHD. Little is written to guide the use or long-term management of multiple psychotropic medications and this practice is reserved for severe, complicated and recalcitrant cases.[30]

Follow-up visits in the MTA trial[22] and studies of Abikoff et al.[23] were monthly. However, in general practice, visits every 3–4 months are reasonable to monitor effectiveness and potential side effects. Blood pressure, pulse, height and weight are followed, because side effects of all medications used for ADHD have the potential to involve these parameters. Reasons for more frequent follow-up visits include the initiation of treatment, titration of dose, changes in medication, and working with difficult behavioural issues or social circumstances. Follow-up visits at 6-month intervals or greater are not recommended because a child might then complete a school year with improperly dosed medication, tolerating side effects that might otherwise be simply alleviated with dose and interval adjustments, or more seriously, fail to gain weight and grow.

BEHAVIOURAL THERAPY

Behavioural therapy is also the subject of the two large, randomised trials with community samples of children. The MTA trial[22] studied behaviour therapy consisting of 35 individual and group sessions over 14 months. These included behaviour management techniques, a summer treatment programme, consultation with each child's teacher, and a behavioural aide in the child's classroom for 12 weeks. This intensive behavioural therapy alone was not as effective as medication alone for improving attention. However, the combination of medication and this behavioural therapy resulted in better outcomes for ADHD related to parent–child conflict and oppositional behaviour.[22] Abikoff et al.[23] examined psychosocial treatment concurrent with medication over 24 months. The weekly sessions in the first year, and monthly in the second year included parent training, family therapy, organisational skill training, individual tutoring, social skills training and individual psychotherapy. No benefit was found for adding psychosocial treatment to medication alone.[23] Psychological interventions are effective in the treatment of frequently co-existing mental health conditions such as depression, anxiety, post-traumatic stress disorder, adjustment reactions, oppositional behaviour and parent–child discord.

Interventions (such as eye and physical exercises, neurofeedback, chelation therapy, systemic antifungal treatment, vitamins, and diet) are often promoted with enticements to parents of quick and 'natural' approaches to treatment. The cost to families may be high. Little evidence supports a role for these interventions in the treatment of ADHD.[31] Such interventions do, however, require a concerted family effort on behalf of the child with ADHD, and it may be this mobilisation of the family which results in positive outcomes sometimes reported anecdotally by families.

THE IMPORTANCE OF COMMUNICATION

Communication between parents, physician and teacher is critical to effective long-term management of ADHD. The MTA studies now document that children whose follow up includes sharing of information between parent, school and physician have the best outcomes.[32] The ADHD Toolkit provides a form to facilitate with this level of communication.[17] The physician can establish the expectation that at each follow-up visit parents will deliver information provided by the school and review it with the physician. This method is efficient and allows parents to control the flow of information between doctor and teacher. As with all chronic conditions of childhood, trust and therapeutic alliance between the doctor, child and parent is the cornerstone of management.

CHALLENGES IN TREATMENT

Very young children and mentally retarded children present a special challenge to the physician. Very young children may exhibit severely disruptive behaviours that jeopardise their own safety and cause great conflict within the family. Parents and other professionals may seek treatment with psychotropic medications.[33–35] However, the best evidence supports parent training as the most effective intervention for improving the behaviour of preschool children. In a study of the Triple P Parenting Program, parents of 87 three-year-olds were randomised to a control group or to 10–12 sessions in which they were taught consistent limit setting and positive interactions. Children in the intervention group were significantly more likely to achieve at least a 30% reduction in negative behaviours (62% versus 28% of controls), and 80% of the intervention children were improved at 1-year follow-up (there was no comparison group at that time).[36] Another 8-week randomised trial involving parents of 3-year-olds likewise showed significant benefit with parent training, and improvement was sustained 15 weeks after the intervention.[37]

Studies examining the effects of medications in the preschool group are few. A short-term study (3–4 weeks) involving 28 children with ADHD, aged 4–5.9 years, showed normalisation of behaviour for 25 children on stimulants, as compared with 3 children taking placebo. Frequent side effects were irritability and decreased appetite.[38] A second study with 27 children yielded similar results.[39] About 1% of children 2–4 years of age in some areas may be treated with psychotropic medications, but there is little evidence to support or guide this treatment. Overuse of medication is a particular concern in this age group. Concern for the safety of the child and others, and failure of parent training, are the most compelling reasons to consider pharmacological management of behaviour in young children.[40]

Mentally retarded children and adults are vulnerable to under-treatment because of difficulty establishing an appropriate developmental context for their behaviour. For these children, attention span and the ability to modulate impulses are not in keeping with their chronological age, as expected, and problems may be incorrectly attributed to an untreatable component of the mental retardation. Several randomised, controlled studies now provide strong evidence to suggest that effective treatment of children and adults with mental retardation may be successfully undertaken.[41] These studies point out important differences, such as lower rates of improvement in behaviour, and more side effects. However, effective treatment of inattention, hyperactivity and impulsivity is possible with stimulant medication.

CONTROVERSIES

Wide geographic and demographic variation in the diagnosis and treatment of ADHD suggests that physicians do not employ a consistent approach.[42,43] Difficulty with implementing consistent and evidenced-based practice patterns should not be confused with the legitimacy of the diagnosis and treatment. Changing social structures, such as family constellations, school and community support systems, unemployment, and difficulty with access to medical care may all contribute to increased behavioural problems and overall distress of families and children. However, it is well documented that treatment options are available for ADHD which, even under the most difficult of social circumstances, help improve the quality of life for a child and family.

The larger conceptualisation of ADHD continues to be discussed. The subtype of predominantly inattentive ADHD may yet emerge as a distinct diagnostic entity rather than a true subtype. In addition, the criteria for hyperkinetic disorder in the *International Classification of Diseases*, 10th edn (*ICD-10*), is more often used in Europe than the *DSM IV TR*. The *ICD-10* definition is more restrictive and results in identification of more severely affected and younger children, whereas the criteria of the *DSM-IV TR* identify a broader range of impairment.[44] As a result, fewer children in Great Britain, for example, are identified as having ADHD, but more are diagnosed with conduct disorder when compared to diagnostic patterns in the US.

Another concern is that treatment with stimulant medications leads to substance abuse. Recent investigations indicate that children who are diagnosed with ADHD and untreated are at higher risk for substance abuse than those who are treated.[45] This is thought to be due to the impulsive nature of behaviour in untreated ADHD and the chronic sense of failure often experienced by young people with persistent academic and social problems.

Key points for clinical practice

- Attention deficit hyperactivity disorder is a common and chronic condition of childhood and persists over a life-time.

- Attention deficit hyperactivity disorder has a strong genetic component.

- Guidelines from international primary and specialty care organisations establish the standard of care and promote consistent practice.

- A thorough history is the most important aspect of the diagnostic process.

- Stimulant medications are the most effective treatment of inattention, hyperactivity and impulsivity.

- Behavioural therapy has an adjunct role in treatment of co-existing disorders and discord between parent and child.

- Monitoring effectiveness and side effects of drug therapy is recommended every 3–4 months.

- Symptoms and impairment vary with developmental age and over time.

References

1. Rappley MD. Clinical practice. Attention deficit-hyperactivity disorder. *N Engl J Med* 2005; **352**: 165–173.
2. Spencer TJ. Adult attention-deficit/hyperactivity disorder. *Psychiatry Clin North Am* 2004; **27**: XI–XII.
3. Durston S. A review of the biological bases of ADHD: what have we learned from imaging studies? *Ment Retard Dev Disabil Res Rev* 2003; **9**: 184–195.
4. Rietveld MJ, Hudziak JJ, Bartels M, van Beijsterveldt CE, Boomsma DI. Heritability of attention problems in children: longitudinal results from a study of twins, age 3 to 12. *J Child Psychol Psychiatry* 2004; **45**: 577–588.

5. Faraone SV, Perlis RH, Doyle AE *et al.* Molecular genetics of attention-deficit/hyperactivity disorder. *Biol Psychiatry* 2005; **57**: 1313–1323.

6. Hille ET, den Ouden AL, Saigal S *et al.* Behavioural problems in children who weigh 1000 g or less at birth in four countries. *Lancet* 2001; **357**: 1641–1643.

7. American Psychiatric Association. *Diagnostic and Statistical Manual of Mental Disorders*, 4th edn, text revision edn. Washington, DC: American Psychiatric Association, 2000.

8. Szatmari P, Offord DR, Boyle MH. Ontario Child Health Study: prevalence of attention deficit disorder with hyperactivity. *J Child Psychol Psychiatry* 1989; **30**: 219–230.

9. Barbaresi WJ, Katusic SK, Colligan RC *et al.* How common is attention-deficit/hyperactivity disorder? Incidence in a population-based birth cohort in Rochester, Minn. *Arch Pediatr Adolesc Med* 2002; **156**: 217–224.

10. American Academy of Pediatrics. Clinical practice guideline: Diagnosis and evaluation of the child with attention deficit/hyperactivity disorder. *Pediatrics* 2000; **105**: 1158–1170.

11. American Academy of Pediatrics, Subcommittee on Attention-Deficit/Hyperactivity Disorder and Committee on Quality Improvement. Clinical practice guideline: Treatment of the school-aged child with attention-deficit/hyperactivity disorder. *Pediatrics* 2001; **108**: 1033–1044.

12. Greenhill LL, Plizka S, Dulcan MK *et al.* Practice parameter for the use of stimulant medications in the treatment of children, adolescents, and adults. *J Am Acad Child Adolesc Psychiatry* 2002; **41(Suppl 2)**: 26S–49S.

13. Taylor E, Sergeant J, Doepfner M *et al.* Clinical guidelines for hyperkinetic disorder. *Eur Child Adolesc Psychiatry* 1998; **7**: 184–200.

14. Guideline No. 52: Attention Deficit and Hyperkinetic Disorders in Children and Young People. 2001. (Accessed at <www.sign.ac.uk>).

15. Remschmidt H. Global consensus on ADHD/HKD. *Eur Child Adolesc Psychiatry* 2005; **14**: 127–137.

16. Owens JA. The ADHD and sleep conundrum: a review. *J Dev Behav Pediatr* 2005; **26**: 312–322.

17. American Academy of Pediatrics, National Initiative for Children's Healthcare Quality. *Caring for Children with ADHD: A Resource Toolkit for Clinicians*. Elk Grove Village: American Academy of Pediatrics, 2002.

18. The revised Conners' Parent Rating Scale (CPRS-R): factor structure, reliability, and criterion validity., 1998.
<http://www.mhs.com/onlineCat/product.asp?productID=CRS-R>).

19. Bussing R, Zima BT, Gary FA *et al.* Social networks, caregiver strain, and utilization of mental health services among elementary school students at high risk for ADHD. *J Am Acad Child Adolesc Psychiatry* 2003; **42**: 842–850.

20. Dixon SD, Stein MT. *Encounters with Children, Pediatric Behavior and Development*, 3rd edn. St Louis, MO: Mosby, 2000.

21. 2003 InfoPOEM Inc. Key Word: Attention deficit hyperactivity disorder. <www.infopoems.com>.

22. National Institute of Mental Health Multimodal Treatment Study of ADHD follow-up: 24-month outcomes of treatment strategies for attention-deficit/hyperactivity disorder. *Pediatrics* 2004; **113**: 754–761.

23. Abikoff H, Hechtman L, Klein RG *et al.* Symptomatic improvement in children with ADHD treated with long-term methylphenidate and multimodal psychosocial treatment. *J Am Acad Child Adolesc Psychiatry* 2004; **43**: 802–811.

24. Tourette's Syndrome Study Group. Treatment of ADHD in children with tics: a randomized controlled trial. *Neurology* 2002; **58**: 527–536.

25. Gross-Tsur V, Manor O, van der Meere J, Joseph A, Shalev RS. Epilepsy and attention deficit hyperactivity disorder: is methylphenidate safe and effective? *J Pediatr* 1997; **130**: 670–674.

26. National Institute of Mental Health Multimodal Treatment Study of ADHD follow-up: changes in effectiveness and growth after the end of treatment. *Pediatrics* 2004; **113**: 762–769.

27. Kelsey DK, Sumner CR, Casat CD *et al.* Once-daily atomoxetine treatment for children with attention-deficit/hyperactivity disorder, including an assessment of evening and morning behavior: a double-blind, placebo-controlled trial. *Pediatrics* 2004; **114**: e1–e8.

28. Michelson D, Buitelaar JK, Danckaerts M *et al*. Relapse prevention in pediatric patients with ADHD treated with Atomoxetine: a randomized, double-blind, placebo-controlled study. *J Am Acad Child Adolesc Psychiatry* 2004; **43**: 896–904.

29. Conners CC, Gualtieri CT, Weller E *et al*. Bupropion hydrochloride in attention deficit disorder associated with hyperactivity. *J Am Acad Child Adolesc Psychiatry* 1996; **35**: 1314–1321.

30. Safer DJ, Zito JM, DosReis S. Concomitant psychotropic medication for youths. *Am J Psychiatry* 2003; **160**: 438–449.

31. Wolraich ML. Addressing behavior problems among school-aged children: traditional and controversial approaches. *Pediatr Rev* 1997; **18**: 266–270.

32. Jensen P, Hinshwa S, Swanson J *et al*. Findings from the NIMH multimodal treatment study of ADHD (MTA): implications and applications for primary care providers. *J Dev Beh Pediatr* 2001; **22**: 60–73.

33. Rappley M, Mullan P, Alvarez F, Eneli I, Wang J, Gardiner J. Diagnosis of attention-deficit/hyperactivity disorder and use of psychotropic medication in very young children. *Arch Pediatr Adolesc Med* 1999; **153**: 1039–1045.

34. Zito JM, Safer DJ, DosReis S, Gardner JF, Boles M, Lynch F. Trends in the prescribing of psychotropic medications to preschoolers. *JAMA* 2000; **283**: 1025–1030.

35. DeBar LL, Lynch F, Powell J, Gale J. Use of psychotropic agents in preschool children: associated symptoms, diagnoses, and health care services in a health maintenance organization. *Arch Pediatr Adolesc Med* 2003; **157**: 150–157.

36. Borr W, Sanders M, Markie-Dadds C. The effects of the triple P-positive parenting program on preschool children with co-occurring disruptive behavior and attentional/hyperactive difficulties. *J Abnormal Child Psychol* 2002; **30**: 571–587.

37. Sonuga-Barke E, Daley D, Thompson M, Laver-Bradbury C, Weeks A. Parent-based therapies for preschool attention-deficit/hyperactivity disorder: a randomized, controlled trial with a community sample. *J Am Acad Child Adolesc Psychiatry* 2001; **40**: 402–408.

38. Firestone P, Musten LM, Pisterman S, Mercer J, Bennett S. Short-term side effects of stimulant medication are increased in preschool children with attention-deficit/hyperactivity disorder: a double-blind placebo-controlled study. *J Child Adolesc Psychopharmacol* 1998; **8**: 13–25.

39. Short EJ, Manos MJ, Findling RL, Schubel EA. A prospective study of stimulant response in preschool children: insights from ROC analyses. *J Am Acad Child Adolesc Psychiatry* 2004; **43**: 251–259.

40. Rappley M, Eneli I, Mullan P *et al*. Patterns of psychotropic medication use in very young children with attention-deficit hyperactivity disorder. *J Dev Behav Pediatr* 2002; **23**: 23–30.

41. Aman M, Buican B, Arnold L. Methylphenidate treatment in children with borderline IQ and mental retardation: analysis of three aggregated studies. *J Child Adolesc Psychopharmacol* 2003; **13**: 29–40.

42. Rappley MD, Gardiner J, Jetton J, Houang R. The use of methylphenidate in Michigan. *Arch Pediatr Adolesc Med* 1995; **149**: 675–679.

43. Brownell MD, Yogendran MS. Attention-deficit hyperactivity disorder in Manitoba children: medical diagnosis and psychostimulant treatment rates. *Can J Psychiatry* 2001; **46**: 264–272.

44. Sorensen MJ, Mors O, Thomsen PH. DSM-IV or ICD-10-DCR diagnoses in child and adolescent psychiatry: does it matter? *Eur Child Adolesc Psychiatry* 2005; **14**: 335–340.

45. Katusic SK, Barbaresi WJ, Colligan RC, Weaver AL, Leibson CL, Jacobsen SJ. Psychostimulant treatment and risk for substance abuse among young adults with a history of attention-deficit/hyperactivity disorder: a population-based, birth cohort study. *J Child Adolesc Psychopharmacol* 2005; **15**: 764–776.

Augusto B. Federici Pier M. Mannucci

Classification, diagnosis and management of von Willebrand disease in childhood

When Erik von Willebrand in 1926 described a novel bleeding disorder in a large family from Foglo on the islands of Aland in the Gulf of Bothnia, he provided an impressive and exhaustive description of its clinical and genetic features. Unlike haemophilia, the epitome of inherited bleeding disorders, both sexes were affected, and mucosal bleeding was the dominant symptom. Prolonged bleeding time with normal platelet count was the most important laboratory abnormality and a functional disorder of the platelets associated with systemic lesion of the vessel wall was suggested as a possible cause of the disorder. However, he called the disease 'hereditary pseudohaemophilia'. To further complicate the issue, some authors subsequently called the disorder 'vascular haemophilia'. Only in the 1950s, was it demonstrated that the

---

Abbreviations and definitions

> VWD, von Willebrand disease; VWF, von Willebrand factor; FVIII, factor VIII; ISTH-SSC on VWF, Scientific Standardization Committees (Sub-Committee on von Willebrand Factor) of the International Society of Thrombosis and Haemostasis; RFLP, restriction fragment length polymorphisms; VWF:RCo, ristocetin co-factor activity of VWF; see also Table 1.

Augusto B. Federici MD (for correspondence)
Associate Professor of Haematology, Angelo Bianchi Bonomi Haemophilia Thrombosis Centre, Department of Internal Medicine and Medical Specialities, IRCCS Maggiore Policlinico Hospital, Mangiagalli, Regina Elena Foundation and University of Milan, Via Pace 9, 20122 Milan, Italy
E-mail: augusto.federici@unimi.it

Pier M. Mannucci MD
Professor of Internal Medicine, Angelo Bianchi Bonomi Haemophilia Thrombosis Centre, Department of Internal Medicine and Medical Specialities, IRCCS Maggiore Policlinico Hospital, Mangiagalli, Regina Elena Foundation and University of Milan, Via Pace 9, 20122 Milan, Italy

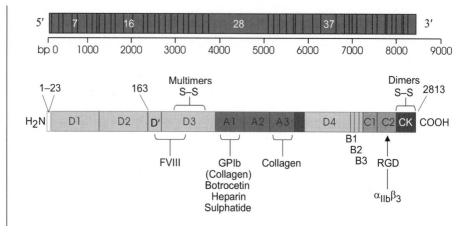

Fig. 1 Schematic representation of the VWF gene located in chromosome 12 together with the pseudogene in chromosome 22. The main exons are indicated with the number of base pairs from 5' to 3' (top). DNA domain structure and pre-pro-VWF polypeptide: the pre-pro-VWF is indicated with amino acids numbered from the amino- (aa 1) to carboxy-terminal portions (aa 2813) of VWF. Note the important CK and D3 domains for formation of VWF dimers and multimers (lower). The native mature subunit of VWF, after the cleaving of the pre-pro VWF, is described with its functional domains: the VWF binding sites for factor VIII (D' and D3), GPIb, botrocetin, heparin, sulfatide, collagen (A1), collagen (A3) and the RGD sequence for binding to $\alpha_{IIb}\beta_3$.

prolonged bleeding time in these patients was associated with reduced factor VIII (FVIII); it was not until the 1970s that the deficiency of another factor, called von Willebrand factor and different from FVIII, was found to be responsible for the disease. Surprisingly, the reduction of this factor caused low FVIII levels, pointing to the close relationship between the two proteins. In the 1980s, cloning of the VWF gene allowed for the characterisation of the molecular basis of the disorder. The history of von Willebrand disease (VWD) has been reviewed.[1] In this chapter, we discuss the progress and the problems of VWD management in childhood today, 80 years after the original description by Erik von Willebrand.

STRUCTURE–FUNCTION AND CHANGES DURING EARLY CHILDHOOD

Von Willebrand factor (VWF) is synthesised by endothelial cells and megakaryocytes.[2] The gene coding for VWF has been cloned and located at chromosome 12p13.2. It is a large gene composed of about 178 kb containing 52 exons. A non-coding, partial, highly homologous pseudogene has been identified in chromosome 22. The pseudogene spans the gene sequence from exons 23 to 34.[3] The primary product of the VWF gene is a 2813 amino acid protein made of a signal peptide of 22 amino acids (also called a pre-peptide), a large pro-peptide of 741 amino acids and a mature VWF molecule containing 2050 amino acids. In keeping with a recently proposed nomenclature,[4] numbering starts from the first amino acid of the signal peptide; thus, 764 is the first amino acid of the mature protein. Different protein regions, corresponding to four types of repeated domains (D1, D2, D', D3, A1, A2, A3,

D4, B, C1, C2) of cDNA, are responsible for the different binding functions of the molecule (Fig. 1). Mature VWF is the result of ordered intracellular processing, leading to the storage and/or secretion of a heterogeneous array of multimeric, multidomain glycoproteins, referred to as VWF.

VWF has two major functions in haemostasis. First, it is essential for platelet–subendothelium adhesion and platelet-to-platelet interactions as well as platelet aggregation in vessels in which rapid blood flow results in elevated shear stress, a function partially explored *in vivo* by measuring the bleeding time. Adhesion is promoted by the interaction of a region of the A1 domain of VWF with GPIbα on the platelet membrane. It is thought that high shear stress activates the A1 domain of the collagen-bound VWF by stretching VWF multimers into their filamentous form. Furthermore, GPIbα and VWF are also necessary for platelet-to-platelet interactions.[2] The interaction between GPIbα and VWF can be mimicked in platelet-rich plasma by addition of the antibiotic ristocetin, which promotes the binding of VWF to GPIbα of fresh or formalin-fixed platelets. Aggregation of platelets within the growing haemostatic plug is promoted by interaction with a second receptor on platelets, GPIIb–IIIa (or integrin $\alpha_{IIb}\beta_3$) which, once activated, binds to VWF and fibrinogen, recruiting more platelets into a stable plug. Both these binding activities of VWF are highly expressed in the largest VWF multimers.

Second, VWF is the specific carrier of FVIII in plasma. VWF protects FVIII from proteolytic degradation, prolonging its half-life in circulation and efficiently localising it at the site of vascular injury. Each VWF monomer has one binding domain, located in the first 272 amino acids of the mature subunit (D′ domain) which can bind one FVIII molecule *in vivo*; however, only 1–2% of available monomers are occupied by FVIII.[5] Therefore, any change in plasma VWF level is usually associated with a corresponding change in FVIII plasma concentration. The correct nomenclature with abbreviations of the different FVIII/VWF activities, as approved by the Scientific Standardization Committees (Sub-Committee on VWF) of the International Society of Thrombosis and Haemostasis (ISTH-SSC on VWF), are summarised in Table 1.[6]

The mature, native VWF circulates in plasma of normal individuals at a concentration of 5–15 μg/ml: subjects with blood group O show lower plasma

Table 1 Recommended nomenclature of factor VIII/von Willebrand factor complex

FACTOR VIII	
Protein	VIII
Antigen	VIII:Ag
Function	VIII:C
VON WILLEBRAND FACTOR	
Mature protein	VWF
Antigen	VWF:Ag
Ristocetin co-factor activity	VWF:RCo
Collagen binding capacity	VWF:CB
Factor VIII binding capacity	VWF:FVIIIB

See Mazurier and Rodeghiero[6] for further information.

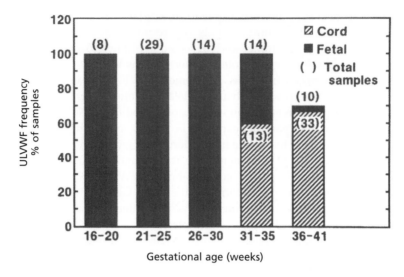

Fig. 2 VWF multimeric pattern evaluated in 75 fetal and 46 cord plasma samples and grouped by gestational age. Note that ultra-large multimers (ULVWF) are present in 100% of samples until week 35 (see Katz et al.[8]).

levels of VWF than those with blood group non-O.[7] During fetal growth, VWF retains ultra-large molecular weight forms (Fig. 2) and plasma levels of VWF are higher in the newborn than in children (Fig. 3): only at 6 months after birth do children show their true levels of VWF and FVIII.[8,9] These data can explain why neonates with severe forms of VWD do not usually bleed but should be also taken into consideration when VWD diagnosis is suspected in young children during their first 6–8 months.

CLASSIFICATION

The revised classification of VWD identifies two major categories, characterised by quantitative (types 1 and 3) or qualitative (type 2) VWF defects.[10] A partial quantitative deficiency of VWF in plasma and/or platelets identifies type 1, whereas type 3 is characterised by the total absence or only trace amounts of VWF in plasma and platelets. Type 1 is easily distinguished from type 3 by the milder VWF deficiency (usually in the range of 10–40 U/dl), the autosomal dominant inheritance pattern and the presence of milder bleeding symptoms.[11] Four type 2 VWD subtypes have been identified, reflecting different pathophysiological mechanisms. Types 2A and 2B VWD are marked by the absence of high molecular weight VWF multimers in plasma; in type 2B, there is increased affinity for the platelet glycoprotein Ib–IX–V complex (GPIbα). The identification of qualitatively abnormal variants with decreased platelet-dependent function and the presence of normal multimers on gel electrophoresis led to the identification of a new subtype, called type 2M. If this definition is followed and more stringent criteria are applied to VWD diagnosis, many cases previously identified as type 1 should now be classified as type 2M because they are caused by single missense mutation affecting VWF function but not its multimeric structure and assembly.

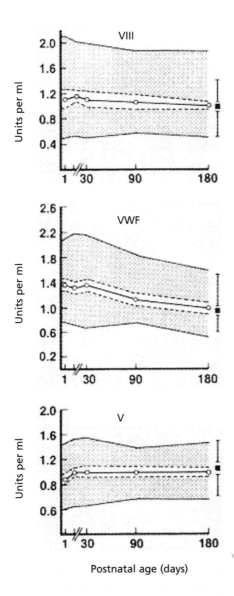

Fig. 3 Plasma factor V, factor VIII and VWF levels in 137 healthy premature infants during the first 6 months of life. Inner line represents mean values, inner clear area is 95% confidence interval and shaded area includes 95% of all values (± 2 SD). Adult values are shown as a bar on the right of each figure (see Andrew et al.[9]).

Furthermore, type 2N (Normandy) also shows a full array of multimers since the defect lies in the N-terminal region of the VWF where the binding domain for FVIII resides. This type is phenotypically identified only by an abnormal FVIII/VWF binding test: in fact, this test is always normal in mild haemophiliacs or carriers of haemophilia A.[12] The current classification of VWD, summarised in Table 2, was proposed by Sadler in 1994 on behalf of the ISTH-SSC on VWF. A working party is preparing an updated classification of VWD to be published within 2006.

Table 2 Classification of von Willebrand disease

QUANTITATIVE DEFICIENCY OF VWF	
Type 1	Partial quantitative deficiency of VWF
Type 3	Virtually complete deficiency of VWF
QUALITATIVE DEFICIENCY OF VWF	
Type 2	Qualitative deficiency of VWF
Type 2A	Qualitative variants with decreased platelet-dependent function associated with the absence of high molecular weight VWF multimers
Type 2B	Qualitative variants with increased affinity for platelet GPIbα
Type 2M	Qualitative variants with decreased platelet-dependent function not caused by the absence of high molecular weight VWF multimers
Type 2N	Qualitative variants with markedly decreased affinity for FVIII

Modified from Sadler[10].

Prevalence and frequency of different types in childhood

VWD is the most frequently inherited bleeding disorder, with a prevalence up to 1% in certain geographic areas according to population studies.[11] On the other hand, prevalence, based on the number of patients registered at specialised centres, ranges from 4–10 cases per 100,000 inhabitants: symptomatic VWD requiring specific treatment occurs in 50–100 cases per million.[11] In the past, type 1 was reported as the most frequent form of VWD (Table 3). A recent, retrospective study based on re-appraisal of type 1 diagnoses after 10 years (1994 versus 2004) in 1234 VWD patients attending 16 Italian Haemophilia Centres found that VWD type 1 was present in only 671 of the 1234 cases (54%); most of the previously diagnosed VWD type 1 patients were re-diagnosed type 2 on the basis of discrepancies in VWF activity (VWF:RCo/Ag ratio < 0.7). The age distribution of the 1234 Italian VWD patients was 5–86 years, with 267 of the 1234 cases (22%) aged below 20 years (Fig. 4). However, the 16 Italian Haemophilia Centres

Table 3 Frequency of von Willebrand disease types

Authors	Number of patients	Type 1 (%)	Type 2 (%)	Type 3 (%)
Tuddenham[11]	134	75	19	6
Lenk et al.[11]	111	76	12	12
Hoyer et al.[11]	116	71	23	6
Awidi[11]	65	59	30	11
Berliner et al.[11]	60	62	9	29
Federici et al.[12,13]	1234	54	40	6

Modified from Castaman et al.[11]

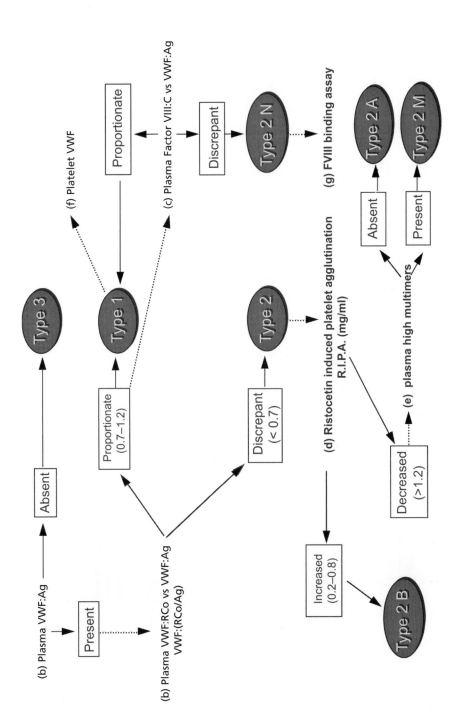

Fig. 4 Distribution of VWD types in 267 paediatric patients (age < 20 years) enrolled into the Italian VWD registry by 16 haemophilia centres. Note that only 73 (6%) of the entire cohort of 1234 VWD patients are children with ages below 10 years.

Table 4 Bleeding score used to evaluate bleeding history in von Willebrand disease

Symptom	−1	0	1	Score 2	3	4
Epistaxis	–	No or trivial (< 5)	> 5 or more than 10	Consultation only	Packing or cauterisation or antifibrinolytic	Blood transfusion or replacement therapy or desmopressin
Cutaneous	–	No or trivial (< 1 cm)	> 1 cm and no trauma	Consultation only		
Bleeding from minor wounds	–	No or trivial (< 5)	> 5 or more than 5	Consultation only	Surgical haemostasis	Blood transfusion or replacement therapy or desmopressin
Oral cavity	–	No	Referred at least one	Consultation only	Surgical haemostasis or antifibrinolytic	Blood transfusion or replacement therapy or desmopressin
Gastrointestinal bleeding	–	No	Associated with ulcer, portal hypertension, haemorrhoids, angiodysplasia	Spontaneous	Surgical haemostasis, blood transfusion, replacement therapy, desmopressin, antifibrinolytic	
Tooth extraction	No bleeding in at least 2 extractions	None done or no bleeding in 1 extraction	Referred in < 25% of all procedures	Referred in > 25% of all procedures, no intervention	Resturing or packing	Blood transfusion or replacement therapy or desmopressin
Surgery	No bleeding in at least 2 surgeries	None done or no bleeding in 1 surgery	Referred in < 25% of all surgeries	Referred in > 25% of all procedures, no intervention	Surgical haemostasis or antifibrinolytic	Blood transfusion or replacement therapy or desmopressin
Menorrhagia	–	No	Consultation only	Antifibrinolytics, pill use	Dilatation and currettage, iron therapy	Blood transfusion or replacement therapy or desmopressin or hysterectomy

Table 4 *(continued)* Bleeding score used to evaluate bleeding history in von Willebrand disease

Symptom	Score					
	−1	0	1	2	3	4
Post-partum haemorrhage	No bleeding in at least 2 deliveries	No deliveries or no bleeding in 1 delivery	Consultation only	Dilatation and currettage, iron therapy, antifibrinolytics	Blood transfusion or replacement therapy or desmopressin	Hysterectomy
Muscle haematomas	–	Never	Post trauma no therapy	Spontaneous, no therapy	Spontaneous or traumatic, requiring desmopressin or replacement therapy	Spontaneous or traumatic, requiring surgical intervention or blood transfusion
Haemarthrosis	–	Never	Post trauma no therapy	Spontaneous, no therapy	Spontaneous or traumatic, requiring desmopressin or replacement therapy	Spontaneous or traumatic, requiring surgical intervention or blood transfusion
CNS bleeding	–	Never	–	–	Subdural, any intervention	Intracerebral, any intervention

Derived from Tosetto *et al.*[16]

followed only 73 (6%) children at ages below 10 years.[13,14] Since most patients enrolled in the study are not located in paediatric hospitals, probably the paediatric population of VWD in Italy is greatly underestimated.

EVALUATION OF BLEEDING HISTORY

Several attempts have been made recently by clinical experts in VWD to evaluate the sensitivity and specificity of bleeding symptoms, which are important especially in the mild cases of type 1 VWD, with VWF:RCo levels > 30 U/dl. In a multicentre study of the clinical presentation of type 1 VWD in obligatory carriers, it has been shown that menorrhagia and epistaxis are not good predictors of type 1 VWD, while cutaneous bleeding and bleeding after dental extractions should be considered the most sensitive symptoms.[15] Therefore, a specific bleeding score has been proposed (Table 5). This bleeding score has been tested in affected and non-affected members of 154 VWD families enrolled prospectively in a large European study, as well as 200 normal individuals.[16]

PATTERNS OF INHERITANCE

The inheritance pattern of VWD type 3 is autosomal recessive. In type 2 VWD patients, the pattern of inheritance is mainly autosomal dominant, even

Table 5 Incidence (%) of bleeding symptoms in patients with von Willebrand disease and in normal subjects

Symptoms	Iranian VWD	Italian VWD (n = 1234)*			Scandinavia	
	Type 3 (n = 348)	Type 1 (n = 671)	Type 2 (n = 497)	Type 3 (n = 66)	VWD (n= 264)	Normals (n = 500)
Epistaxis	77	61	63	66	62	5
Menorrhagia	69	32	32	56	60	25
Post-extraction bleeding	70	31	39	53	51	5
Haematomas	NR	13	14	33	49	12
Bleeding from minor wounds	NR	36	40	50	36	0.2
Gum bleeding	NR	31	35	56	35	7
Post-surgical b leeding	41	20	23	41	28	1
Post-partum bleeding	15	17	18	26	23	19
Gastrointestinal bleeding	20	5	8	20	14	1
Joint bleeding	37	3	4	45	8	0
Haematuria	1	2	5	12	7	1
Cerebral bleeding	NR	1	2	9	NR	0

Adapted from Federici et al.,[12,13] Silwer[19] and Lak et al.[20]
NR, not reported
*Bleeding symptoms in Italian patients have been recently recalculated according to the updated results of the Italian Registry of VWD and, therefore, are different from previously reported.[13,14]

though rare cases with recessive pattern have been reported.[11] The inheritance of the mild type 1 VWD is usually autosomal dominant, with variable phenotype and penetrance. Despite its high prevalence, the precise genetic cause of type 1 VWD is still elusive in most cases, especially those with a mild phenotype. In type 1 VWD, in fact, a number of genetic and non-genetic factors are likely to contribute to the wide variability of the clinical and laboratory phenotype. About 60% of the variation in VWF plasma is due to genetic factors, with ABO group accounting for only about 30%. In type O subjects, the VWF level is 25–35% lower than in non-O individuals.[7] Other factors outside the VWF gene, such as platelet polymorphisms, have been proposed to modify the bleeding tendency of type 1 VWD.[18]

CLINICAL FEATURES AND BLEEDING SYMPTOMS IN DIFFERENT TYPES

The clinical expression of VWD is usually mild in most type 1 cases, increasing in severity in types 2 and 3. In general, the severity of bleeding correlates with the degree of the reduction of VWF:RCo and FVIII:C activities, but not with the magnitude of bleeding time prolongation or with the patient ABO blood type. Mucocutaneous bleeding (epistaxis, menorrhagia) is a typical manifestation of the disease and may even affect the quality of life. VWD may be highly prevalent in patients with isolated menorrhagia.[11] To date, only a few detailed descriptions of symptoms in VWD patients have been provided[19,20] but only one study took into account the differentiation according to the VWD types.[13,14] Table 5 shows the relative frequency of bleeding symptoms in three large series of patients with VWD diagnosed at specialised centres.

LABORATORY DIAGNOSIS

The diagnosis of VWD, particularly type 1, may require several laboratory tests to be repeated on different occasions. These tests are usually applied to patients with suspected bleeding disorders; Table 6 summarises the different steps for VWD diagnosis. The bleeding time is usually prolonged, though it may be normal in patients with mild forms of VWD such as those with type 1 and normal platelet VWF content.[21] Evaluation of closure time with the Platelet Function Analyzer (PFA-100) gives a rapid and simple measure of VWF-dependent platelet function at high shear stress: it can be performed in whole blood and, therefore, has been proposed instead of bleeding time in children. This system is sensitive and reproducible for VWD screening, but is not always specific and must always be performed together with other VWF tests.[11] Differential diagnosis of VWD types can be done by using these laboratory tests, following the flow chart proposed by the guidelines for diagnosis and treatment of VWD in Italy (Fig. 5). Type 3 VWD can be diagnosed in case of unmeasurable VWF:Ag. A proportionate reduction of both VWF:Ag and VWF:RCo with a RCo/Ag ratio > 0.7 suggests type 1 VWD. If the VWF:RCo/Ag ratio is < 0.7, type 2 is diagnosed. Type 2B VWD can be identified in case of an enhanced RIPA (< 0.8 mg/ml) while types 2A and 2M cause low RIPA (>1.2 mg/ml). Multimeric analysis in plasma is necessary to distinguish between type 2A VWD (lack of the largest and intermediate

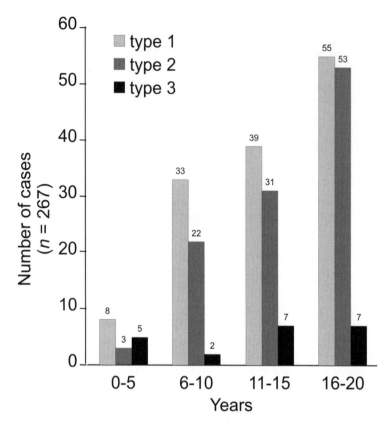

Fig. 5 Flow chart proposed in diagnosis of different VWD types. Type 3 VWD can be diagnosed in cases of unmeasurable VWF:Ag (a). A proportionate reduction of both VWF:Ag and VWF:RCo with a RCo/Ag ratio > 0.7 suggests type 1 VWD (b). If the VWF:RCo/Ag ratio is < 0.7, type 2 is diagnosed. Type 2B VWD (d) can be identified in cases of an enhanced RIPA (< 0.8 mg/ml) while types 2A and 2M cause low RIPA (> 1.2 mg/ml). Multimeric analysis in plasma (e) is necessary to distinguish between type 2A VWD (lack of the largest and intermediate multimers) and type 2M VWD (all the multimers present as in normal plasma). Type 2N VWD can be suspected in case of discrepant values for factor VIII (c) and VWF:Ag (ratio < 1) and diagnosis should be confirmed by the specific test (g) of VWF:FVIII binding capacity. In type 1 VWD, the ratio between FVIII and VWF:Ag is always ≥ 1 and the severity of type 1 VWD phenotype can usually be evaluated from platelet VWF (f) measurements.[13]

multimers) and type 2M VWD (all the multimers present). Type 2N VWD can be suspected in case of discrepant values for FVIII and VWF:Ag (ratio <1) and diagnosis should be confirmed by the specific test of VWF:FVIIIB. In type 1 VWD, the ratio between FVIII and VWF:Ag is always > 1 and the severity of type 1 VWD phenotype can usually be evaluated from platelet VWF measurements.[13]

MOLECULAR AND PRENATAL DIAGNOSIS IN CHILDHOOD

Cloning the VWF gene has allowed the identification of several suitable restriction fragment length polymorphisms (RFLP) which demonstrate the co-segregation of VWD phenotype with haplotype-specific RFLP patterns in family members of different kindred with VWD.[11] Knowledge of the crucial

Table 6 Clinical and laboratory parameters used for von Willebrand disease diagnosis

Patients at risk for VWD
- Clinical history: life-long mucocutaneous and postoperative bleeding; symptoms are sometimes present in other family members
- Screening tests: prolonged bleeding time (may be normal); normal platelet count; prolonged PTT (may be normal)

Diagnosis and definition of VWD
- VWF antigen [a]
- VWF:ristocetin co-factor activity [b]
- Factor VIII [c]
- VWF multimeric structure on low resolution gels [e]

Diagnosis of VWD types
- Ristocetin-induced platelet agglutination (RIPA) [d]
- VWF multimeric structure on high resolution gels [e]
- Platelet VWF content [f]
- Factor VIII binding assay [g]

For the use of these tests see the diagnostic flow-chart reported in Figure 5 and also Federici et al.[13]

segments of VWF involved in the interaction with GPIbα initially prompted the fruitful search for mutations in exon 28 of the VWF gene which encodes for the A1 and A2 domains of mature VWF as shown in Figure 1 (for review, see Castaman et al.[11]). The search for mutations has been extended to additional VWF exons encoding for the other functional domains of VWF. The most frequent mutations reported in types 2A, 2B, 2M, 2N are listed in Table 7 according to the specific VWF domains and are currently updated in the web site organised on behalf of the ISTH-SSC on VWF (<www.shef.ac.uk/vwf>). Most type 2A cases are due to missense mutations in the A1 domain, with R1597W or Q or Y and S1506L accounting for about 60%.[22] The majority of type 2B cases are due to missense mutations in the A1 domain, about 90% being caused by R1306W, R1308C, V1316M and R1341Q mutations (Table 7). A few heterogeneous mutations are responsible for type 2M cases and are also located within the A1 domain. Therefore, most mutations are expressed and the mutated recombinant VWF have been compared with others found within the same domain.[23] A recurrent mutation in type 2M Vicenza has been recently reported in families from Europe (R1205H), associated with a second nucleotide change (M740I) exclusively identified in some families from the Vicenza area.[24,25] Missense mutations in the FVIII-binding domain at the amino-terminal portion of VWF are responsible for type 2N (for review, see Mazurier et al.[12]). Despite its high prevalence, the precise genetic cause of type 1 VWD is still elusive in most cases, especially those with a mild phenotype. The molecular defects are distributed within the entire VWF gene. More information about molecular diagnosis of VWD type 1 will be available as soon as the data of the European project entitled *Molecular and Clinical Markers for Diagnosis and Management of Type 1 VWD* is published within 2006. In type 3 VWD, partial or total gene deletions have been initially reported (for review, see Eikenboom[26]). Notably, homozygous states for gene deletion may be

Table 7 List of most frequent mutations in types 2A, 2B, 2M and 2N according to von Willebrand factor domains

Localisation of VWF defects	VWD types	VWF mutations associated with specific types
D2 domain	Type 2A (formerly IIC)	F404insNP, R436del6, N528S, G550R, C623W, A625insG
D'–D3 domains	Type 2N	R782W, G785E, E787K, C788R, C788Y, T791M, Y795C, M800V, R816W, R816Q, H817Q, R854Q, R854W, C858F, D879N, Q1053H, C1060R, C1225G
D3 domain	Type 2M (formerly 1 Vicenza)	R1205H, Y1146C
	Type 2A (formerly IIE)	C1143Y, C1173R
A1 domain	Type 2B (formerly IIB)	P1266L, H1268D, C1272G, C1272R, M1304insM, R1306Q, R1306L, R1306W, R1308C, R1308P, I1309V, S1310F, W1313C, V1314F, V1314L, V1316M, P1337L, R1341L, R1341Q, R1341W, L1460V, A1461V
	Type 2M	G1324S, G1324A, E1359K, F1369I, I1425F, Q1191del1, K1408delK
	Type 2M/2A	L1276P, R1374C, R1374H, C1458Y, R1374R
A2 domain	Type 2A (formerly IIA)	G1505E, G1505R, S1506L, F1514C, K1518E, L1540P, S1543F, Q1556R, L1562P, R1597G, R1597Q, R1597W, V1604F, V1607D, V1609R, P1627H, I1628T, G1629R, V1630F, E1638K, L1639P, P1648S, L1657I, V1665E, G1672R
CK domain	Type 2A (formerly IID)	C2773R

For an updated list of VWF mutations according to VWD type see <www.shef.ac.uk/vwf>.

associated with the appearance of allo-antibodies against VWF, which may render replacement therapy ineffective and stimulate anaphylactic reactions to treatment.[11] Gene defects of type 3 VWD patients from different populations have now been studied, but there was no founder effect and mutations were distributed throughout the entire VWF gene.[27] Compared to haemophilia, most VWD patients show relatively mild bleeding symptoms. Therefore, prenatal diagnosis is required mainly in case of parents already known to be carriers of VWD type 3, with gene defects identified in their first affected child. Neonatal diagnosis can be performed in case of children born from parents with VWF defects already characterised, but phenotypic diagnosis of VWD should be always confirmed later on in the child and compared with the other affected members within the same family. Since young children with VWD type 3 might carry deletions of VWF gene that predispose to the allo-antibodies to VWF, every new child with VWD type 3 should be intensively investigated by searching deletions by Southern blot analysis,[28] before starting extensive therapy with exogenous VWF concentrates.

MANAGEMENT

The goal of therapy for VWD is to correct the dual defects of haemostasis, *i.e.* abnormal platelet adhesion due to low VWF activities and the abnormal intrinsic coagulation pathway due to low FVIII levels.[29] Two therapeutic approaches are available to manage VWD patients: (i) desmopressin that releases endogenous VWF from endothelial compartments; and (ii) the transfusion of exogenous VWF contained in FVIII/VWF plasma-derived concentrates.

Desmopressin

Desmopressin (1-deamino-8-D-arginine vasopressin, desmopressin) is a synthetic analogue of vasopressin originally designed for the treatment of diabetes insipidus. The first successful clinical trial with desmopressin was in 1977, its aim being to avoid the use of blood products in mild haemophilia and VWD patients who needed dental extractions and other surgical procedures.[30] Following these early observations, desmopressin has been widely used for the treatment of these diseases. The obvious advantage is that desmopressin is relatively inexpensive and carries no risk of transmitting blood-borne viruses. Desmopressin is usually injected intravenously at a dose of 0.3 μg/kg diluted in 50 ml saline, infused over 30 min. This increases plasma FVIII/VWF 3–5 times above the basal levels within 30–60 min and, in general, high FVIII/VWF concentrations last for 6–8 h. Since the responses in a given patient are consistent on different occasions,[11] a test dose of desmopressin at the time of diagnosis helps to establish the individual response pattern.[13] The protocol of the desmopressin infusion test with the clinical and laboratory parameters to be used to assess the biological response in each patient are summarised in Table 8; the definition of biological response to desmopressin has also been reported.[13,31] This test infusion has also been recommended in children.[32] Infusions can be repeated every 12–24 h depending on the type and severity of the bleeding episode. However, most patients treated repeatedly with desmopressin become less responsive to therapy.[33] The drug is also available

Table 8 Recommendations for the infusion test with desmopressin

---

Infusion protocol
Administer in 30 min 0.3 μg/kg of desmopressin in 50 ml of saline. The same dosage can be administered also subcutaneously

Clinical and laboratory parameters
Factor VIII/VWF activities must be measured before and 0.5, 1, 2 and 4 h after the administration of desmopressin; bleeding time must be performed at least before and after 2 h. Check platelet count before and at least 2 h after infusion

Definition of responsiveness
VWD patients should be considered responsive to desmopressin if after 2 h they show increases of baseline levels of FVIII:C and VWF:RCo by at least 3-fold, with levels of at least 30 U/dl and bleeding time of 12 min or less, when prolonged

See Mazurier *et al.*[12] and Federici.[33]

---

in concentrated forms for subcutaneous and intranasal administration, which can be convenient for home treatment.[11] Side effects of desmopressin are usually mild, such as transient tachycardia and headache. Hyponatraemia and volume overload due to the antidiuretic effects of desmopressin are also relatively rare in adults and children. Despite the wide-spread use of desmopressin in the clinical management of VWD patients, there are no large prospective studies on efficacy and safety aimed to determine the benefits and the limits of this therapeutic approach in VWD. A large observational study evaluating both biological response and clinical efficacy in more than 150 patients with VWD types 1 and 2 has been organised on behalf of ISTH-SSC on VWF. For the first time, VWD patients will be enrolled not only to evaluate their biological response to desmopressin but also to test efficacy and safety during repeated injections required for bleeding episodes and major/minor surgery, with a prospective clinical evaluation during the following 24 months.

Other non-transfusional therapies for VWD

Antifibrinolytic amino acids are synthetic drugs that interfere with the lysis of newly formed clots by saturating the binding sites on plasminogen, thereby preventing its attachment to fibrin and making plasminogen unavailable within the forming clot. Epsilon aminocaproic acid (50 mg/kg, 4 times a day) and tranexamic acid (15–25 mg/kg, 3 times a day) are the most frequently used antifibrinolytic amino acids. Both can be administered orally, intravenously or topically and are useful alone or as adjuncts in the management of oral cavity bleeding, epistaxis, gastrointestinal bleeding and menorrhagia. They should be avoided in the management of urinary tract bleeding.

Oestrogens raise plasma VWF levels, but the response is variable and unpredictable, so they are not widely used for therapeutic purposes. It is common clinical experience that the continued use of oral contraceptives is very useful in reducing the severity of menorrhagia in women with VWD, even in those with type 3, despite the fact that FVIII/VWF levels are not modified.

Transfusional therapies

FVIII/VWF concentrates are indicated in type 3 VWD, in type 2B because desmopressin can induce transient thrombocytopenia, and in all types 1 and 2 patients who are not responsive to desmopressin or who may have contra-indications to its use. Minimal requirements for plasma-derived FVIII/VWF concentrates in VWD management are the following: (i) they must contain VWF and some FVIII:C; (ii) they should be treated by virucidal methods; and (iii) before clinical use, they should be tested for pharmacokinetic profile and efficacy in retrospective and prospective clinical trials in relatively large numbers of VWD patients. Among several concentrates containing VWF, only four have been extensively evaluated in pharmacokinetic trials as well as in retrospective or prospective efficacy studies in VWD.[34] The Alphanate Study Group published results of pharmacokinetics and clinical efficacy studies in 2002 This was the first study to enrol not only type 3 ($n = 12$), but also type 2A ($n = 5$) and type 1 ($n = 18$) VWD patients. An important finding in this study was that, in VWD type 3, the half-life of FVIII:C was twice that of VWF:Ag due to the endogenous FVIII:C. Efficacy results showed that 75% of bleeding episodes were controlled with one or two infusions, and 71% of patients who received prophylactic treatment for surgery or invasive procedures had good clinical responses. In another retrospective study, 22 VWD patients in Italy received Fanhdi, a concentrate similar to Alphanate. Excellent-to-good clinical responses were seen in 92% of bleeding episodes and in 93% of surgical procedures, despite the relative loss of high molecular weight VWF multimers in the product.

Haemate P/Humate-P, an intermediate-purity FVIII/VWF concentrate, has been widely used in VWD and has been considered the gold standard in the management of this disorder. This product was introduced into clinical practice in Europe (Haemate P) in 1984 and in the US (Humate-P) in 1999. The first pharmacokinetic study of Haemate P, published in 1998, was a single-centre evaluation involving 6 type 3 VWD patients. Clinical efficacy data were collected retrospectively, and showed excellent-to-good responses for 99% of surgery cases ($n = 73$) and for 97% of bleeding episodes ($n = 3440$). Results of a large retrospective study organised by the Canadian Hemophilia Centers were published in 2002.[34] Other published studies include a retrospective analysis of Haemate P/Humate-P efficacy and safety in preventing bleeding during surgery or invasive procedures in 26 Italian VWD patients, as well as two prospective, multicentre, open-label, non-randomised studies conducted in the US on Haemate P/Humate-P used in urgent bleeding and urgent surgical events.[34] Another plasma-derived VWF concentrate with low FVIII:C levels was introduced in France in 1992 and the first pharmacokinetic study in type 3 VWD was published in 1996.[34] An improved version of this concentrate, which is almost devoid of FVIII:C, was evaluated in two large French and European studies and data on pharmacokinetics are now available.[34] Results in type 3 VWD show no major differences in VWF:RCo and VWF:Ag for the concentrates that did or did not contain FVIII:C: as expected, the only difference was an approximate 6-h delay in FVIII:C increase with the concentrate devoid of FVIII:C; therefore, administration of exogenous FVIII:C is recommended in type 3 VWD cases of acute life-threatening bleeding episodes or emergency surgeries.[34] Clinical efficacy results of the French and European studies are expected in 2006. Data derived from pharmacokinetic and clinical studies have contributed to more appropriate use of FVIII/VWF concentrates. The specific activity of concentrates is important to derive the degree of FVIII/VWF product purity, while VWF:RCo/Ag and VWF:RCo/FVIII ratios can be considered markers of VWF/FVIII protein activity. The accumulation of FVIII:C that is exogenously infused together with that endogenously synthesised and stabilised by the infused VWF may cause very high FVIII levels when multiple infusions are given to cover major surgery. There is some concern that sustained high FVIII levels may increase risk of postoperative deep vein thrombosis: however, deep vein thromboses are rare events that have been reported only in VWD patients receiving repeated FVIII/VWF concentrate infusions to maintain clinical haemostasis after surgery.[35] Therefore, when using repeated injections of FVIII/VWF concentrates for recurrent bleeding episodes and especially after major surgery, we suggest daily monitoring of FVIII:C levels and adjusting the FVIII/VWF

Table 9 Doses of FVIII-VWF concentrates recommended in von Willebrand disease patients unresponsive to desmopressin

Type of bleeding	Dose (IU/kg)	Number of infusions	Objective
Major surgery	50	Once a day or every other day	Maintain FVIII > 50 U/dl for at least 7 days
Minor surgery	30	Once a day or every other day	FVIII > 30 U/dL for at least 5–7 days
Dental extractions	20–40	Single	FVIII >30 U/dl for up to 6 h
Spontaneous or post-traumatic bleeding	20–40	Single	

concentrate dose to keep the patient's FVIII:C levels at 50–150 U/dl. The minimal VWF:RCo level to maintain sufficient haemostasis in VWD has not yet been determined in prospective studies; however, preliminary retrospective data from a large cohort of well-characterised Italian VWD patients suggest that VWF:RCo levels > 30 U/dl are associated with a low incidence of spontaneous mucosal bleedings.[14] The dosages of concentrates with the most correct therapeutic approaches according to VWD types are summarised in Tables 9 and 10.

Treatment of patients with allo-antibodies to von Willebrand factor

For the rare patients with type 3 VWD who develop anti-VWF allo-antibodies after multiple transfusions, the use of VWF concentrates not only is ineffective, but may even cause postinfusion anaphylaxis due to the formation of immune complexes.[36] These reactions may be life-threatening. To overcome this drawback, a patient undergoing emergency abdominal surgery was treated with recombinant FVIII, because this product, that contains no VWF, could not cause anaphylactic reactions. In view of the very short half-life of FVIII without its VWF carrier, recombinant FVIII had to be administered by

Table 10 Management of different types and subtypes of von Willebrand disease

	Treatment of choice	Alternative and adjunctive therapy
Type 1	Desmopressin	Antifibrinolytics, oestrogens
Type 2A	FVIII/VWF concentrates	
Type 2B	FVIII/VWF concentrates	
Type 2M	Desmopressin	FVIII/VWF concentrates
Type 2N	Desmopressin	FVIII/VWF concentrates
Type 3	FVIII/VWF concentrate	Desmopressin, platelet concentrates
Type 3 with allo-antibodies	Recombinant FVIII	Recombinant activated FVII

continuous i.v. infusion, at very large doses, to keep FVIII levels above 50 U/dl for 10 days after surgery.[37] Another possible therapeutic approach is recombinant activated factor VII (rFVIIa) that can be used in VWD with allo-antibodies according to the same dosage and regimens as for haemophilia A patients with inhibitors.[38] Since only few data on efficacy and safety on the use of recombinant FVIII and VIIa are available, prospective cross-over studies should be designed to determine the best therapeutic approach in these cases.

The use of FVIII/VWF concentrates in the secondary long-term prophylaxis of von Willebrand's disease

Patients with severe forms of VWD may have frequent haemarthrosis, especially in cases with FVIII levels below 20 IU. Mucosal bleedings are the most frequent in VWD because they can occur not only in VWD type 3, but also in types 1, 2A, 2B and 2M, all characterised by VWF:RCo below 10 IU.[13,14] There are rare patients with chronic gastrointestinal bleeds, with or without demonstrated vascular lesions localised in the gastrointestinal tract, who have been treated on demand every day or every other day for more than a year in an attempt to stop such bleeding. In several cases, the identification and local intervention at the site of vascular angiodysplasia and Dieulafoy's lesions could stop bleeding and resolve the problem.[11] Unfortunately, in most cases, the site of bleeding cannot be found and, therefore, large doses of FVIII/VWF concentrates are required to control the bleeding and reduce the need of packed red blood cells transfused to maintain physiological levels of haemoglobin. Compared to patients with haemophilia A and B who have been exposed to secondary long-term prophylaxis mainly to prevent degeneration of the joints, little retrospective or prospective data on secondary long-term prophylaxis in VWD are available. The largest experience on secondary long-term prophylaxis has been collected in VWD in Sweden in 35 patients with severe forms of VWD.[39] Another experience of secondary long-term prophylaxis was performed in a large cohort of VWD patients by our group. This is a cohort study on 452 VWD patients regularly followed up at our institute for at least 3 years. Overall, 89 of 452 cases (20%) have been treated with FVIII/VWF concentrates during the last 2 years because of one or more bleedings; 11 of 89 (12%) were included in a long-term prophylaxis programme because of frequent recurrence of bleeds at the same sites. Effectiveness of prophylaxis was based on resolution/reduction of bleeding as well as on numbers of transfused packed red blood cells and days of hospitalisation. Safety was measured by monitoring side effects and FVIII levels before and after every injection during the first 3 weeks of prophylaxis.[40] Prophylaxis was started because of gastrointestinal bleeds in 7 patients with VWD type 3 ($n = 1$), 2A ($n = 4$), 2M ($n = 1$) and 1 ($n = 1$) and for joint bleeds only in VWD type 3 ($n = 4$). Prophylaxis stopped bleeding in 8 patients and largely reduced hospitalisation for packed red blood cell transfusions in the remaining 3. When prophylaxis was compared with the previous on-demand regimen in all 11 cases, the annual total FVIII IU of concentrate as well as number of packed red blood cells used and days in hospital were significantly reduced. As far as safety, FVIII levels were always < 180 U/dl in all VWD and no side effects, including thrombosis, were observed. These two retrospective studies suggest that cost-effectiveness of these prophylaxis regimens versus on-demand therapy should be further investigated in large prospective studies.

Key points for clinical practice

- von Willebrand disease (VWD) is the most frequent inherited disorder of haemostasis and is due to quantitative (VWD type 1 and 3) or qualitative (VWD type 2) defects of von Willebrand factor (VWF).

- Due to the large heterogeneity of VWF defects and to the external variables (blood groups and other physiological modifiers) influencing VWF levels in the circulation, VWD diagnosis can be difficult in children especially in its relatively mild forms.

- Three criteria should be always satisfied for a correct VWD diagnosis: (i) a positive bleeding history in the patient; (ii) reduced levels of VWF activity in plasma; and (iii) a positive family history suggestive of VWD.

- According to the most recent clinical prospective studies, bleeding history in the patients and in their family members should be now derived from a detailed questionnaire on 11 bleeding symptoms and a bleeding score can be calculated.

- The ristocetin co-factor activity of VWF (VWF:RCo) is the most useful test for VWD screening in the general population because it reproduces *in vitro* the first VWF interactions with its platelet receptor: however, other assays are required to identify and classify the different VWD types.

- The current classification into different VWD types (1, 2A, 2B, 2M, 2N, 3) is important to understand the basic mechanisms of VWF defects, to determine the risk of bleeding and to select the best therapeutic approach.. Molecular screening can be important to confirm phenotypic diagnosis.

- Compared to haemophilia, most VWD patients show relatively mild bleeding symptoms. Therefore, prenatal diagnosis is required mainly in case of parents already known to be a carrier of VWD type 3, with gene defects identified in their first affected child. No major bleeding problems usually occur at birth also in severe type 3 VWD.

- Neonatal diagnosis can be performed in case of children born from parents with previously characterised VWF defects, but phenotypic diagnosis of VWD should always be confirmed and compared with the other affected members within the same family.

- Since young children with VWD type 3 might carry deletions of the VWF gene that predispose to the allo-antibodies to VWF, every new child with VWD type 3 should be intensively investigated by searching deletions using Southern blot analysis, before starting extensive therapy with exogenous VWF concentrates.

- Desmopressin is the first line treatment in most VWD types 1 and 2. All children at diagnosis should be exposed to an infusion trial with desmopressin to determine their responsiveness to this drug.

Key points for clinical practice (continued)

- Plasma-derived FVIII/VWF concentrates are safe and effective in the management of most bleeding episodes and in preventing bleeding during surgery. They are indicated in all children proven to be unresponsive to desmopressin.

- Plasma-derived FVIII/VWF can be used also in secondary, long-term prophylaxis. In case of repeated injections of concentrates especially during surgery, FVIII levels should be carefully observed before deciding on an additional dose.

References

1. Lee CA, Kessler CM. (eds) Proceedings of a Nordic von Willebrand symposium. *Haemophilia* 1999; **5 (Suppl 2)**.
2. Ruggeri ZM. Structure of von Willebrand factor and its function in platelet adhesion and thrombus formation. *Best Practice Res Clin Haematol* 2001; **14**: 257–79.
3. Mancuso DJ, Tuley EA, Westfield LA *et al.* Human von Willebrand factor gene and pseudogene: structural analysis and differentiation by polymerase chain reaction. *Biochemistry* 1991; **30**: 253–269.
4. Goodeve A, Eikenboom JCJ, Ginsburg D *et al.* A standard nomenclature for von Willebrand factor gene mutations and polymorphisms. On behalf of the ISTH SSC Subcommittee on von Willebrand factor. *Thromb Haemost* 2001; **85**: 929–931.
5. Vlot AJ, Koppelman SJ, Bouma BN, Sixma JJ. Factor VIII and von Willebrand Factor. *Thromb Haemost* 1998; **79**: 456–465.
6. Mazurier C, Rodeghiero F. Recommended abbreviations for von Willebrand factor and its activities. *Thromb Haemost* 2001; **85**: 929–931.
7. Gill JC, Endres-Brooks J, Bauer PJ, Marks WJ, Montgomery RR. The effect of ABO blood group on the diagnosis of von Willebrand disease. *Blood* 1987; **69**: 1691–1695.
8. Katz JA, Moake JL, McPherson PD *et al.* Relationship between human development and disappearance of unusually large von Willebrand factor multimers from plasma. *Blood* 1989; **73**: 1851–1858
9. Andrew M, Paes B, Milner R *et al.* Development of the human coagulation system in the healthy premature infant. *Blood* 1988; **72**: 1651–1657.
10. Sadler JE. A revised classification of von Willebrand disease. *Thromb Haemost* 1994; **71**: 520–523.
11. Castaman G, Federici AB, Rodeghiero F, Mannnucci PM. von Willebrand's disease in the year 2003: towards the complete identification of gene defects for correct diagnosis and treatment. *Haematologica* 2003; **88**: 94–108.
12. Mazurier C, Goudemand J, Hilbert L, Caron C, Fressinaud E, Meyer D. Type 2N von Willebrand disease: clinical manifestations, pathophysiology, laboratory diagnosis and molecular biology. *Best Practice Res Clin Haematol* 2001; **14**: 337–348.
13. Federici AB, Castaman G, Mannucci PM. Guidelines for the diagnosis and management of VWD in Italy. *Haemophilia* 2002; **8**: 607–621.
14. Federici AB. Clinical diagnosis of von Willebrand disease. *Haemophilia* 2004; **10**: 169–176.
15. Rodeghiero F, Castaman G, Tosetto A *et al.* The discriminant power of bleeding history for the diagnosis of von Willebrand disease type 1: an international multicenter study. *J Thromb Hemost* 2005; **3**: 2619–2626.
16. Tosetto A, Rodeghiero F, Castaman G *et al.* A quantitative analysis of bleeding symptoms in type 1 of von Willebrand disease: results from a multicenter European Study (MCMDM-1VWD). *J Thromb Hemost* 2006; In press.
17. Mohlke KL, Ginsburg D. von Willebrand disease and quantitative variation in von Willebrand factor. *J Lab Clin Med* 1997; **130**: 252–261.

18. Kunicki TJ, Federici AB, Salamon DR *et al.* An association of candidate gene haplotypes and bleeding severity in von Willebrand disease type 1 pedigree. *Blood* 2004; **104**: 2359–2367.

19. Silwer J. von Willebrand's disease in Sweden. *Acta Paediatr Scand* 1973; **238**: 1–159.

20. Lak M, Peyvandi F, Mannucci PM. Clinical manifestations and complications of childbirth and replacement therapy in 348 Iranian patients with type 3 von Willebrand disease. *Br J Haematol* 2000; **111**: 1223–1229.

21. Mannucci PM, Lombardi R, Bader R *et al.* Heterogeneity of type I von Willebrand's disease: evidence for a subgroup with an abnormal von Willebrand factor. *Blood* 1985; **66**: 796–802.

22. Meyer D, Fressinaud E, Hilbert L *et al.* Type 2 von Willebrand disease causing defective von Willebrand factor-dependent platelet function. *Best Practice Res Clin Haematol* 2001; **14**: 349–364.

23. Lyons SE, Bruck ME, Bowie EJW *et al.* Impaired cellular transport produced by a subset of type IIA von Willebrand disease mutations. *J Biol Chem* 1992; **267**: 4424–4430.

24. Schneppenheim R, Federici AB, Budde U *et al.* von Willebrand disease type 2M 'Vicenza' in Italian and German patients: identification of the first candidate mutation (G3864A; R1205H) in 8 families. *Thromb Haemost* 2000; **83**: 136–140.

25. Castaman G, Missiaglia E, Federici AB, Schneppenheim R, Rodeghiero F. An additional candidate mutation (G2470A; M740I) in the original families with von Willebrand disease type 2M Vicenza and the G3864A (R1205H) mutation. *Thromb Haemost* 2000; **84**: 350–35-1.

26. Eikenboom JCJ. Congenital von Willebrand disease type 3: clinical manifestations, pathophysiology and molecular biology. *Best Practice Res Clin Haematol* 2001; **14**: 365–379.

27. Shelton-Inloes BB, Chebab FF, Mannucci PM *et al.* Gene deletion correlates with the development of alloantibodies in von Willebrand disease. *J Clin Invest* 1987; **79**: 1459–1465.

28. Baronciani L, Cozzi G, Canciani MT *et al* Molecular characterization of a multiethnic group of 21 patients with type 3 von Willebrand disease. *Thromb Haemost* 2000; **84**: 536–540.

29. Mannucci PM. Treatment of von Willebrand disease. *N Engl J Med* 2004; **351**: 683–694.

30. Mannucci PM, Ruggeri ZM, Pareti FI, Capitanio A. A new pharmacological approach to the management of haemophilia and von Willebrand disease. *Lancet* 1977; **1**: 869–872.

31. Federici AB, Mazurier C, Berntorp E *et al.* Biological response to desmopressin in patients with severe type 1 and type 2 von Willebrand disease: results of a multicenter European study. *Blood* 2004; **103**: 2032–2038.

32. Revel-Vilk S, Schmugge M, Carcao MD *et al.* Desmopressin (DDAVP) responsiveness in children with von Willebrand disease. *J Pediatr Hematol Oncol* 2003; **25**: 874–879.

33. Federici AB. Management of von Willebrand disease with factor VIII/von Willebrand factor concentrates: results from current studies and surveys. *Blood Coagul Fibrinol* 2005; **16**: XX–XX.

34. Mannucci PM. Venous thromboembolism in von Willebrand disease. *Thromb Haemost* 2002; **88**: 378–379.

35. Mannucci PM, Federici AB. Antibodies to von Willebrand factor in von Willebrand disease. *Adv Exp Med Biol* 1995; **125**: 348–355.

36. Bergamaschini L, Mannucci PM, Federici AB *et al.* Posttransfusion anaphylactic reaction in a patient with severe von Willebrand disease: role of complement and alloantibodies to von Willebrand factor. *J Lab Clin Med* 1995; **125**: 348–355.

37. Ciavarella N, Schiavoni M, Valenzano E *et al.* Use of recombinant factor VIIa (Novoseven) in the treatment of two patients with type III von Willebrand disease and an inhibitor against von Willebrand factor. *Haemostasis* 1996; 26: 150–154.

38. Boyer-Neumann C, Dreyfus M, Wolf M *et al.* Multi-therapeutic approach to manage delivery in an alloimmunized patient with type 3 von Willebrand disease. *J Thromb Haemost* 2003; **1**: 190–192.

39. Berntorp E, Petrini P. long-term prophylaxis in von Willebrand disease. *Blood Coagul Fibrinol* 2005; **16**: S23–S26.

40. Federici AB, Gianniello F, Canciani MT, Mannucci PM. Secondary long-term prophylaxis in severe patients with von Willebrand disease: An Italian cohort study [abstract 1782]. *Blood* 2005; **106**: 507a.

Timothy J. David

Paediatric literature review – 2004

ALLERGY

Bahna SL. You can have fish allergy and eat it too! J Allergy Clin Immunol 2004; 114: 125–126. *Review. See also pp. 159–165.*

Bateman B *et al.* The effects of a double blind, placebo controlled, artificial food colourings and benzoate preservative challenge on hyperactivity in a general population sample of preschool children. Arch Dis Child 2004; 89: 506–511. *Possible adverse effect of additives, but not detectable by clinic assessment.*

Breitenender H *et al.* A classification of plant food allergens. J Allergy Clin Immunol 2004; 113: 821–830. *Review.*

Breuer K *et al.* Late eczematous reactions to food in children with atopic dermatitis. Clin Exp Allergy 2004; 34: 817–824. *Isolated late eczematous reactions were seen in 12% of all positive challenges.*

Eigenmann PA *et al.* Food colourings and preservatives – allergy and hyperactivity. Lancet 2004; 364: 823–824. *Review.*

Fleischer DM *et al.* Peanut allergy: recurrence and its management. J Allergy Clin Immunol 2004; 114: 1195–1201. *Children who outgrow peanut allergy are at risk for recurrence.*

Holgate ST. The epidemic of asthma and allergy. J R Soc Med 2004; 97: 103–110. *Review.*

Timothy J. David MB ChB MD PhD FRCP FRCPCH DCH
Professor of Child Health and Paediatrics, Booth Hall Children's Hospital, Charlestown Road,
Blackley, Manchester M9 7AA, UK
E-mail: t.david@netcomuk.co.uk

Hu W *et al.* Making clinical decisions when the stakes are high and the evidence unclear. BMJ 2004; 329: 852–854. *Debate about need for adrenaline auto-injectors in children with peanut allergy.*

Johansson SGO *et al.* Revised nomenclature for allergy for global use: report of the nomenclature review committee of the World Allergy Organization, October 2003. J Allergy Clin Immunol 2004; 113: 832–836. *Review.*

Lack G. New developments in food allergy: old questions remain. J Allergy Clin Immunol 2004; 114: 127–130. *Review.*

Laubereau B *et al.* Effect of breast-feeding on the development of atopic dermatitis during the first 3 years of life – results from the gini–birth cohort study. J Pediatr 2004; 144: 602–607. *Does not support the hypothesis that exclusive breast-feeding is a risk factor for development of atopic dermatitis. See also pp. 564–567.*

Perry TT *et al.* Risk of oral food challenges. J Allergy Clin Immunol 2004; 114: 1164–1168. *No children required hospitalisation, and there were no deaths.*

Perry TT *et al.* Distribution of peanut allergen in the environment. J Allergy Clin Immunol 2004; 113: 973–976. *Relatively easily cleaned from hands and tabletops.*

Rosenthal M. How a non-allergist survives an allergy clinic. Arch Dis Child 2004; 89: 238–243. *Review.*

Sampson HA. Update on food allergy. J Allergy Clin Immunol 2004; 113: 805–819. *Review.*

Sicherer SH *et al.* Advances in allergic skin disease, anaphylaxis, and hypersensitivity reactions to foods, drugs, and insect stings. J Allergy Clin Immunol 2004; 114: 118–124. *Review.*

Sopo SM *et al.* Sublingual immunotherapy in asthma and rhinoconjunctivitis; systematic review of paediatric literature. Arch Dis Child 2004; 89: 620–624. *Low-to-moderate clinical efficacy.*

Stabbell Benn C *et al.* Cohort study of sibling effect, infectious disease, and risk of atopic dermatitis during first 18 months of life. BMJ 2004; 328: 1223–1226. *Early infections do not seem to protect against allergic diseases.*

Turunen S *et al.* Lymphoid nodular hyperplasia and cow's milk hypersensitivity in children with chronic constipation. J Pediatr 2004; 145: 606–611. *No evidence of cow's milk allergy in children with chronic constipation. See also pp. 578–580.*

Velissariou I *et al.* Management of adrenaline (epinephrine) induced digital ischaemia in children after accidental injection from an EpiPen. Emerg Med J 2004; 21: 387–388. *Report of 3 cases seen in a 6-month period.*

CARDIOLOGY

Andrews RE *et al.* Interventional cardiac catheterisation in congenital heart disease. Arch Dis Child 2004; 89: 1168–1173. *Review.*

Fu YC *et al.* Cardiac complications of enterovirus rhombencephalitis. Arch Dis Child 2004; 89: 368–373. *Acute heart failure was noted in 19% of patients with enterovirus rhombencephalitis, which had a fatality rate of 77%.*

COMMUNITY

Baddock SA *et al.* Bed-sharing and the infant's thermal environment in the home setting. Arch Dis Child 2004; 89: 1111–1116. *Bed-share infants experience warmer thermal conditions than those of cot-sleeping infants.*

Barnett AL *et al.* Can the Griffiths scales predict neuromotor and perceptual–motor impairment in term infants with neonatal encephalopathy? Arch Dis Child 2004; 89: 637–643. *A poor score on the Griffiths scales at 1 and/or 2 years is a good predictor of impairment at school age.*

Black D *et al.* Babies behind bars revisited. Arch Dis Child 2004; 89: 896–898. *Review.*

Blair PS *et al.* The prevalence and characteristics associated with parent–infant bed-sharing in England. Arch Dis Child 2004; 89: 1106–1110. *Bed sharing strongly related to breast feeding. See also pp. 1082–1083.*

Bu'Lock FA. Dummies. Arch Dis Child 2004; 89: 1081–1082. *Review.*

Frankowski BL. Sexual orientation and adolescents. Pediatrics 2004; 113: 1827–1832. *Review.*

Mather M. Community paediatrics in crisis. Arch Dis Child 2004; 89: 697–699. *Review. See also pp. 695–696.*

McArdle P. Substance abuse by children and young people. Arch Dis Child 2004; 89: 701–704. *Review.*

Roo MR *et al.* Long term cognitive development in children with prolonged crying. Arch Dis Child 2004; 89: 989–992. *Excessive uncontrolled crying that persists beyond 3 months of age may be a marker for cognitive deficits.*

ACCIDENTS

Dunning J *et al.* The implications of NICE guidelines on the management of children presenting with head injury. Arch Dis Child 2004; 89: 763–767. *In place of skull radiography and admission, computed tomography is advocated.*

Dunning J *et al.* A meta-analysis of variables that predict significant intracranial injury in minor head trauma. Arch Dis Child 2004; 89: 653–659. *Significant correlation between intracranial haemorrhage and skull fracture, focal neurology, loss of consciousness, and GCS abnormality.*

Martin BW *et al.* Patterns and risks in spinal trauma. Arch Dis Child 2004; 89: 860–865. *Study of 662 patients.*

Norton C *et al.* Head injury and limb fracture in modern playgrounds. Arch Dis Child 2004; 89: 152–153. *Impact absorbing surfaces help.*

Norton C *et al.* Playground injuries to children. Arch Dis Child 2004; 89: 103–108. *Review.*

Osterhoudt KC. Risk factors for emesis after therapeutic use of activated charcoal in acutely poisoned children. Pediatrics 2004; 113: 806–810. *Previous vomiting or nasogastric tube administration were risk factors.*

CHILD ABUSE

Adams G *et al.* Update from the Ophthalmology Child Abuse Working Party: Royal College Ophthalmologists. Eye 2004; 18: 795–798. *Review.*

Bechtel K *et al.* Characteristics that distinguish accidental from abusive injury in hospitalized young children. Pediatrics 2004; 114: 165–168. *Retinal haemorrhage covering the macula and extending to the periphery of the retina, abnormal mental status and seizures were associated with abuse.*

Chan L *et al.* When is an abnormal frenulum a sign of child abuse? Arch Dis Child 2004; 89: 277. *There can be non-traumatic abnormalities of the frenulum.*

Craft AW *et al.* Munchausen syndrome by proxy and sudden infant death. BMJ 2004; 328: 1309–1312. *Review.*

Ellaway BA *et al.* Are abused babies protected from further abuse? Arch Dis Child 2004; 89: 845–846. *Of the 49 babies who returned home following child protection investigations, 15 were further abused in the 3-year period.*

Ellaway BA *et al.* Are abused babies protected from further abuse? Arch Dis Child 2004; 89: 845–846. *Re-abuse rate was 31%.*

Harding B *et al.* Shaken baby syndrome. BMJ 2004; 328: 720–721. *Review. See also pp. 719–720.*

Hymel KP. Traumatic intracranial injuries can be clinically silent. J Pediatr 2004; 144: 701–702. *Review. See also pp. 719–722.*

Johnson CF. Child sexual abuse. Lancet 2004; 364: 462–470. *Review.*

Lantz PE *et al.* Perimacular retinal folds from childhood head trauma. BMJ 2004; 328: 754–756. *Retinal haemorrhages, retinoschisis and perimacular folds resulted from massive crush injury to head.*

Malnick S *et al.* Pattern of prescription of the shaken baby syndrome. Four types of inflicted brain injury predominate. BMJ 2004; 328: 766–769. *Divides cases into four categories according to the pattern of presentation.*

Reijneveld SA *et al.* Infant crying and abuse. *Lancet* 2004; 364: 1340–1342. *In infants aged 6 months, 5.6% of parents reported having smothered, slapped, or shaken their baby at least once. See also pp. 1295–1296.*

Starling SP *et al.* Analysis of perpetrator admissions to inflicted traumatic brain injury in children. Arch Pediatr Adolesc Med 2004; 158: 454–458. *The symptoms of inflicted head injury in children are immediate.*

Stewart–Brown S. Legislation on smacking. BMJ 2004; 329: 1195–1196. *A complete ban would help improve parenting practices.*

Williams RL *et al.* In children undergoing chest radiography what is the specificity of rib fractures for non-accidental injury? Arch Dis Child 2004; 89: 490–492. *Rib fractures under age of 3 years highly predictive of abuse.*

CEREBRAL PALSY

Caulton JM *et al.* A randomised controlled trial of standing programme on bone mineral density in non-ambulant children with cerebral palsy. Arch Dis Child 2004; 89: 131–135. *Might reduce risk of vertebral fractures but unlikely to reduce risk of lower limb fractures.*

Koman LA *et al.* Cerebral palsy. Lancet 2004; 363: 1619–1631. *Review.*

Sleigh G *et al.* Gastrostomy feeding in cerebral palsy: a systematic review. Arch Dis Child 2004; 89: 534–539. *Review.*

IMMUNISATION

Bedford H *et al.* Misconceptions about the new combination vaccine. BMJ 2004; 329: 411–412. *New pentavalent vaccine is better in many ways.*

Fine PEM. Non-specific 'non-effects' of vaccination. BMJ 2004; 329: 1297–1298. *Literature does not support either beneficial or detrimental effects. See also pp. 1309–1311.*

Horton R. A statement by the editors of *The Lancet*. Lancet 2004; 363: 820–821. *Editorial associated with retraction of paper suggesting a link between MMR and autism. See also pp. 750.*

Levitsky LL. Childhood immunizations and chronic illness. N Engl J Med 2004; 350: 1380–1382. *Review.*

Moylett EH *et al.* Mechanistic actions of the risks and adverse events associated with vaccine administration. J Allergy Clin Immunol 2004; 114: 1010–1020. *Review.*

Robinson MJ *et al.* Antibody response to diphtheria–tetanus–pertussis immunization in preterm infants who receive dexamethasone for chronic lung disease. Pediatrics 2004; 113: 733–737. *Antibody responses are reduced but clinical significance is unclear.*

Trotter CL *et al.* Effectiveness of meningococcal serogroup C conjugate vaccine 4 years after introduction. Lancet 2004; 364: 365–367. *Rapid waning of vaccine effectiveness in routinely vaccinated infants is worrying. See also pp. 309–310.*

INFANT FEEDING

Collins CT *et al.* Effect of bottles, cups, and dummis on breast feeding in preterm infants: randomised controlled trial. BMJ 2004; 329: 193–196. *Dummies do not affect breast feeding.*

Wright CM *et al.* Postnatal weight loss in term infants: what is 'normal' and do growth charts allow for it? Arch Dis Child 2004; 89: F254–F257. *Neonatal weight loss is brief, with few children remaining more than 10% below birth weight after 5 days.*

SCREENING

Comeau AM *et al.* Population-based newborn screening for genetic disorders when multiple mutation DNA testing is incorporated: a cystic fibrosis newborn screening model demonstrating increased sensitivity but more carrier detections. Pediatrics 2004; 113: 1573–1581. *110 of 112 cystic fibrosis affected infants were detected by screening. See also pp. 1811–1812.*

Kennedy C *et al.* Universal neonatal hearing screening moving from evidence to practice. Arch Dis Child 2004; 89: F378–F383. *Review.*

Olusanya BO *et al.* Infant hearing screening: route to informed choice. Arch Dis Child 2004; 89: 1039–1040. *Review.*

Russ SA *et al.* Qualitative analysis of parents' experience with early detection of hearing loss. Arch Dis Child 2004; 89: 353–358. *Parents need greater support during the testing and at the time of diagnosis.*

Taylor HA *et al.* Ethical issues in newborn screening research: lessons from The Wisconsin cystic fibrosis trial. J Pediatr 2004; 145: 292–296. *Review.*

SUDDEN INFANT DEATH SYNDROME

Byard RW. Unexpected infant death: lessons from the Sally Clark case. Med J Aust 2004; 181: 52–54. *Review.*

Carpenter RG *et al.* Sudden unexplained infant death in 20 regions in Europe: case control study. Lancet 2004; 363: 185–191. *Suggests a basis for further substantial reductions in SIDS incidence rates.*

de Jonge GA *et al.* Sudden infant death syndrome in child care settings in The Netherlands. Arch Dis Child 2004; 89: 427–430. *Over 10% of cases of SIDS took place during some type of child care.*

Horne RSC *et al.* Comparison of evoked arousability in breast and formula fed infants. Arch Dis Child 2004; 89: 22–25. *Breast-fed infants are more easily aroused at 2–3 months of age than formula-fed infants. This age co-incided with the peak incidence of SIDS.*

Krous HF *et al.* Sudden infant death syndrome and unclassified sudden infant deaths: a definitional and diagnostic approach. Pediatrics 2004; 114: 234–238. *Review.*

Levene S *et al.* Sudden unexpected death and covert homicide in infancy. Arch Dis Child 2004; 89: 443–447. *Review.*

Mooney JA *et al.* Higher incidence of SIDS at weekends, especially in younger infants. Arch Dis Child 2004; 89: 670–672. *The excess of SIDS at weekends still appears to be present.*

Opdal SH *et al.* The sudden infant death syndrome gene: does it exist? Pediatrics 2004; 114: e506–e512. *Review.*

Opdal SH *et al.* New insight into sudden infant-death syndrome. Lancet 2004; 364: 825–826. *Explains the newly identified TSPYL gene.*

Smith GCS *et al.* Second-trimester maternal serum levels of alpha-fetoprotein and the subsequent risk of sudden infant death syndrome. N Engl J Med 2004; 351: 978–986. *Direct association which may be mediated through impaired fetal growth and preterm birth.*

DERMATOLOGY

Beattie PE *et al.* A pilot study on the use of wet wraps in infants with moderate atopic eczema. Clin Exp Dermatol 2004; 29: 348–353. *Wet wraps are no more useful than conventional therapy.*

Flohr C *et al.* Evidence based management of atopic eczema. Arch Dis Child 2004; 89: ep35–ep39. *Review.*

Sladden MJ *et al.* Common skin infections in children. BMJ 2004; 329: 95–99. *Review.*

Ahmed SF *et al.* Intersex and gender assignment; the third say? Arch Dis Child 2004; 89: 847–850. *Review.*

Birrell G *et al.* Juvenile thyrotoxicosis; can we do better? Arch Dis Child 2004; 89: 745—750. *Review.*

Conrad SC *et al.* Soy formula complicates management of congenital hypothyroidism. Arch Dis Child 2004; 89: 37–40. *May need increased levothyroxime doses to achieve normal thyroid function tests.*

Crofton PM *et al.* Cortisol and growth hormone response to spontaneous hypoglycaemia in infants and children. Arch Dis Child 2004; 89: 472–478. *Young infants mount a poor cortisol response compared with older infants and children.*

Eugster EA *et al.* Definitive diagnosis in children with congenital hypothyroidism. J Pediatr 2004; 144: 643–647. *A significant percentage of children have a transient requirement for thyroid hormone.*

Ogilvy–Stuart AL *et al.* Early assessment of ambiguous genitalia. Arch Dis Child 2004; 89: 401–407. *Review.*

DIABETES

Dunger DB *et al.* ESPE/LWPES consensus statement on diabetic ketoacidosis in children and adolescents. Arch Dis Child 2004; 89: 188–194. *Review.*

Ehtisham S *et al.* First UK survey of paediatric type 2 diabetes and MODY. Arch Dis Child 2004; 89: 526–529. *UK children still have a low prevalence of type 2 diabetes.*

Greenhalgh S *et al.* Forearm blood glucose testing in diabetes mellitus. Arch Dis Child 2004; 89: 516–518. *An acceptable alternative to finger prick testing.*

Hviid A *et al.* Childhood vaccination and Type 1 diabetes. N Engl J Med 2004; 350: 1398–1404. *Do not support a causal relation.*

Lowes L *et al.* Management of newly diagnosed diabetes: home or hospital? Arch Dis Child 2004; 89: 934–937. *Review.*

Porter JR *et al.* Acquired non-type 1 diabetes in childhood: subtypes, diagnosis, and management. Arch Dis Child 2004; 89: 1138–1144. *Review.*

Weill J *et al.* Understanding the rising incidence of type 2 diabetes in adolescence. Arch Dis Child 2004; 89: 502–505. *Review.*

GROWTH

Dattani M *et al.* Growth hormone deficiency and related disorders: insights into causation, diagnosis, and treatment. Lancet 2004; 363: 1977–1987. *Review.*

Mills JL *et al.* Long-term mortality in the United States cohort of pituitary-derived growth hormone recipients. J Pediatr 2004; 144: 430–436. *Hypoglycaemia and adrenal insufficiency accounted for far more mortality than Creutzfeldt–Jakob disease.*

Wright CM *et al.* Postnatal weight loss in term infants: what is 'normal' and do growth charts allow for it? Arch Dis Child 2004; 89: F254–F257. *Growth charts are misleading in the first 2 weeks, because they make no allowance for neonatal weight loss.*

ENT

Lieberthal AS *et al.* Diagnosis and management of acute otitis media. Pediatrics 2004; 113: 1451–1465. *Review.*

van Staaij BK *et al.* Effectiveness of adenotonsillectomy in children with mild symptoms of throat infections or adenotonsillar hypertrophy: open, randomised controlled trial. BMJ 2004; 329: 651–654. *No major clinical benefits over watchful waiting.*

GASTROENTEROLOGY

Bonamco M *et al.* Tissue transglutaminase autoantibody detection in human saliva: a powerful method for celiac disease screening. J Pediatr 2004; 144: 632–636. *A non-invasive, simple to perform, reproducible and sensitive method.*

Burnett CA *et al.* Nurse management of intractable functional constipation: a randomised controlled trial. Arch Dis Child 2004; 89: 717–722. *Important role for clinic nurse specialists.*

Hoffenberg EJ *et al.* Clinical features of children with screening-identified evidence of celiac disease. Pediatrics 2004; 113: 1254–1259. *Screening-identified children demonstrate mild alterations in growth and nutrition.*

Marion AW *et al.* Fatty liver disease in children. Arch Dis Child 2004; 89: 648–652. *Review.*

Naser SA *et al.* Culture of *Mycobacterium avium* subspecies *paratuberculosis* from the blood of patients with Crohn's disease. Lancet 2004; 364: 1039–1044. *Viable mycobacteria were detected and might be causal. See also pp. 1013–1014.*

Quiros-Tejeira RE *et al.* Long-term parenteral nutritional support and intestinal adaptation in children with short bowel syndrome: a 25 year experience. J Pediatr 2004; 145: 157–163. *Report of 78 patients.*

Rosen R *et al.* Incidence of spinal cord lesions in patients with intractable constipation. J Pediatr 2004; 145: 409–411. *8 (9%) had spinal cord abnormalities.*

Russell RK *et al.* Unravelling the complex genetics of inflammatory bowel disease. Arch Dis Child 2004; 89: 598–603. *Review.*

COELIAC DISEASE

Hogberg L *et al.* Oats to children with newly diagnosed coeliac disease: a randomised double blind study. Gut 2004; 53: 649–654. *Oats are tolerated.*

Tommasini A *et al.* Mass screening for coeliac disease using antihuman transglutaminase antibody assay. Arch Dis Child 2004; 89: 512–515. *Two-thirds of cases were asymptomatic. See also pp. 499–500.*

HAEMATOLOGY

Bolton-Maggs PHB. Hereditary spherocytosis; new guidelines. Arch Dis Child 2004; 89: 809–812. *Review.*

Chakravorty S *et al.* Sickle cell disease pain in London and the Caribbean. Arch Dis Child 2004; 89: 272–273. *A simple diary can provide useful clinical information.*

Juwah AI *et al.* Types of anaemic crises in paediatric patients with sickle cell anaemia seen in Enugu, Nigeria. Arch Dis Child 2004; 89: 572–576. *Hyper-haemolytic crises were the commonest types.*

Revel-Vilk S *et al.* Effect of intracranial bleeds on the health and quality of life of boys with hemophilia. J Pediatr 2004; 144: 490–495. *Of 172 patients with haemophilia A or B, 18 (10%) had at least one episode.*

Stuart MJ *et al.* Sickle-cell disease. Lancet 2004; 364: 1343–1360. *Review.*

Thomas AE. The bleeding child; is it NAI? Arch Dis Child 2004; 89: 1163–1167. *Review.*

INFECTIOUS DISEASE

Boxall EH *et al.* Natural history of hepatitis B in perinatally infected carriers. Arch Dis Child 2004; 89: F456–F460. *Asymptomatic carriers remain infectious with notable liver pathology.*

Davison KL *et al.* Clusters of meningococcal disease in school and preschool settings in England and Wales: what is the risk? Arch Dis Child 2004; 89: 256–260. *There was a higher risk of further cases of meningococcal disease in schools and especially in preschool settings.*

Dobie D *et al.* Fusidic acid resistance in *Staphylococcus aureus*. Arch Dis Child 2004; 89: 74–77. *Review.*

Kirkwood C. Viral gastroenteritis in Europe: a new norovirus variant? Lancet 2004; 363: 671–672. *Review.*

Ladhani S *et al.* Bacteraemia due to *Staphylococcus aureus*. Arch Dis Child 2004; 89: 568–571. *Children most at risk of death with bacteraemia are least likely to have clinical features traditionally associated with this infection.*

Pathan N *et al.* Role of interleukin 6 in myocardial dysfunction of meningococcal septic shock. Lancet 2004; 363: 203–209. *Interleukin 6 is a mediator of myocardial depression in meningococcal disease.*

Plowe CV *et al.* Sustained clinical efficacy of sulfadoxine–pyrimethamine for uncomplicated falciparum malaria in Malawi after 10 years as first line treatment: five year prospective study. BMJ 2004; 328: 545–548. *Sulfadoxine–pyrimethamine has retained good efficacy in Malawi.*

Rao BL *et al.* A large outbreak of acute encephalitis with high fatality rate in children in Andhra Pradesh, India, in 2003, associated with Chandipura virus. Lancet 2004; 364: 869–874. *An important emerging pathogen. See also pp. 821 822.*

MEDICINE IN THE TROPICS

Chintu C *et al.* Co-trimoxazole as prophylaxis against opportunistic infections in HIV-infected Zambian children (CHAP): a double-blind randomised placebo-controlled trial. Lancet 2004; 364: 1865–1871. *Children of all ages should receive prophylaxis irrespective of local resistance to this drug.*

Dillingham R *et al.* Childhood stunting: measuring and stemming the staggering costs of inadequate water and sanitation. Lancet 2004; 363: 94–95. *Review.*

Manary MJ *et al.* Home based therapy for severe malnutrition with ready-to-use food. Arch Dis Child 2004; 89: 557–561. *Home-based therapy was successful.*

Puthucheary J *et al.* Severe acute respiratory syndrome in Singapore. Arch Dis Child 2004; 89: 551–556. *The diagnosis is suggested by the paucity of clinical signs with an abnormal chest radiograph, leukopenia, lymphopenia, thrombocytopenia.*

Solomon AW *et al.* Mass treatment with single-dose azithromycin for trachoma. N Engl J Med 2004; 351: 1962–1971. *Can interrupt the transmission of ocular* Chlamydia trachomatis *infection. See also pp. 2004–2007.*

Thapar N *et al.* Diarrhoea in children: an interface between developing and developed countries. Lancet 2004; 363: 641–653. *Review.*

Thomas JE *et al.* Early *Helicobacter pylori* colonisation: the association with growth faltering in The Gambia. Arch Dis Child 2004; 89: 1149–1154. *Predisposes to the development of malnutrition and growth faltering.*

MALARIA

Kremsner PG *et al.* Antimalarial combinations. Lancet 2004; 364: 285–294. *Review.*

Rosen JB *et al.* Malaria intermittent preventive treatment in infants, chemo-prophylaxis, and childhood vaccinations. Lancet 2004; 363: 1386–1388. *Review.*

METABOLIC

Allgrave J. Is nutritional rickets returning? Arch Dis Child 2004; 89: 699–701. *Review. See also pp. 781–784.*

Bosch AM *et al.* High tolerance for oral galactose in classical galactosaemia: dietary implications. Arch Dis Child 2004; 89: 1034–1036. *Attempts to exclude trace amounts of galactose from the diet are not justified.*

James J *et al.* Preventing childhood obesity by reducing consumption of carbonated drinks: cluster randomised controlled trial. BMJ 2004; 328: 1237–1239. *Schools can have an important role in preventing obesity in children.*

Kishnani PS *et al.* Pompe disease in infants and children. J Pediatr 2004; 144: S35–S43. *Review.*

Melis D *et al.* Brain damage in glycogen storage disease type 1. J Pediatr 2004; 144: 637–642. *Probably caused by recurrent severe hypoglycaemia.*

Sedlak TW *et al.* Bilirubin benefits: cellular protection by a biliverdin reductase antioxidant cycle. Pediatrics 2004; 113: 1776–1782. *Review.*

Wilcox WR. Lysomal storage disorders: the need for better pediatric recognition and comprehensive care. J Pediatr 2004; 144: S3–S14. *Review.*

Wraith JE *et al.* Enzyme replacement therapy for mucopolysaccharidosis I: a randomized, double-blinded, placebo-controlled, multinational study of recombinant human α-L-iduronidase (laronidase). J Pediatr 2004; 144: 581–588. *Definite benefit.*

MISCELLANEOUS

Armon K *et al.* The impact of presenting problem based guidelines for children with medical problems in an accident and emergency department. Arch Dis Child 2004; 89: 159–164. *Improved documentation; reduced invasive investigations; more appropriate treatment, and reduced time spent in A&E.*

Boisen KA *et al.* Difference in prevalence of congenital cryptorchidism in infants between two Nordic countries. Lancet 2004; 363: 1264–1269. *Much higher prevalence in Denmark than in Finland.*

Burns JC *et al.* Kawasaki syndrome. Lancet 2004; 364: 533–544. *Review.*

Christakis DA *et al.* Early television exposure and subsequent attentional problems in children. Pediatrics 2004; 113: 708–713. *Early television exposure is associated with attentional problems at age 7.*

De Inocencio J. Epidemiology of musculoskeletal pain in primary care. Arch Dis Child 2004; 89: 431–434. *A common presenting complaint.*

Dummer TJB *et al.* Hospital accessibility and infant death risk. Arch Dis Child 2004; 89: 232–234. *No evidence of an increased risk of infant death with greater travel time to hospitals.*

Evans AM *et al.* Prevalence of 'growing pains' in young children. J Pediatr 2004; 145: 255–258. *Prevalence was 36.9%.*

Friedman JN *et al.* Development of a clinical dehydration scale for use in children between 1 and 36 months of age. J Pediatr 2004; 145: 201–207. *A 4-item, 8-point, rating scale.*

Gatrad AR *et al.* Hindu birth customs. Arch Dis Child 2004; 89: 1094–1097. *Review.*

Gould J *et al.* Health needs of children in prison. Arch Dis Child 2004; 89: 549–550. *Review.*

Greenes DS *et al.* When body temperature changes, does rectal temperature lag? J Pediatr 2004; 144: 824–826. *When body arterial temperature changes rapidly, changes in rectal temperature may lag.*

Grigg J. Environmental toxins; their impact on children's health. Arch Dis Child 2004; 89: 244–250. *Review.*

Hagger LE. *The Human Rights Act 1998* and medical treatment: time for re-examination. Arch Dis Child 2004; 89: 460–463. *Review.*

Miura M *et al.* Coronary risk factors in Kawasaki disease treated with additional gammaglobulin. Arch Dis Child 2004; 89: 776–780. *An additional γ-globulin infusion, if administered early, may prevent coronary artery lesions in initial γ-globulin non-responders.*

Otieno H *et al.* Are bedside features of shock reproducible between different observers? Arch Dis Child 2004; 89: 977–979. *Not very.*

Rothenberg SP *et al.* Autoantibodies against folate receptors in women with a pregnancy complicated by a neural-tube defect. N Engl J Med 2004; 350: 134–142. *It is not yet known if these antibodies cause neural tube deficits. See also pp. 101–103.*

Stewart B *et al.* Validation of the Alder Hey Triage Pain Score. Arch Dis Child 2004; 89: 625–630. *Useful for triage.*

Tan M *et al.* Parents' attitudes toward performance of lumbar puncture on their children. J Pediatr 2004; 144: 400–402. *Parents can tolerate watching this procedure.*

Thomas AJ. Beneath the surface. Arch Dis Child 2004; 89: ep15–ep22. *Management of vulvo-vaginitis.*

Watson AR. Hospital youth work and adolescent support. Arch Dis Child 2004; 89: 440–442. *Review.*

White J *et al.* Parents measuring pulses; an observational study. Arch Dis Child 2004; 89: 274–275. *Parents can be taught to measure the pulse in school age children, but have difficulty with preschool children.*

NEONATOLOGY

Acharya AB *et al.* Oral sucrose analgesia for preterm infant venepuncture. Arch Dis Child 2004; 89: F17–F18. *Clear benefit of sucrose.*

Ahlfors CE. Effect of ibuprofen on bilirubin–albumin binding. J Pediatr 2004; 144: 386–388. *Ibuprofen interferes with bilirubin–albumin binding.*

Baud O. Postnatal steroid treatment and brain development. Arch Dis Child 2004; 89: F96–F100. *Review.*

Becher JC *et al.* The Scottish perinatal neuropathology study: clinicopathological correlation in early neonatal deaths. Arch Dis Child 2004; 89: F399–F407. *In a large proportion of neonatal deaths, brain injury predates the onset of labour.*

Bell R *et al.* Changing patterns of perinatal death, 1982–2000: a retrospective cohort study. Arch Dis Child 2004; 89: F531–F536. *No reduction in neonatal mortality from prematurity or mortality from congenital anomalies.*

Cartwright DW. Central venous lines in neonates: a study of 2186 catheters. Arch Dis Child 2004; 89: F504–F508. *One case of non-lethal pericardial effusion occurred in a baby whose catheter was inappropriately left coiled in the right atrium.*

Cornette L. Contemporary neonatal transport: problems and solutions. Arch Dis Child 2004; 89: F212–F214. *Review.*

Cuttini M *et al.* Should euthanasia be legal? An international survey of neonatal intensive care units staff. Arch Dis Child 2004; 89: F19–F24. *Opinions vary.*

Danielsson N *et al.* Intracranial haemorrhage due to late onset vitamin K deficiency bleeding in Hanoi province, Vietnam. Arch Dis Child 2004; 89: F546–F550. *Major public health problems in Hanoi.*

Davis PG *et al.* Resuscitation of newborn infants with 100% oxygen or air: a systematic review and meta-analysis. Lancet 2004; 364: 1329–1333. *Air should be used initially. See also pp. 1293–1294.*

Davis PJ *et al.* Long-term outcome following extracorporeal membrane oxygenation for congenital diaphragmatic hernia: the UK experience. J Pediatr 2004; 144: 309–315. *Long-term physical and neurodevelopmental morbidity remains in the majority of survivors.*

Di Lorenzo C et al. Gastric suction in newborns: guilty as charged or innocent bystander? J Pediatr 2004; 144: 417–420. *Review. See also pp. 449–454.*

Fenton AC *et al.* Optimising neonatal transfer. Arch Dis Child 2004; 89: F215–F219. *Review.*

Hallman M. Lung surfactant, respiratory failure, and genes. N Engl J Med 2004; 350: 1278–1280. *Review. See also pp. 1296–1303.*

Hameed B *et al.* Trends in the incidence of severe retinopathy of prematurity in a geographically defined population over a 10 year period. Pediatrics 2004; 113: 1653–1657. *The incidence of severe retinopathy of prematurity increased in the latter half of the last decade.*

Hofman PL *et al.* Premature birth and later insulin resistance. N Engl J Med 2004; 351: 2179–2186. *May be a risk factor for type 2 diabetes mellitus. See also pp. 2229–2231.*

Hussain K *et al.* Hyperinsulinaemic hypoglycaemia in preterm neonates. Arch Dis Child 2004; 89: F65–F67. *Report of 7 infants.*

Hussey SG *et al.* Comparison of three manual ventilation devices using an intubated mannequin. Arch Dis Child 2004; 89: F490–F493. *The anaesthetic bag with manometer and Neopuff device both facilitate accurate and reproducible manual ventilation.*

Inwald D *et al.* Enterovirus myocarditis as a cause of neonatal collapse. Arch Dis Child 2004; 89: F461–F462. *Of 7 cases, 3 died.*

Jackson GL *et al.* Are complete blood cell counts useful in the evaluation of asymptomatic neonates exposed to suspected chorioamnionitis? Pediatrics 2004; 113: 1173–1180. *No.*

Jackson L *et al.* A randomised controlled trial of morphine versus phenobarbitone for neonatal abstinence syndrome. Arch Dis Child 2004; 89: F300–F304. *Opiate replacement therapy helpful for management when maternal opiate use is prevalent.*

Jain A *et al.* Project 27/18. Arch Dis Child 2004; 89: F14–F16. *An enquiry into the quality of care and its effect on the survival of babies born at 27–28 weeks.*

Joyce R *et al.* Associations between perinatal interventions and hospital stillbirth rates and neonatal mortality. Arch Dis Child 2004; 89: F51–F56. *Stillbirth rates were significantly lower in units that took a more interventionalist approach and in those with higher levels of consultant obstetric staffing.*

Konduri GG *et al.* A randomized trial of early versus standard inhaled nitric oxide therapy in term and near-term newborn infants with hypoxic respiratory failure. Pediatrics 2004; 113: 559–564. *Improves oxygenation but does not reduce the incidence of ECMO/mortality.*

Kuschel CA *et al.* Can methadone concentrations predict the severity of withdrawal in infants at risk of neonatal abstinence syndrome? Arch Dis Child 2004; 89: F390–F393. *May be a useful predictor of severe withdrawal.*

Maayan–Metzger A *et al.* Characteristics of neonates with isolated rectal bleeding. Arch Dis Child 2004; 89: F68–F70. *Outcome was excellent.*

Marlow N. Neurocognitive outcome after very preterm birth. Arch Dis Child 2004; 89: F224–F228. *Review.*

McGuire W *et al.* Systematic review of transpyloric versus gastric tube feeding for preterm infants. Arch Dis Child 2004; 89: F245–F248. *Review.*

Menakaya J *et al.* A randomized comparison of resuscitation with an anaesthetic rebreathing circuit or an infant ventilator in very preterm infants. Arch Dis Child 2004; 89: F494–F496. *Very preterm infants can be safely and effectively resuscitated using a ventilator.*

Mercuri E *et al.* Neonatal cerebral infarction and neuromotor outcome at school age. Pediatrics 2004; 113: 95–100. *The involvement of the internal capsule on neonatal MRI is a good predictor for motor abnormalities.*

Modi N. Management of fluid balance in the very immature neonate. Arch Dis Child 2004; 89: F108–F111. *Review.*

Mohan PV *et al.* Can polyclonal intravenous immunoglobulin limit cytokine mediated cerebral damage and chronic lung disease in preterm infants? Arch Dis Child 2004; 89: F5–F8. *Review.*

Ng PC *et al.* Transient adrenocortical insufficiency of prematurity and systemic hypotension in very low birthweight infants. Arch Dis Child 2004; 89: F119–F126. *Results provide the centiles of serum cortisol for hypotensive patients and infants with normal blood pressure.*

Ng PC. Diagnostic markers of infection in neonates. Arch Dis Child 2004; 89: F229–F235. *Review.*

Nock ML *et al.* Relationship of the ventilatory response to hypoxia with neonatal apnea in preterm infants. J Pediatr 2004; 144: 291–295. *Apnoea of prematurity may be associated with enhanced peripheral chemoreceptor activity.*

Omari T *et al.* Paradoxical impact of body positioning on gastroesophageal reflux and gastric emptying in the premature neonate. J Pediatr 2004; 145: 194–200. *Right-side positioning is associated with increased reflux despite accelerating gastric emptying.*

Patra K *et al.* Adverse events associated with neonatal exchange transfusion in the 1990s. J Pediatr 2004; 144: 626–631. *The majority of adverse events are laboratory abnormalities, asymptomatic and treatable.*

Petrou S *et al.* Cost effectiveness analysis of neonatal extracorporeal membrane oxygenation based on four year results from the UK Collaborative ECMO Trial. Arch Dis Child 2004; 89: F263–F268. *Rigorous evidence of the cost effectiveness.*

Rennie JM *et al.* Non-expert use of the cerebral function monitor for neonatal seizure detection. Arch Dis Child 2004; 89: F37–F40. *Half of all neonatal seizures may be missed.*

Robertson NJ *et al.* The magnetic resonance revolution in brain imaging: impact on neonatal intensive care. Arch Dis Child 2004; 89: F193–F197. *Review.*

Shinwell ES *et al.* Effect of birth order on neonatal morbidity and mortality among very low birthweight twins: a population based study. Arch Dis Child 2004; 89: F145–F148. *Second twins are at increased risk for acute and chronic lung disease.*

Simpson JH *et al.* Reducing medication errors in the neonatal intensive care unit. Arch Dis Child 2004; 89: F480–F482. *Errors are common but actual harm is rare. See also pp. F483–F484.*

Steer P *et al.* High dose caffeine citrate for extubation of preterm infants: a randomised controlled trial. Arch Dis Child 2004; 89: F499–F503. *Short-term benefits.*

Stoll BJ *et al.* To tap or not to tap: high likelihood of meningitis without sepsis among very low birth weight infants. Pediatrics 2004; 113: 1181–1186. *Meningitis may be under-diagnosed.*

Strunk T *et al.* Does erythropoietin protect the preterm brain? Arch Dis Child 2004; 89: F364–F366. *Review.*

Theilen U *et al.* Infection with *Ureaplasma urealyticum*: is there a specific clinical and radiological course in the preterm infant? Arch Dis Child 2004; 89: F163–F167. *Less acute lung disease but early onset chronic lung disease.*

Trevisanuto D *et al.* The laryngeal mask airway: potential applications in neonates. Arch Dis Child 2004; 89: F485–F489. *Review.*

Tucker J *et al.* Epidemiology of preterm birth. BMJ 2004; 329: 675–678. *Review.*

Van Overmeire B *et al.* Prophylactic ibuprofen in premature infants: a multicentre, randomised, double–blind, placebo–controlled trial. Lancet 2004; 364: 1945–1949. *Does decrease occurrence of patient ductus arteriosus.*

Wright C *et al.* Investigating perinatal death: a review of the options when autopsy consent is refused. Arch Dis Child 2004; 89: F285–F288. *Review.*

Yeh TF *et al.* Outcomes at school age after postnatal dexamethasone therapy for lung disease of prematurity. N Engl J Med 2004; 350: 1304–1313. *Leads to substantial adverse effects on neuromotor and cognitive function at school age.*

NEPHROLOGY

Anonymous. Management of bedwetting in children. Drug Ther Bull 2004; 42: 33–37. *Review.*

Anonymous. Treating nocturnal enuresis in children. Effective Health Care 2004; 8: 1–7. *Review.*

Craig JC *et al.* Treatment of acute pyelonephritis in children. BMJ 2004; 328: 179–180. *Evidence favours a short course of appropriate antibiotics.*

Ismaili K *et al.* Long-term clinical outcome of infants with mild and moderate fetal pyelectasis: validation of neonatal ultrasound as a screening tool to detect significant nephrouropathies. J Pediatr 2004; 144: 759–765. *39% incidence of significant nephrouropathies.*

Leonard MB *et al.* Long-term, high-dose glucocorticoids and bone mineral content in childhood glucocorticoid-sensitive nephrotic syndrome. N Engl J Med 2004; 351: 868–875. *Did not demonstrate the expected deficits in the bone mineral content of the spine or whole body. See also pp. 924–926.*

McDonald SP *et al.* Long-term survival of children with end-stage renal disease. N Engl J Med 2004; 350: 2654–2662. *Increasing the proportion of children treated with renal transplantation rather than dialysis can improve survival further. See also pp. 2637–2639.*

Rao S *et al.* An improved urine collection pad method: a randomised clinical trial. Arch Dis Child 2004; 89: 773–775. *Changing the pad every 30 min reduces contamination.*

Zamir G *et al.* Urinary tract infection: is there a need for routine renal ultrasonography? Arch Dis Child 2004; 89: 466–468. *Questionable.*

NEUROLOGY

Anonymous. Managing migraine in children. Drug Ther Bull 2004; 42: 25–28. *Review.*

Baumer JH. Guidelines for the establishment and operation of human milk banks in the UK. Arch Dis Child 2004; 89: ep27–ep28. *Guidelines.*

Baumer JH. Childhood arterial stroke. Arch Dis Child 2004; 89: ep50–ep53. *Guideline review.*

Campbell C *et al.* Congenital myotonic dystrophy: assisted ventilation duration and outcome. Pediatrics 2004; 113: 811–816. *Prolonged ventilation was followed by greater morbidity and developmental delay.*

Church AJ *et al.* Anti-basal ganglia antibodies: a possible diagnostic utility in idiopathic movement disorders? Arch Dis Child 2004; 89: 611–614. *Potentially useful diagnostic marker in post-streptococcal neurological disorders. See also pp. 595–597.*

Goodkin HP *et al.* Intracerebral abscess in children: historical trends at Children's Hospital Boston. Pediatrics 2004; 113: 1765–1770. *Congenital heart disease was the most common predisposing factor.*

Harris RJ. Nutrition in the 21st century: what is going wrong. Arch Dis Child 2004; 89: 154–158. *Review.*

Hughes RAC. Treatment of Guillain–Barré syndrome with corticosteroids: lack of benefit? Lancet 2004; 363: 181–182. *Review. See also pp. 192–196.*

Mennella JA *et al.* Flavor programming during infancy. Pediatrics 2004; 113: 840–845. *Early exposure to hydrolysate formulae may be associated with greater acceptance later.*

Miller C *et al.* The epidemiology of subacute sclerosing panencephalitis in England and Wales 1990–2002. Arch Dis Child 2004; 89: 1145–1148. *Average annual decline of 14% consistent with the decline in notified measles.*

EPILEPSY

Baumer JH. Evidence based guideline for post-seizure management in children presenting acutely to secondary care. Arch Dis Child 2004; 89: 278–280. *Review.*

Lux AL *et al.* The United Kingdom Infantile Spasms Study comparing vigabatrin with prednisolone or tetracosactide at 14 days: a multicentre, randomised controlled trial. Lancet 2004; 364: 1773–1778. *Steroids more effective than vigabatrin.*

Newton RW. When is drug treatment not necessary in epilepsy? Factors that should influence the decision to prescribe. J R Soc Med 2004; 97: 15–19. *Review.*

O'Callaghan FJK *et al.* Epilepsy related mortality. Arch Dis Child 2004; 89: 705–707. *A decreasing problem?*

Warrington M. Living with reflex anoxic seizure. Arch Dis Child 2004; 89: 682. *Parental description of the problem.*

Waruiru C *et al.* Febrile seizures: an update. Arch Dis Child 2004; 89: 751–756. *Review.*

Wilson MT *et al.* Nasal/buccal midazolam use in the community. Arch Dis Child 2004; 89: 50–51. *20/24 (83% families) preferred using midazolam to rectal diazepam.*

NUTRITION

Miller Perrin E *et al.* Body mass index charts: useful yet underused. J Pediatr 2004; 144: 455–460. *BMI charting prompted greater recognition of a weight problem than height and weight charting.*

O'Callaghan FJK *et al.* The relation of infantile spasms, tubers, and intelligence in tuberous sclerosis complex. Arch Dis Child 2004; 89: 530–533. *Significant relation between the number of tubers and IQ.*

Silberstein SD. Migraine. Lancet 2004; 363: 381–391. *Review.*

Vaccarino FM *et al.* Injury and repair in developing brain. Arch Dis Child 2004; 89: F190–F192. *Review.*

Wyldes M *et al.* Isolated mild fetal ventriculomegaly. Arch Dis Child 2004; 89: F9–F13. *Review.*

Yates K *et al.* Outcome of children with neuromuscular disease admitted to paediatric intensive care. Arch Dis Child 2004; 89: 170–175. *Most recover.*

Zelnik N *et al.* Range of neurologic disorders in patients with celiac disease. Pediatrics 2004; 113: 1672–1676. *Patients were more prone to develop neurological disorders than control subjects.*

OPHTHALMOLOGY

Quinn GE *et al.* Recent advances in the treatment of amblyopia. Pediatrics 2004; 113: 1800–1802. *Review.*

ORTHOPAEDICS

Engelbert RHH *et al.* Pediatric generalized joint hypomobility and musculoskeletal complaints: a new entity? Clinical, biochemical, and osseal characteristics. Pediatrics 2004; 113: 714–719. *Increased stiffness of connective tissue as a result of higher amounts of collagen with increased cross-linking.*

Rauch F *et al.* Osteogenesis imperfecta. Lancet 2004; 363: 1377–1385. *Review.*

PSYCHIATRY

Coghill D *et al.* Use of stimulants for attention deficit hyperactivity disorder. BMJ 2004; 329: 907–909. *Debate.*

Hultman CM *et al.* Autism – prenatal insults or an epiphenomenon of a strongly genetic disorder? Lancet 2004; 364: 485–488. *Review.*

Jansen I *et al.* Associations between overweight and obesity with bullying behaviours in school-aged children. Pediatrics 2004; 113: 1187–1194. *Children are more likely to be the victims and perpetrators of bullying.*

Macleod J *et al.* Psychological and social sequelae of cannabis and other illicit drug use by young people: a systematic review of longitudinal, general population studies. Lancet 2004; 363: 1579–1588. *Better evidence is needed.*

Murray ML *et al.* A drug utilisation study of antidepressants in children and adolescents using the General Practice Research Database. Arch Dis Child 2004; 89: 1098–1102. *SSRLs have gained popularity for the treatment.*

Ramchandani P. Treatment of major depressive disorder in children and adolescents. BMJ 2004; 328: 3–4. *Most selective serotonin re-uptake inhibitors are no longer recommended.*

Roberts H *et al.* Mentoring to reduce antisocial behaviour in childhood. BMJ 2004; 328: 512–514. *Review.*

Vitiello B *et al.* Antidepressant medications in children. N Engl J Med 2004; 350: 1489–1491. *Review.*

Whittington CJ *et al.* Selective serotonin reuptake inhibitors in childhood depression: systematic review of published versus unpublished data. Lancet 2004; 363: 1341–1345. *Risks could outweigh benefits. See also pp. 1335–1336.*

RESPIRATORY

Bjornson CL *et al.* A randomized trial of a single dose of oral dexamethasone for mild croup. N Engl J Med 2004; 351: 1306–1313. *Consistent and small but important clinical and economic benefits. Long-term effects not known. See also pp. 1283–1284.*

Edwards EA *et al.* Sending children home on tracheostomy dependent ventilation: pitfalls and outcomes. Arch Dis Child 2004; 89: 251–255. *Review.*

Lakhanpaul M *et al.* Community acquired pneumonia in children: a clinical update. Arch Dis Child 2004; 89: ep29–ep34. *Review.*

Michelow IC *et al.* Epidemiology and clinical characteristics of community-acquired pneumonia in hospitalized children. Pediatrics 2004; 113: 701–707. *Bacteria found in 60% (pneumococcus 73% of these).*

Murphy SM *et al.* Burns caused by steam inhalation for respiratory tract infections in children. BMJ 2004; 328: 757. *Report of 7 cases.*

Pope CA. Air pollution and health – good news and bad. N Engl J Med 2004; 351: 1057–1067. *Editorial. See also pp. 1057–1064.*

Russell G. The use of inhaled corticosteroids during childhood: plus ca change.... Arch Dis Child 2004; 89: 893–895. *Review*.

Samuels MP. The effects of flight and altitude. Arch Dis Child 2004; 89: 448–455. *Review*.

Smith VC *et al*. Rehospitalization in the first year of life among infants with bronchopulmonary dysplasia. J Pediatr 2004; 144: 799–803. *Bronchopulmonary dysplasia substantially increases the risk of rehospitalisation during the first year of life*.

Whiteford L *et al*. Who should have a sleep study for sleep related breathing disorders? Arch Dis Child 2004; 89: 851–855. *Review*.

Williams JV *et al*. Human metapneumovirus and lower respiratory tract disease in otherwise healthy infants and children. N Engl J Med 2004; 350: 443–450. *Leading cause of respiratory tract infection in the first years of life. See also pp. 431–433*.

ASTHMA

Bacharier LB *et al*. Long-term effect of budesonide on hypothalmic–pituitary–adrenal axis function in children with mild to moderate asthma. Pediatrics 2004; 113: 1693–1699. *Absence of a comulative effect on hypothalmic–pituitary–adrenal axis function over a 3-year period*.

Doull IJM. The effect of asthma and its treatment on growth. Arch Dis Child 2004; 89: 60–63. *Review*.

Dunlop KA *et al*. Monitoring growth in asthmatic children treated with high dose inhaled glucocorticoids does not predict adrenal suppression. Arch Dis Child 2004; 89: 713–716. *Both growth and adrenal function should be monitored in patients on high-dose inhaled glucocorticoids*.

Hayden JT *et al*. A randomised crossover trial of facemask efficacy. Arch Dis Child 2004; 89: 72–73. *The choice of facemask can affect the drug dose delivered to the child*.

Mahachoklertwattana P *et al*. Decreased cortisol response to insulin induced hypoglycaemic in asthmatics treated with inhaled fluticasone proprionate. Arch Dis Child 2004; 89: 1055–1058. *Half the children had evidence of adrenal suppression*.

Massie J *et al*. Implementation of evidence based guidelines for paediatric asthma management in a teaching hospital. Arch Dis Child 2004; 89: 660–664. *No effect on re-attendance or re-admission to hospital, asthma, morbidity or quality of life*.

Sunderland RS *et al*. Continuing decline in acute asthma episodes in the community. Arch Dis Child 2004; 89: 282–285. *No causative factor has been identified*.

BRONCHIOLITIS

Handforth J *et al.* Prevention of respiratory syncytial virus infection in infants. BMJ 2004; 328: 1026–1027. *Palivizumab is effective but too expensive.*

Muething S *et al.* Decreasing overuse of therapies in the treatment of bronchiolitis by incorporating evidence at the point of care. J Pediatr 2004; 144: 703–710. *Evidence-based point-of-care instruments can have a significant effect on unwarranted treatment variation.*

CYSTIC FIBROSIS

Balfour-Lynn IM *et al.* Intravenous immunoglobulin for cystic fibrosis lung disease: a case series of 16 children. Arch Dis Child 2004; 89: 315–319. *May be worth considering.*

Borowitz D *et al.* Use of fecal elastase–1 to classify pancreatic status in patients with cystic fibrosis. J Pediatr 2004; 145: 322–326. *Accurate screening test. See also pp. 285–286.*

Brody AS. Early morphologic changes in the lungs of asymptomatic infants and young children with cystic fibrosis. J Pediatr 2004; 144: 145–146. *Review. See also pp. 154–161.*

Button BM *et al.* Chest physiotherapy, gastro-oesophageal reflux, and arousal in infants with cystic fibrosis. Arch Dis Child 2004; 89: 435–439. *Physiotherapy is associated with gastro-oesophageal reflux, distressed behaviour, and lower oxygen saturation.*

Koscik RL *et al.* Cognitive function of children with cystic fibrosis: deleterious effect of early malnutrition. Pediatrics 2004; 113: 1549–1558. *Prevention of prolonged malnutrition by early diagnosis is associated with better cognitive functioning.*

Maiya S *et al.* Cough plate versus cough swab in patients with cystic fibrosis; a pilot study. Arch Dis Child 2004; 89: 577–579. *Cough plates were more sensitive than cough swabs.*

Taccetti G *et al.* Sweat testing in newborns positive to neonatal screening for cystic fibrosis. Arch Dis Child 2004; 89: F463–F464. *Centiles of sweat chloride concentrations are presented.*

SURGERY

Burch M *et al.* Current status of paediatric heart, lung, and heart–lung transplantation. Arch Dis Child 2004; 89: 386–389. *Review.*

THERAPEUTICS

Avci Z *et al*. Nephrolithiasis associated with ceftriaxone therapy: a prospective study in 51 children. Arch Dis Child 2004; 89: 1069–1072. *4 of 51 developed small stones.*

Gray JE *et al*. Medication errors in the neonatal intensive care unit: special patients, unique issues. Arch Dis Child 2004; 89: F472–F473. *Review.*

Hoorn EJ *et al*. Acute hyponatremia related to intravenous fluid administration in hospitalized children: an observational study. Pediatrics 2004; 113: 1279–1284. *Caution needed when giving hypotonic fluid.*

Mahachoklertwattania P *et al*. Suppression of adrenal function in children with acute lymphoblastic leukemia following induction therapy with corticosteroid and other cytotoxic agents. J Pediatr 2004; 144: 736–740. *About 50% developed adrenal suppression 2 weeks after a 4-week therapy with prednisolone.*

Mann NP. What routine intravenous maintenance fluids should be used? Arch Dis Child 2004; 89: 411–414. *Debate. See pp. 411–414.*

Moghal NE *et al*. Ibuprofen and acute renal failure in a toddler. Arch Dis Child 2004; 89: 276–277. *The patient information sheet lacks advice on the importance of maintaining good fluid intake.*

Pashankar DS *et al*. Polyethylene glycol 3350 without electrolytes: a new safe, effective, and palatable bowel preparation for colonoscopy in children. J Pediatr 2004; 144: 358–362. *Effective and safe.*

Perondi MBM *et al*. A comparison of high-dose and standard-dose epinephrine in children with cardiac arrest. N Engl J Med 2004; 350: 1722–1730. *High-dose therapy may be worse than standard-dose therapy. See also pp. 1708–1709.*

Shields CH *et al*. Sleep deprivation for pediatric sedated procedures: not worth the effort. Pediatrics 2004; 113: 1204–1208. *No effect in reducing the sedation failure rate.*

Turner S *et al*. Role of the selective cyclo-oxygenase-2 (Cox-2) inhibitors in children. Arch Dis Child 2004; 89: ep46–ep49. *Review.*

Index

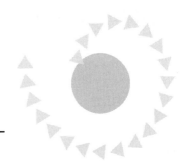

Note: references relating to the Literature Review chapter are indicated by an * after the page number.

Recent Advances in Paediatrics 21
Edited by T.J. David

ISBN 1-85315-572-1

ISSN 0-309-0140

Recent Advances in Paediatrics 20
Edited by T.J. David

Noisy breathing in children
Heather Elphick, Mark L. Everard

Sinusitis in children: diagnosis and management
Ellen R. Wald

Recognition and treatment of atypical forms of cystic fibrosis
Colin Wallis

Positive expiratory pressure (PEP) masks, flutter devices and other mechanical aids
to physiotherapy in cystic fibrosis
A. George F. Davidson, Maggie McIlwaine

Nitrous oxide in alleviating pain and anxiety during painful procedures in children
Jonathan H. Smith, Suchitra A. Kanagasundaram

The investigation of easy bruising
Kate Khair, Ian M. Hann, Ri Liesner

Management of feeding disorders in children with developmental disabilities
Steven M. Schwarz

Management of diabetic ketoacidosis
Eric I. Felner, Perrin C. White

The assessment and management of genital and anal warts
Carole Jenny

Diagnosis and management of Stevens Johnson syndrome
Christine Léauté-Labrèze, Alain Taïeb

Understanding Muslim customs: a practical guide for health professionals
A. Rashid Gatrad, Aziz Sheikh

Management of a potential organ donor
Harish Vyas, Jonathan H.C. Evans

Learning and staying up-to-date – advice for trainees and career paediatricians
Helena A. Davies, Vin Diwakar

Paediatric literature review – 2001
Tim J. David

Index

ISBN 1-85315-509-8

ISSN 0-309-0140